HAMSTER IMMUNE RESPONSES IN INFECTIOUS AND ONCOLOGIC DISEASES

ADVANCES IN EXPERIMENTAL MEDICINE AND BIOLOGY

Recent Volumes in this Series

Volume 129
AGING PHENOMENA: Relationships among Different Levels of Organization
Edited by Kunio Oota, Takashi Makinodan, Masami Iriki, and Lynn S. Baker

Volume 130
THE RENIN–ANGIOTENSIN SYSTEM
Edited by J. Alan Johnson and Ralph R. Anderson

Volume 131
THE CEREBRAL MICROVASCULATURE: Investigation of the Blood–Brain Barrier
Edited by Howard M. Eisenberg and Robert L. Suddith

Volume 132
ALCOHOL AND ALDEHYDE METABOLIZING SYSTEMS–IV
Edited by Ronald G. Thurman

Volume 133
SEROTONIN: Current Aspects of Neurochemistry and Function
Edited by Bernard Haber, Sabit Gabay, M. R. Issidorides, and S. G. A. Alivisatos

Volume 134
HAMSTER IMMUNE RESPONSES IN INFECTIOUS AND ONCOLOGIC DISEASES
Edited by J. Wayne Streilein, David A. Hart, Joan Stein-Streilein, William R. Duncan,
and Rupert E. Billingham

Volume 135
DIET AND RESISTANCE TO DISEASE
Edited by Marshall Phillips and Albert Baetz

HAMSTER IMMUNE RESPONSES IN INFECTIOUS AND ONCOLOGIC DISEASES

Edited by

J. Wayne Streilein
David A. Hart
Joan Stein-Streilein
William R. Duncan
and
Rupert E. Billingham

The University of Texas
Southwestern Medical School at Dallas
Dallas, Texas

PLENUM PRESS • NEW YORK AND LONDON

Library of Congress Cataloging in Publication Data

Symposium on Hamster Immune Responsiveness and Experimental Models of Infectious and Oncologic Diseases, Dallas, 1980.
Hamster immune responses in infectious and oncologic diseases.

(Advances in experimental medicine and biology; v. 134)
"Proceedings of a Symposium on Hamster Immune Responsiveness and Experimental Models of Infectious and Oncologic Diseases, held June 3-5, 1980, in Dallas, Texas."
Includes index.
1. Cancer—Immunological aspects—Animal models—Congresses. 2. Communicable diseases—Immunological aspects—Animal models—Congresses. 3. Immune response—Congresses. 4. Hamsters—Physiology—Congresses. 1. Streilein, Jacob Wayne. II. Title. III. Series. [DNLM: 1. Allergy and immunology—Congresses. 2. Infection—Immunology—Congresses. 3. Neoplasms—Immunology—Congresses. 4. Disease models, Animal—Congresses. W1 AD559 v. 134/QW 504 H232 1980]
RC268.3.S96 1980   616.99'2079   80-29639
ISBN 0-306-40642-X

Proceedings of a symposium on Hamster Immune Responsiveness
and Experimental Models of Infectious and Oncologic Diseases,
held June 3—5, 1980, in Dallas, Texas

© 1981 Plenum Press, New York
A Division of Plenum Publishing Corporation
227 West 17th Street, New York, N.Y. 10011

PREFACE

     This volume comprises the written contributions of participants in a symposium held in Dallas, Texas, June 3-5, 1980, entitled "HAMSTER IMMUNE RESPONSIVENESS AND EXPERIMENTAL MODELS OF INFECTIOUS AND ONCO-LOGIC DISEASES". This meeting followed its predecessor, "Hamster Immune Responses: Experimental Models Linking Immunogenetics, Oncogenesis and Viral Immunity" by three years. This more recent meeting was more pointed in its focus and the contributions appeared to be more tightly associated. These meetings are part of an extended effort by experimentalists using the Syrian hamster as an animal model system to bring together workers in potentially related areas for the exchange of ideas and information. The success of the symposia derives partly from the scientific excellence of the contributing scientists, and partly from the financial support of the National Institutes of Health through the Fogarty International Center. The administration of the University of Texas Health Science Center at Dallas, under President Charles C. Sprague, also donated time, facilities, and financial support.

     Preparation of the manuscripts in this volume, as camera-ready copy for the publisher, was the diligent and dedicated effort of Ms. Sara Howard. Copy editing was expertly performed by Ms. Sandra Schulte and proof-reading was the responsibility of Dr. Patricia Fultz and Ms. Alix Gerboth. However, final responsibility for any errors and omissions in the published volume is taken by the five local editors:

J. Wayne Streilein

David A. Hart

Joan Stein-Streilein

William R. Duncan

R. E. Billingham

CONTENTS

INTRODUCTION 1
   R. E. Billingham and J. Wayne Streilein

SECTION I

IMMUNE RESPONSES IN VITRO AND IN VIVO

Chairpersons: R. E. Billingham and James Forman

Hamster Lymphoid Cell Responses in Vitro 7
   David A. Hart and Joan Stein-Streilein

Syrian Hamsters Express Polymorphism at an MHC Equivalent. . 23
   William R. Duncan and J. Wayne Streilein

IgE-Dependent Release of Inflammatory Mediators from
     Hamster Mast Cells in Vitro 33
   Timothy J. Sullivan, David A. Hart and J. Wayne Streilein

Induction and Regulation of Contact Hypersensitivity in
     Syrian Hamsters 43
   J. Wayne Streilein, Pamela Witte, Kim Burnham
   and Paul R. Bergstresser

Allergic Contact Dermatitis in the Hamster and Other
     Rodents 59
   Henry C. Maguire, Jr.

SECTION II

MOLECULAR IMMUNOLOGY

Chairpersons: David A. Hart and J. Donald Capra

Immunochemical Characterization of Syrian Hamster Major
    Histocompatiblity Complex Homologues 69
  J. Theodore Phillips, J. Wayne Streilein, Diane A. Proia,
  and William R. Duncan

Immunoglobulins on the Surfaces of Hamster Lymphocytes . . . 87
  Claire P. Robles, Richard L. Proia, David A. Hart
  and Leon Eidels

Comparative Immunology of Old World Hamsters - Cricetinae. . 95
  John E. Coe

Hemolytic Complement and Its Components in Syrian Hamsters:
    A Study of Five Strains Uninfected and Infected with
    Brugia Pahangi 103
  Ota Barta, Priscilla P. Oyekan, John B. Malone
  and Thomas R. Klei

Isolation and Characterization of Hamster Alpha$_2$
    Macroglobulin 111
  Joan Stein-Streilein and David A. Hart

SECTION III

EFFECTOR CELLS IN VIRAL AND TUMOR IMMUNITY

Chairpersons: Joan Stein-Streilein and John J. Trentin

Functional Analysis of Lymphoid Cell Subpopulations
    Involved in Rejection of Tumors Induced by Simian
    Virus 40 123
  John W. Blasecki

Natural Cytotoxicity by Hamster Lymphoid Cells for Virus-
    Infected and Transformed Cells 135
  Robert N. Lausch, Nancy Patton, and Donna Walker

The Hamster Major Histocompatibility Complex and Alternate
    Mechanisms of Cell-Mediated Anti-Viral Cytotoxic
    Activity in the Syrian Hamster 143
  Mitchell J. Nelles and J. Wayne Streilein

Natural Killer (NK) Cells in Hamsters and Their
    Modulation in Tumorigenesis 153
  John J. Trentin and Surjit K. Datta

Prevention of Primary Simian Adenovirus Type 7 (SA$_7$) Tumors
    in Hamsters by Adoptive Transfer of Lymphoid Cells:
    Role of Different Cell Types 165
    Surjit K. Datta, John J. Trentin and Kenneth J. McCormick

Relationship between SV40-transformed Cell Susceptibility
    to Macrophage Killing and Tumor Induction in
    Rodents 177
    James T. Cook, J. B. Hibbs, Jr., and Andrew M. Lewis, Jr.

SECTION IV

PULMONARY IMMUNOLOGY

Chairpersons: Joan Stein-Streilein and Timothy Sullivan

Immune Responses Related to the Hamster Lung 191
    Joan Stein-Streilein, Mary F. Lipscomb, and David A. Hart

Functional Heterogeneity of Alveolar Macrophages 205
    Bruce S. Zwilling and Laura B. Campolito

Anti-Viral Cytotoxic Lymphocyte Response in Hamsters
    with Parainfluenza Virus Type 3 Infection. 215
    Frederick W. Henderson

Mechanisms of Inflammation in Lung Tissue. 221
    Donald L. Kreutzer, Usha Desai, William H.J. Douglas,
    and Mark Blazka

SECTION V

RESPONSES TO NON-VIRAL PATHOGENS

Chairpersons: David A.Hart and John A. Shadduck

Immune Response of the Hamster to Experimental Mycoplasma
    Pneumoniae Disease 233
    Wallace A. Clyde, Jr. and Gerald W. Fernald

Hemadsorption and Virulence of Mycoplasma Pneumoniae 241
    Eric J. Hansen, Richard M. Wilson, and Joel B. Baseman

Experimental Filariasis in Hamsters; Immunological
    Aspects of Complex Host-Parasite Interactions 253
    Niklaus Weiss and Marcel Tanner

Transmissible Ileal Hyperplasia 267
    Robert O. Jacoby and Elizabeth A. Johnson

LSH Hamster Model of Syphilitic Infection and Transfer
    of Resistance with Immune T Cells 291
    Ronald F. Schell, Jack L. LeFrock, John K. Chan,
    and Omar Bagasra

SECTION VI

RESPONSES TO VIRAL INFECTIONS

Chairpersons: John A. Shadduck and Kenneth P. Johnson

Experimental Subacute Sclerosing Panencephalitis (SSPE)
    in the Hamster. 303
    Kenneth P. Johnson

Enhanced Intrauterine Transmission of Herpes Simplex
    Virus Infection in Immunosuppressed Hamsters. 311
    Takeshi Kurata, K. Kurata, and Y. Aoyama

Susceptiblity to Fatal Pichinde Virus Infection in the
    Syrian Hamster. 327
    Sidney R. Gee, Marcia A. Chan, David A. Clark, and
    William E. Rawls

Genetically Determined Resistance to Lethal Vesicular
    Stomatitis Virus in Syrian Hamsters 339
    Patricia N. Fultz, J. Wayne Streilein, John A. Shadduck
    and C. Yong Kang

Defective Interfering Virus Particles and Their Biological
    Functions 353
    C. Yong Kang

SECTION VII

INFECTIONS WITH UNCONVENTIONAL AGENTS

Chairpersons: William R. Duncan and Richard F. Marsh

Effect of Vaccinia-Activated Macrophages on Scrapie In-
        fection in Hamsters   359
    Richard F. Marsh

Use of the Golden Syrian Hamster in Study of Scrapie
        Virus   365
    Paul Brown, Robert G. Rohwer, Marie-Claude Moreau-
        Dubois, Ernest M. Green, and D. Carleton Gajdusek

Hamster Scrapie: Evidence for Alterations in Serotonin
        Metabolism   375
    Robert G. Rohwer, Jaap Goudsmit, Leonard M. Neckers,
        and D. Carleton Gajdusek

Determination of Scrapie Agent Titer from Incubation
        Period Measurements in Hamsters   385
    Stanley B. Prusiner, S. Patricia Cochran,
        Deborah E. Downey, and Darlene F. Groth

Toward Development of Assays for Scrapie-Specific
        Antibodies   401
    Kenneth C. Kapser, Karen Bowman, Daniel P. Stites,
        and Stanley B. Prusiner

SECTION VIII

VIRAL ONCOGENESIS AND IMMUNE RESPONSES

Chairperson: William R. Duncan

An Immune- and Hormone-dependent Phase During the Latency
        Period of SV40 Oncogenesis in Syrian Hamsters   417
    Sachi Ohtaki

The Implications of the Different Tumor-Inducing Capacities
        of Adenovirus-2 and SV40-Transformed Hamster Cells. . .   433
    Andrew M. Lewis, Jr., James L. Cook,
        C. H. Kirkpatrick, and A. S. Rabson

Modifications of the Lymphoid B and T Cell Populations in
        Spleen and Thymus of Tumor-Bearing Hamsters   445
    H. Haddada, Ch. de Vaux Saint Cyr, F. Louisillier,
        and J. Zuinghedau

C-Type Particles in Thymic Development: A Correlation
    with Thymus Function. 455
  Pamela L. Witte, J. Wayne Streilein, and
  W. A. Shannon, Jr.

Summation 463
  J. Wayne Streilein

Index 469

INTRODUCTION

R. E. Billingham and J. Wayne Streilein

Departments of Cell Biology and Internal Medicine,
University of Texas Health Science Center at Dallas
Dallas, TX 75235

A symposium devoted to hamsters as experimental animals was held
in Dallas, Texas, May 31–June 2, 1977. In those early hamster days,
when it came to Grant Winning, those of us who wished to work on this
relatively late arrival from the wilds of Syria felt ourselves at some
disadvantage. It was essential to make a strong case why we needed to
work on hamsters rather than mice, because, as we were told so often
by overzealous Site Visitors, "that has already been done in the mouse,"
or "it would be much easier to do in the mouse." Those who chose to
work on rats have had similar problems with the "mouse lobby."

The response to our decision to hold this Second Dallas Hamster
Symposium may be taken firstly as a gratifying vote of confidence that
hamsters do indeed have some unique qualifications to help solve some
specific problems, and secondly as evidence of an incipient "hamster
lobby."

The purpose of this introduction is to provide some pertinent background information about hamster immunobiology to enable readers to fit
into a general conceptual framework or perspective the contents of the
many excellent papers presented in this volume.

Even within the first year of its domestication, the potential
usefulness of the hamster as a host or model for studying certain parasitic diseases was established with kala-azar or Leishmaniasis by the
late Saul Adler in Jerusalem. Then followed evidence that hamsters
are valuable hosts for viral as well as bacterial pathogens, and especially for xenogeneic-specific viruses. These animals also proved
to be remarkably susceptible to chemical carcinogenesis, and both induced and spontaneous tumors were found to be relatively easy to propa-
gate even in non-inbred stocks, in part at least because of lack of

segregating histocompatibility antigens. In certain genetic contexts,
however, there was no doubt about the hamsters' ability to develop
immune responses against tumors.

This pioneering work on hamsters led to two important conclusions:

1.   They are very susceptible to infection with xenogeneic
viruses and to the induction of tumors with a variety of agents;
2.   They appear to be highly resistant to natural enzootic viruses. No pathogenic virus unique to the hamster has ever been reported. (This might simply be the consequence of the small sample,
three litter-mate origin, of nearly all currently available hamsters.)
On the basis of empirical observations, hamsters appear to be highly
resistant to the development of spontaneous neoplasms.

In general, susceptibility both to infections and to oncologic
agents is intimately related to immune responsiveness. On this basis
it is the general thesis of this symposium that, since immunity plays
such an important role in the host response to infection and oncogenic
agents, an understanding of the immune response faculty and immune response apparatus of the hamster might bring to light some general
principles of both clinical and biological importance.

We can summarize the "classic" knowledge of hamster immunobiology
as follows:

1.   Hamsters do have the requisite apparatus to mount immune responses: (a) thymus, spleen (relatively small), lymph nodes and mu-
cosa-associated lymphoid tissue, e.g., GALT, BALT, and possibly SALT.
It has been found that BALT is only rudimentary in hamsters. (b) T-
lymphocytes, B-lymphocytes, macrophages, immunoglobulins and complement components.
2.   Hamsters can develop humoral immunity to various exogenous
antigens, including xenografts, and they can develop cellular immunity,
rejecting skin allografts and manifesting graft-versus-host reactivity.
3.   Their gestation period is short--only 16 days. The ontogeny
of their thymic system, and therefore their cellular immunity, is delayed as compared with that of other rodents.

Questions pertinent to hamster immune responsiveness addressed at
the first day's sessions included:

1.   Do hamsters have a major histocompatibility complex and, if
so, how is it organized genetically?
2.   Do antigen-presenting cells (Langerhans cells, alveolar macrophages, splenic and peritoneal macrophages) function in the familiar
manner in this species?
3.   What types of effector mechanisms do hamsters employ to destroy allogeneic, parasitic, virus-infected, and neoplastic tissues?
4.   How do hamsters regulate their immune responses initiated
systemically, via the skin, within the pulmonary tree, and during oncogenesis?

Questions addressed at the second day's sessions related to:

1.   The immune response of hamsters, as experimental hosts, to various pathogens including Mycoplasma, a filarial parasite, Treponema pallidum, and an unidentified enzootic agent that causes ileal hyperplasia in weanlings;

2.   The basis of the susceptibility and resistance of hamsters to certain viral agents, and the pathogenesis of some of the diseases they cause;

3.   The importance of the hamster as an experimental host in the study of the enigmatic scrapie agent;

4.   Viral induction of tumors in hamsters and the manner in which these animals respond immunologically to tumors of viral origin.

SECTION I

IMMUNE RESPONSES IN VITRO AND IN VIVO

Chairpersons:

R. E. Billingham

James Forman

HAMSTER LYMPHOID CELL RESPONSES IN VITRO

David A. Hart and Joan Stein-Streilein

Department of Microbiology
The University of Texas Health Science Center at Dallas
Dallas, TX   75235

INTRODUCTION

Lymphoid cells localized to different areas within an animal appear to perform specific immune functions. Their reactivity in vivo is dependent on the microenvironment within a particular tissue as well as the ability of a tissue to attract and accumulate specific re-circulating elements. While in vitro culturing of lymphoid cells does not accurately approximate the in vivo situation, information regarding differences among lymphoid tissues in responsiveness to a variety of specific and non-specific stimulants can be useful in assessing the potential of different tissues. That is, the responsiveness of lymphoid tissues (lymph node, spleen, thymus, bone marrow, peripheral blood) to non-specific mitogens such as concanavalin A (Con A), phyto-hemagglutinin (PHA), lipopolysaccharide (LPS), dextran sulfate (DxS), proteases, anti-immunoglobulin (anti-Ig) or mitogenic ions (Zn^{+2} and Hg^{+2}) can yield information concerning the compartmentalization of subpopulations of lymphocytes or accessory cells. Similarly, charac-terization of antigen-driven responses in vitro can yield information concerning compartmentalization as well as information on the regula-tion of activation and differentiation of lymphoid cells which may differ from those employed for mitogen activation. In vitro culture of lymphoid cells also permits evaluation of agents that can modulate the activity of lymphoid cells.

In the present report, we have analyzed lymphoid tissues of MHA hamsters for both mitogen and antigen responsiveness, and investigated susceptibility of the lymphoid tissues to reagents potentially capable of modulating in vivo responsiveness. The reagents studied were Li^+ (a biologically active ion known to modify the activity of cellular enzymes), and proteases and protease inhibitors, ubiquitous regulators of several humoral and cellular functions.

7

MATERIALS AND METHODS

Lymphoid tissues from female MHA hamsters (Charles River), 7 to 12 weeks of age, were removed aseptically and single-cell suspensions prepared (1). Lymphocyte stimulation assays (^{3}H-TdR incorporation) were performed under serum-free conditions for 72 hours with 5×10^6 cells per assay (1). For determination of the development of antibody-forming cells (AFC), the modified Mishell-Dutton procedure described previously was employed (2-4). Normal, non-immune cells were cultured for 4 or 5 days in the presence or absence of either sheep erythrocytes (SRBC) or trinitrophenylated <u>Brucella</u> <u>abortus</u> (TNP-B) and then direct AFC were counted utilizing the slide modification of the Jerne plaque assay.

Sources and optimal concentrations of most reagents employed have been described (1-8). Reagents not previously described are the rabbit anti-hamster (IgG or F(ab')$_2$ fraction) reagents from Cappel Laboratories (Downington, Pa.). These reagents have IgG heavy and light chain activity.

RESULTS AND DISCUSSION

Mitogen Responses of Different Lymphoid Tissues

When dissociated lymphoid cells from thymus, spleen, lymph nodes, and bone marrow were analyzed for their responsiveness to reagents which have been shown to be mitogenic in one or more other species, the pattern of tissue responsiveness to Con A, PHA, LPS, DxS and the proteases (9, 10) was not unexpected (Table 1) and is similar to responsiveness patterns obtained with cells from other species such as the mouse (11,12). In addition, responsiveness is consistent with the plant lectins (Con A, PHA) being T-cell mitogens and LPS, DxS and the proteases being B-cell mitogens. In contrast, the finding that stimulation by the mitogenic ions, Zn^{+2} and Hg^{+2}, was restricted to the lymph node cell (LNC) population was unexpected (13, 14). These ions have been shown to be mitogenic for human peripheral blood lymphocytes (15, 16). While the target cell for Hg^{+2} stimulation has not been characterized, Zn^{+2} is believed to be a macrophage-dependent T-cell mitogen (17). If this ion has similar stimulation characteristics in the hamster, then there may be something unique about the T-cells and/ or macrophages localized in the lymph nodes. Interestingly, Zn^{+2} does not appear to be a mitogen for either LNC or splenocytes from BDF$_1$ mice (Hart, unpublished) but is a weak mitogen for both LNC and splenocytes of Hartley guinea pigs (13).

Another reagent, theoretically a B-cell mitogen, which has also yielded unexpected results was rabbit anti-hamster Ig. This reagent apparently has the potential to interact with cell-surface immunoglobulin on both LNC and splenocytes (18), but is mitogenic for LNC and

Table 1. Distribution of Mitogen Reactivity of Lymphoid Tissues

Stimulant	Responsive tissue(s)[1]	Reference
Concanavalin A	Spleen, thymus, lymph node	1, 7
Phytohemagglutin-P	Spleen, thymus, lymph node	1, 7
Lipopolysaccharide	Spleen, lymph node	1, 7, 9
Dextran sulfate	Spleen, bone marrow, lymph node (mesenteric only)	1, 7, 9
Proteases[2]	Spleen, bone marrow, lymph node	9, 10, UP[3]
Zinc ions	Lymph node	13, 14
Mercuric ions	Lymph node	14
Rab A-Hamster Ig (IgG)	Lymph none	UP
Rab A-Hamster Ig (F(ab')$_2$)	Lymph node	UP

[1]Lymphoid tissues tested were spleen, lymph node, bone marrow and thymus.

[2]Proteases tested were trypsin, chymotrypsin and papain.

[3]UP = unpublished.

not splenocytes (Table 2), thymocytes or bone marrow cells (data not shown). Normal rabbit IgG was not mitogenic. Additional experiments with the F(ab')$_2$ fragments of rabbit anti-hamster Ig revealed that these reagents were also mitogenic for LNC (data not shown). Since no qualitative differences were observed when cell-surface Ig from LNC and splenocytes were analyzed (18), the reason for the tissue restriction for mitogenesis by these reagents may reside in an accessory cell population rather than the B lymphocytes themselves. Resolution of this question, however, as well as that of Zn^{+2} and Hg^{+2} stimulation, must await further investigation.

Responses to Multiple Mitogens

While mitogens may be classed as T-cell or B-cell mitogens, different mitogens within each class may stimulate separate subpopulations of cells (11,12). For instance, LPS stimulated cells in the LNC (peripheral and mesenteric LN) and splenocyte populations, whereas DxS stimulation was restricted primarily to spleen and to a lesser extent, bone marrow and mesenteric LN. While both of these reagents are B-cell mitogens, they may stimulate different subpopulations of cells (12), possibly by delivering different signals (19). In the mouse system, LPS + DxS has a synergistic effect on the stimulation of a single B lymphocyte (19). Multiple mitogen experiments could therefore provide

Table 2.   Effect of Anti-Ig Reagents on LNC and Splenocytes

Experiment	Stimulation index[1] µg Rab A-hamster Ig (IgG)				
	0	50	100	200	250
LNC					
2	1.0		3.5	11.5	
3	1.0	1.7	7.9	11.5	12.3
Peripheral	1.0		5.0	6.3	
Mesenteric	1.0		7.5	8.9	
Spleen					
1	1.0		1.2	1.5	
2	1.0			1.0	
3	1.0	1.2	1.3		

[1]Indicated values are the ratio of the mean ^{3}H-TdR cpm incorporated in the presence of rabbit anti-hamster Ig/^{3}H-TdR cpm incorporated into the unstimulated control cultures. All assays performed in triplicate.

interesting information concerning mitogenic activation of subpopulations of cells. Therefore, hamster splenocytes or LNC were cultured with various combinations of two mitogens (Table 3). There are several interesting points that can be made from these data. The first point is that, as in the mouse system, DxS + LPS yielded a synergistic response as determined by ^{3}H-TdR incorporation, but only with spleen cells. In the lymph node cells, where DxS is minimally mitogenic, no potentiation of the LPS response was observed. In contrast to this finding was the observation that Zn^{+2} and anti-Ig, neither of which is mitogenic for splenocytes, could potentiate LPS responses of splenocytes but did not potentiate DxS or Con A responses. These findings with anti-Ig reagents are shown in more detail in Table 4. Anti-Ig not only failed to potentiate DxS responses in the spleen, but anti-Ig responses in the LNC also were inhibited by DxS. A similar effect of DxS on Zn^{+2} stimulation of LNC was also found (data not shown). The protease, trypsin, also appears to differentially yield a synergistic response with LPS (Table 3). The finding that DxS, trypsin, Zn^{+2} and anti-Ig all seem to yield a potentiated or synergistic response only when cultured with LPS may indicate that there is a unique mechanism by which LPS activates B lymphocytes.

Activation of Hamster Lymphoid Cells by Antigen

Two different assays have been utilized to evaluate antigen-dependent activation. The first is ^{3}H-TdR incorporation utilizing LNC

Table 3.   Responses of Splenocytes or LNC to Multiple Mitogens

Mitogens	Synergy or potentiation[1]		Reference
	Spleen	LNC	
Zn^{+2} + LPS	+	+	13
Zn^{+2} + DxS	−	−	13
Zn^{+2} + Con A	−	−	13
Trypsin + LPS	+	+	9
Trypsin + DxS	−	−	9
Trypsin + Con A	−	−	UP[2]
Anti-Ig + LPS	+	+	
Anti-Ig + DxS	−	−	
Anti-Ig + Con A	−	−	
DxS + LPS	+	−	UP

[1]Synergy defined as ^{3}H-TdR incorporation of (A+B) > A+B. Potentiation defined as ability of a non-mitogenic agent to enhance the response of a mitogen.

[2]UP = unpublished.

primed in vivo with a soluble antigen such as DNP-BSA, KLH or ovalbumin and the second assay is the primary in vitro development of antibody-forming cells (AFC) in response to particulate antigens such as SRBC or TNP-B. In the mouse, SRBC is a thymus-dependent (T-D) antigen and TNP-B is a thymus-independent (T-I) antigen (20).

When LNC and splenocytes were assayed in proliferation studies, non-immune LNC or splenocytes from animals injected with complete Freund's adjuvant (CFA), incomplete Freund's adjuvant (ICFA) or Ag in saline did not yield detectable proliferation (^{3}H-TdR incorporation) when cultured with soluble antigens (Table 5). A detectable response, however, could be obtained with lymphoid cells from animals immunized in the footpads with 1 to 100 µg Ag in either CFA or ICFA (Table 5). The response was maximal in the draining LN 12 to 15 days post immunization and was restricted to these nodes even after 21 days post immunization. While in vivo injection of Ag in ICFA could induce antigen-reactive cells that were detectable in vitro, ICFA was less effective than CFA (Table 6). Therefore in vivo priming is required for generation of in vitro proliferation responses to soluble antigens.

In contrast to the above studies, it was possible to generate primary in vitro AFC responses to the particulate antigens, SRBC and TNP-B with spleen or LN cells but not BM or thymus cells (2, 3, and unpublished). Utilizing a slightly modified Mishell-Dutton culture system, specific AFC to either antigen could be readily detected by day 4 or 5 in cultures of LNC. In contrast, the response of spleno-

Table 4.   Effect of Anti-Ig Reagents on Mitogen Stimulation of LNC or
           Splenocytes

Experiment	Stimulation index[1]		
	μg Rabbit anti-hamster Ig (IgG)[2]		
	0	100	200
LNC			
1			
Control	1.0	3.5	11.5
10 λ LPS	4.2	7.6	24.6
50 λ LPS	20.1	33.0	48.4
2			
Control	1.0	7.9	11.5
2 λ Con A	73.7	71.7	70.9
25 λ LPS	14.4	44.9	50.3
3			
Control	1.0	5.0	6.3
2 λ Con A	72.3	74.4	66.7
50 λ DxS	0.8	2.8	2.8
Spleen			
1			
Control	1.0	1.3	
100 λ DxS	9.2	4.7	
50 λ LPS	10.1	22.2	
2			
Control	1.0		1.0
2 λ Con A	137.0		133.0
25 λ LPS	17.3		25.5

[1,2]Same as Table 2.

cytes to SRBC, but not TNP-B, was quite low and variable. Interestingly, the number of AFC developing in the LNC cultures in response
to an optimal concentration of SRBC (10^6) was consistently 3- to 10-
fold greater than the TNP-B response. The number of AFC developing
in response to SRBC in the spleen cell cultures was usually 10-fold
less than found in parallel LNC cultures. In contrast, the number of
TNP-B AFC was always greater in the spleen cell cultures than in the
LNC cultures. This finding with the putative thymus-independent antigen, TNP-B, is consistent with the hypothesis that such antigens stimulate a less mature population of B lymphocytes, which are concentrated in the spleen. It is interesting to note that the response to DxS,
a mitogen believed to stimulate a less mature population of B lymphocytes, also was concentrated in the spleen cell populations. The

Table 5. Detection of Antigen Reactive Cells in Hamster Lymphoid
          Tissues

Treatment	Tissue hypertrophy			Ag reactivity[1]		
	D-LN[2]	ND-LN[2]	Spl	D-LN	ND-LN	Spl
Normal	−	−	−	−	−	−
CFA	+	−	−	−	−	−
ICFA	+	−	−	−	−	−
100 μg Ag in saline	−	−	−	−	−	−
100 μg Ag in CFA	+	−	−	+	−	−
100 μg Ag in ICFA	+	−	−	+	−	−
1 μg Ag in ICFA	+	−	−	+	−	−

[1]Lymphoid cells cultured with DNP-BSA or KLH for three days and
[3]HTdR incorporation determined. Where appropriate, hamsters were
injected in all four footpads with antigen, adjuvant or antigen and
adjuvant 14 days prior to in vitro culture.

[2]The lymph nodes draining (D-LN) the sites of injection (popliteal,
axial and brachial) were kept separate from the non-draining nodes
(ND-LN) which included the mesenteric, cervical, hepatic,and inguinal
nodes.

reason for the difference in responsiveness of the LNC and spleen cell
cultures to SRBC does not appear to be related to the numbers of B
lymphocytes in the two tissues. By fluorescence analysis with anti-Ig
reagents, there are fewer B lymphocytes in the LNC population than in
the spleen (5) and there does not appear to be any qualitative difference in the cell-surface Ig of the two tissues (5,18). Therefore, the
difference may not reside in the B lymphocytes but could reside in
the T cell or accessory cell (macrophage?) populations. Whatever the
mechanism, these results are additional evidence for compartmentalization of cells in different lymphoid tissues of hamsters.

Modulation of In Vitro Responses by Proteases and Protease Inhibitors

Proteases and protease inhibitors modulate a large number of
humoral and cellular functions (21,22). One of the postulated areas
of protease involvement in cellular regulation is cell proliferation.
As discussed earlier, proteases such as trypsin, chymotrypsin and
papain are mitogens for subpopulations of hamster LNC and splenocytes,
most likely B lymphocytes. In addition, it was reported that LPS
stimulation was uniquely influenced by co-culture of the cells with
trypsin (Table 3). Therefore, it was of interest to determine whether

Table 6.   Comparison of CFA and ICFA in the Induction of In Vitro
           Antigen Reactivity·

| DNP-BSA | Net CPM ^{3}H-TdR incorporated[1] | | | |
| | ICFA | | CFA | |
(μg/ml)	1 μg Ag	100 μg Ag	1 μg Ag	100 μg Ag
0.01	5710	2840	17580	10420
0.1	8690	5700	22320	15700
1.0	10770	8520	29920	24130
10.5	19050	18480	34830	40440
50.0	27640	23640	34160	39210

[1]Animals were immunized 14 days earlier with 1 μg DNP-BSA in ICFA or
CFA or 100 μg DNP-BSA in ICFA or CFA. Cells were obtained from the
draining LN and cultured in vitro for 72 hours in the presence of
the indicated quantities of DNP-BSA.

proteases could modulate antigen-driven activation of hamster B lymphocytes, i.e., AFC development. Previous reports of others have indicated that proteases can modulate AFC development in cultures of mouse
splenocytes (23).

Six proteases were tested for their ability to enhance or potentiate in vitro responses to either SRBC or TNP-B. Of the six tested
(trypsin, papain, chymotrypsin, thermolysin, thrombin and submaxil-
lary gland endopeptidase), only papain and trypsin enhanced AFC responses (3,4). Chymotrypsin, previously shown to be mitogenic, did
not enhance AFC development when tested at concentrations of 1-50 μg/
assay. While papain and trypsin both enhanced AFC development, some
differences between the effectiveness of the proteases on LNC or
splenocytes and SRBC or TNP-B responses were noted (Table 7). First,
the enhancement of the SRBC response induced by either protease in
the LNC cultures was always less than that seen in the cultures of
splenocytes. As discussed previously, the SRBC AFC response was
greater in the LNC than in the splenocyte cultures, so a two-fold increase in the LNC cultures involved a larger actual number of AFC. A
second point from these experiments is that both proteases enhanced
the splenocyte response to the T-D antigen (SRBC) to a greater degree
than the response to the putative T-I antigen, TNP-B. A third point
raised by the splenocyte data is the finding that trypsin was consistently less effective than papain in enhancing the SRBC response and
did not enhance the T-I, TNP-B, response. Additional experiments have
revealed that papain is only effective if added within the first 48
hours of culture (3). The observed enhancement by papain appears to
be an effect on the lymphoid cells involved and is probably not due
to modification of either the antigen (SRBC) or fetal calf serum components (3). From these data we conclude that specific cell-surface

Table 7.   Effect of Proteases on AFC Development In Vitro

Experiment	Effective conc. (μg/ml)	Ratio of AFC (Ag+Protease)/AFC(Ag)[1]	
		SRBC	TNP–B
LNC			
Trypsin	25–50	1.5–2.0	ND[2]
Papain	10–25	1.5–2.5	
Spleen			
Trypsin	25–50	≤3.0	≤1.1
Papain	10–25	4.0–7.0	2.0

[1]Numbers represent the enhancement usually observed in the presence of protease. The number of experiments involved was greater than 10 (for more details see ref. 3 and 4).

[2]Not done.

or extracellular proteolytic events may be involved in the proliferative rather than the differentiation stages of AFC development. In the hamster, in contrast to the mouse (23), the proteolytic events must be in association with the presentation of specific antigen since neither trypsin nor papain induced a polyclonal response in the absence of SRBC.

Protease Inhibitors

As discussed above, cell surface or extracellular proteases may play a role in the activation of hamster lymphoid cells. Specific exogenous proteases can serve as mitogens and can potentiate both mitogen and antigen-dependent responses. This approach provided circumstantial evidence for the involvement of proteases in the activation process. If essential activation events were indeed mediated by endogenous proteases, then the activation process should be inhibited by protease inhibitors. Several protease inhibitors have been tested for their effectiveness in modulating stimulation by mitogens (^{3}H-TdR incorporation) as well as modulating the development of AFC. Utilizing a single lot of soybean trypsin inhibitor (SBTI), it has been possible to demonstrate that stimulation of LNC by PHA or Con A was uniquely sensitive to inhibition by this inhibitor (Table 8). However, stimulation of splenocytes or thymocytes by these lectins was not inhibited by SBTI. Therefore stimulation of cells by these lectins appeared to involve a proteolytic event(s) only in the lymph node population; and the peripheral LNC were more sensitive than the mesenteric LNC. In contrast to the T-cell lectins, stimulation of both LNC and splenocytes by LPS was partially inhibited by SBTI. The reason for the tissue distribu-

tion of SBTI-sensitive T-cell stimulation is unknown since SBTI-sensitive proteases have been detected on both LNC and thymocytes (8). It
has also been reported that SBTI as well as SBTI-Sepharose can inhibit
activation of human peripheral blood lymphocytes (HPBL) by several
agents (24). Perhaps the situation in the hamster LNC is similar to
that in another study (25), which found that proteases from non-lym-
phoid cells in a culture of HPBL could potentiate lectin responses.
If this explanation is correct, then SBTI-sensitive proteolytic events
may not be absolutely required for lectin stimulation of hamster LN
lymphocytes and the observed inhibition may have been due to the participation of proteases from an accessory cell which is apparently
uniquely distributed to the LN.

While proteolytic events may not be required for activation
of T cells, there is some evidence that proteolytic events may be important for the activation of B lymphocytes by LPS or antigen (Table
8). Stimulation of hamster LNC or splenocytes by LPS was inhibited
by SBTI. In addition, stimulation of splenocytes by LPS was differentially inhibited by the plasma protease inhibitor α_2-macroglobulin
(α_2M). However, the mechanism of this suppression remains to be elucidated (Stein-Streilein and Hart, this volume).

Two additional protease inhibitors have also been utilized for
these studies. Antipain and leupeptin are low molecular weight compe-
titive inhibitors of trypsin- and papain-like enzymes. Proteases sensitive to inhibition by these inhibitors have been found on the surface of both hamster LNC and thymocytes (8). Addition of a non-toxic
concentration of these inhibitors, 250 µg/ml, leads to suppression of
the in vitro AFC response of LNC to either SRBC or TNP-B by 70-90%
and 30-70%, respectively, and the ^{3}H-TdR incorporation induced by LPS
by approximately 40% (Table 8). Suppression of the AFC responses was
observed only if the inhibitors were added within the first 24 hours
of culture (4), results consistent with previously discussed findings
implicating the involvement of proteolytic events during the proliferative phase of activation rather than the differentiation phase.

In conclusion, these studies, utilizing proteases and protease
inhibitors in vitro, have provided insights into the biochemical mechanisms of activation of hamster lymphoid cells and raise the possibility that in vivo immune responses could be modulated by specific
protease inhibitors.

Modulation of In Vitro Responses with Ions

Lymphoid cells, like most mammalian cells, require certain inor-
ganic ions (Ca^{+2}, Mg^{+2}, K^+, Na^+, etc.) to perform specific cell functions. In many instances, the maintenance of the concentration differential of specific ions between the intracellular and extracellular space is dependent on the integrity of plasma membrane localized

Table 8.   Effect of Protease Inhibitors on Lymphoid Activation

Inhibitor	Conc. tested[1]	Maximum percent inhibition			Ref.
		Spl	LN	Thy	
SBTI	500 µg/ml				
Con A		0	76	0	7
PHA		0	73	0	7
LPS		64	93		9
DxS		0			9
$\alpha_2 M$[2]	7.5 µg/ml				
Con A		25			
LPS		75			
Antipain	250 µg/ml				
LPS		44			UP[3]
SRBC			90		4
TNP-B			70[4]		4
Leupeptin	250 µg/ml				
LPS		38			UP
SRBC			83		4
TNP-B			70[4]		4

[1]Inhibitors were added to the cultures one hour prior to the stimulant.

[2]This volume (Stein-Streilein and Hart).

[3]Unpublished.

[4]Variable inhibition observed.

transport systems. In addition to the previously discussed mitogenic ions (Zn^{+2}, Hg^{+2}), we have examined the effect of divalent cations (Ca^{+2}, Mg^{+2}) and their antagonists (Sr^{+2}, Mn^{+2}) on in vitro activation of hamster lymphoid cells. The effect of the biologically active ion Li^+ on mitogen and antigen activation has also been investigated.

Divalent Cations

Calcium and Mg^{+2} are important for cellular function and lymphocyte activation (reviewed in 26, 27). Manganese ions are also important for the activity of specific cellular enzymes. At high concentrations, Mn^{+2} can apparently antagonize Ca^{+2} -dependent events, possibly by displacement of the latter ion (28). Addition of 100µM Mn^{+2} to serum-free cultures of hamster lymphoid cells (containing 0.4mM Ca^{+2}) leads to the differential suppression of T cell activa-

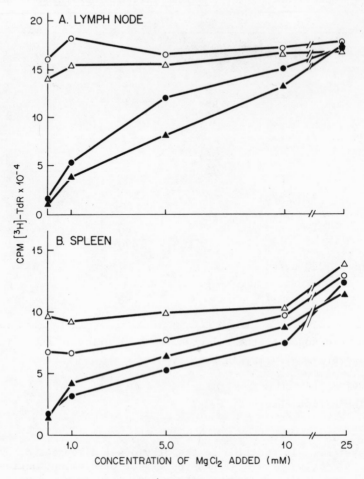

Fig. 1: Reversal of 100μM Mn^{+2} inhibition of Con A stimulation by MgCl$_2$. Lymph node cells (A) or splenocytes (B) were stimulated with 1 μg Con A (0,0) or 2 μg Con A (Δ,Δ) in the presence (closed symbols) or absence (open symbols) of 100μM MnCl$_2$. The indicated concentrations of MgCl$_2$ were added to appropriate cultures 30 minutes prior to the MnCl$_2$. All cultures were performed in triplicate and the indicated values represent the mean incorporation of ^{3}H-TdR. Variation from the reported mean was less than 10%.

Table 9.   Modulation of In Vitro Lymphoid Cell Responses by LiCl

Stimulant	Conc. of LiCl (mM)[1]	Effect Enhance	Suppress	Ref.
^{3}H-TdR Incorp.				
PHA (1-100 µg)	1-10	Yes	No	6
Con A (0.1-0.5 µg)	1-10	Yes	No	29
Con A (1-2 µg)	5-10	No	Yes	29
Zn^{+2}, Hg^{+2}	5-10	Yes	No	14
Soluble Ag	5-10	Yes	No	30

AFC formation		Percent of control AFC response[2]				
Antigen	Cell Source		LiCl concentration (mM)[1]			
		0.5	1.0	2.5	5	10
10^6 SRBC	LN	153	177	128	92	21
		(±27)	(±56)	(±20)	(±58)	(±0)

[1]LiCl added one hour prior to the stimulant.

[2]Average of four experiments. Cultures performed as described in Materials and Methods.

tion, with little or no suppression of LPS activation of B lymphocytes (28). The events inhibited are early events of activation since Mn^{+2} is ineffective if added 24 hours after initiation of the cultures. In addition, the effect of 100µM Mn^{+2} could be reversed in cultures of splenocytes and thymocytes, but not LNC, by supplementing the medium with 1.5mM $CaCl_2$ or $SrCl_2$. Not only did these latter results indicate that Mn^{+2} was interfering with Ca^{+2}-dependent results, they also indicated, again, that events occurring in the LNC population were unique. Again, the molecular basis of this tissue difference is not known, but it could reside in the T cells or in the accessory cell populations.

Manganese can also substitute for Mg^{+2} in many enzyme systems. Therefore it was of interest to investigate the possibility that the reason for the finding in the LNC was due to the fact that a unique Mg-dependent event was inhibited. Experiments have indicated that Ca^{+2} and Mg^{+2} apparently modulate different events during lectin stimulation of hamster LNC (6,29). Lectin stimulation of hamster cells (6, 29) will tolerate high concentrations of Mg^{+2}, while antigen stimulation will not (14); therefore the ability of Mg^{+2} to reverse Mn^{+2} inhibition of lectin stimulation was investigated. As depicted in Fig. 1, addition of 1 to 25mM Mg^{+2} to cultures of either LNC or splenocytes lead to a dose-dependent reversal of Mn^{+2} inhibition of the Con A response. The high concentration of Mg^{+2} (25mM) required to completely reverse Mn^{+2} inhibition (Mg/Mn=250) would indicate that Mg^{+2} can reverse Mn^{+2} inhibition, but it does so relatively inefficiently. The important point, however, is that Mg^{+2} can reverse Mn^{+2} inhibition in both lymphoid tissues.

In conclusion, Mn^{+2} appears to interfere uniquely with stimulation events in the LNC populations that are not reversed by Ca^{+2} but may be Mg^{+2} dependent. These findings are another indication of compartmentalization of subpopulations of cells in various lymphoid tissues.

Modulation of Responses by LiCl

Lithium is a biologically active ion which has been used in the treatment of human manic-depression states (6,29). This ion has also been shown to modulate the in vitro activity of human PBL (6,14,29). We have also demonstrated an effect of this ion on activation of hamster lymphoid cells in vitro.

Addition of Li^+ to cultures stimulated with either mitogens or antigens revealed a specific potentiating effect of this ion on all responses (Table 9). Proliferation responses (^3H-TdR incorporation) by all of the agents tested, with the exception of optimal concentrations of Con A, were enhanced 30% to 400% by addition of 5 to 10mM LiCl to the cultures. Mitogen responses were enhanced to a greater degree by Li^+ than were the responses to soluble antigens, which were only enhanced 30% to 90%, and the enhancement was quite variable. Higher concentrations (25mM) of LiCl were inhibitory to all responses. Like the previously discussed effects of Mn^{+2} on stimulation and the effect of proteases and protease inhibitors on AFC development, LiCl was only effective if added within the first 24 hours of culture, again indicating that early events of activation were being modulated.

In contrast to the ^3H-TdR incorporation experiments, 5 to 50mM LiCl did not enhance the AFC response to the T-D antigen, SRBC (Table 9). In a series of four experiments, optimal enhancement of the AFC response occurred at 1mM LiCl and 10mM LiCl was very inhibitory to AFC development. The difference could be due to an effect of the Li^+ on the differentiation stage of AFC development, or it could be due to the presence of fetal calf serum in the AFC cultures.

Lithium ions are believed to exert an effect on human lymphoid cells by modulating either cyclic nucleotide metabolism (inhibition of adenylate cyclase) or the activity of the plasma membrane Na-K ATPase (6,29,30). Recent experiments have indicated that the effect of Li^+ on PHA and DNP-BSA induced proliferation may also be related to altered cyclic nucleotide metabolism (31 and unpublished), while the effect of Li^+ on Con A stimulation may be more related to an alteration of the activity of the Na-K ATPase (31). This finding may be the basis for the suppression noted with high concentrations of Con A in the presence of 5 to 10mM LiCl (Table 9;31). If LiCl enhances antigen driven proliferation by inhibiting adenylate cyclase, then the observed suppression of AFC formation by 10mM LiCl may be due to an insufficient supply of cAMP to induce the appropriate differentiation sequence leading to antibody secretion.

Whether or not Li^+ could be used to modulate hamster immune responses in vivo is not known. Preliminary experiments, however, have revealed that daily IP injection of MHA hamsters with 5 mEq Li^+/kg, led to death within five days. Animals seemed to tolerate 1 to 2 mEq/kg, a dose range used to treat human disease states. Some gross changes were noted, however, in the kidneys and there was a decrease in thymic weight even when animals were treated with 1 to 2 mEq Li/kg.

CONCLUSIONS

The in vitro response of hamster lymphoid cells to a variety of antigens and mitogens has revealed a pattern of responsiveness similar to that seen with lymphoid cells from other species. The results indicate, however, that some of the characteristics of the cells that populate the lymph nodes are different from those populating other tissues (thymus, spleen, BM). These findings point to compartmentalized functions for subpopulations of hamster lymphoid cells. Interestingly, some of the unique LNC characteristics (Hg^{+2} and Zn^{+2} stimulation, SBTI inhibition) are similar to those found for human PBL. In addition, the findings concerning the modulation of in vitro responses by protease inhibitors and Li^+ have provided insights into the biochemical mechanisms of activation of hamster lymphoid cells and raise the possibility that these reagents may be useful tools to modulate in vitro immune responses as well.

ACKNOWLEDGMENTS

These studies were supported in part by United States Public Health Service Grants CA-24444, AI-11851, and CA-26842. The technical assistance of Janet Frazier, Nanette Broyles and Cheryl Hendricks during the course of these investigations is gratefully acknowledged. The authors thank Sara Howard for secretarial assistance in the preparation of this manuscript.

REFERENCES

1.   Streilein, J.S.; Hart, D.A.   Infect Immun 14 (1976) 463.
2.   Stein-Streilein, J.; Hart, D.A.   Cell Immunol 45 (1979) 241.

3.   Stein-Streilein, J.; Hart, D.A.   Cell Immunol, in press.
4.   Stein-Streilein, J.; Hart, D.A.   J Supramol Struct, suppl 4
     (1980) Abst. 500.
5.   Hart, D.A. et al.   Fed Proc 37 (1978) 2039.
6.   Hart, D.A.   Exp Cell Res 119 (1979) 47.
7.   Hart, D.A.   Cell Immunol 32 (1977) 146.
8.   Fulton, R.J.; Hart, D.A.   Cell Immunol, in press.
9.   Hart, D.A.; Streilein, J.S.   Exp Cell Res 107 (1977) 434.
10. Hart, D.A.; Streilein, J.S.   Exp Cell Res 102 (1976) 246.
11. Moller, G., ed.   Transplant Rev 11 (1972).
12. Moller, G., ed.   Transplant Rev 25 (1975).
13. Hart, D.A.   Infect Immun 19 (1978) 457.
14. Hart, D.A.   Exp Cell Res 121 (1979) 419.
15. Kirchner, H.; Rühl, H.   Exp Cell Res 61 (1970) 229.
16. Caron, G.A. et al.   Int Arch Allergy Appl Immunol 37 (1970) 76.
17. Rühl, H.L.; Kircher, H.   Fed Proc 36 (1977) 1284.
18. Eidels, L. et al.   Mol Immunol 16 (1979) 541.
19. Wetzel, G.D.   Ph.D. Thesis, Univ. of Texas Health Science Center
     at Dallas (1980).
20. Cambier, J.C. et al. J Exp Med 145 (1977) 778.
21. Clarkson, R.; Baserga, R., eds.   Control of Proliferation of
     Animal Cells.   Cold Spring Harbor Laboratory, Cold Spring Harbor,
     N.Y. (1974).
22. Gisler, R. et al.   J Immunol 116 (1976) 1354.
23. Moreau, P. et al.   Can J Biochem 53 (1975) 1337.
24. Arend, P. et al.   Immunology 144 (1972) 366.
25. Oppenheim, J.; Rosenstreich, D.   Prog Allergy 20 (1976) 65.
26. Wedner, H.; Parker, C.W.   Prog Allergy 20 (1976) 195.
27. Hart, D.A.   Exp Cell Res 113 (1978) 139.
28. Hart, D.A.   Exp Cell Res 43 (1979) 113.
29. Hart, D.A.   In: The Molecular Basis of Immune Cell Function,
     ed. J. G. Kaplan.Elsevier-North Holland (1979) 408.
30. Hart, D.A.   Cell Immunol, in press.

SYRIAN HAMSTERS EXPRESS POLYMORPHISM AT AN MHC EQUIVALENT

W. R. Duncan and J. W. Streilein

Departments of Cell Biology and Internal Medicine
University of Texas Health Science Center at Dallas
5323 Harry Hines Blvd.
Dallas, TX 75235

INTRODUCTION

The classical inbred strains of Syrian hamsters, MHA, LSH, CB, and PD4, display strong cellular alloimmune reactions as indicated by acute skin graft rejection (1,2), strong mixed lymphocyte reactivity (1), and potent graft-vs-host reactivity (1,3); they are unable, however, to develop detectable alloantibody responses to strong histocompatibility determinants (4-6). This quality of the immune response to transplantation alloantigens appears to be unique in hamsters, since in all other species, strong transplantation alloantigens elicit potent alloantibody responses (7-12). Several hypotheses have been advanced to explain this paradox: 1. domesticated Syrian hamsters display a rather limited genetic polymorphism, i.e., because of their derivation from a restricted gene pool, they may differ only at several minor histocompatibility loci but not at a major histocompatibility complex (MHC) equivalent; 2. hamster B cells fail to recognize or respond to MHC-like determinants; 3. Syrian hamsters as a species display little or no polymorphism at their MHC equivalent, Hm-1.

Previous studies from our laboratory have suggested that the classical inbred strains of Syrian hamsters exhibit polymorphism at an MHC equivalent, Hm-1; Hm-1 disparity, however, only induces cell-mediated alloreactivity (7). This lack of serologically detectable polymorphism at Hm-1 is reminiscent of the disparities represented among the murine K^b mutants as well as disparities exhibited between congenic strains of mice differing only at some Ia determinants (8-11).

23

Recently, we have reported that wild Syrian hamsters from a new source possess new histocompatibility determinants which induce strong, mutual cellular alloimmune reactions; and for the first time we could detect alloantibody responses to transplantation alloantigens (13). In this report, we present evidence suggesting that Syrian hamsters possess a polymorphic MHC, Hm-1, but the extent of polymorphism as detected serologically appears to be limited.

MATERIALS AND METHODS

Syrian hamsters (Mesocricetus auratus) of the domestic inbred strains MHA, LSH, CB, PD4, and LHC were either purchased from Charles River/Lakeview Hamster Colony, Vineland, N.J., or obtained from our inbred hamster colony. The recently-wild and semi-inbred hamster lines were obtained from Dr. William Nixon, Massachusetts Institute of Technology (14). Eight partially inbred lines: MIT, UT2, UT1, TX, DFW, GS, ZO, and SYR were obtained and some of these lines are now in the process of further inbreeding.

Alloantisera were produced as previously described (13). Briefly, $20-30 \times 10^6$ donor lymphoid cells were mixed with complete Freund's adjuvant and injected into the recipients' front and rear footpads. Two weeks later an intraperitoneal (IP) booster injection was given, followed by weekly IP injections. Sera were harvested at weekly intervals, tested for cytotoxicity and stored at -70°C.

The two-stage microcytotoxicity assay was carried out as described (15). Normal rabbit serum was used as a source of complement (Pell Freeze, Inc., Ark.).

In vitro absorptions were performed as follows. Lymphocytes from spleen and lymph nodes (minus erythrocytes) were washed twice in cold balanced salt solution; 1×10^8 packed lymphocytes were mixed with 50 µl antiserum and incubated for 30 minutes at 4°C. The cells were removed by centrifugation and the procedure was repeated using fresh lymphocytes.

Mixed lymphocyte reactions (MLR) were performed as previously described (1). We mixed 0.5×10^6 responder lymph node cells (LNC) with 0.5×10^6 irradiated (3000 rads, gamma Cell 40, Atomic Energy of Canada, Ltd.) stimulator LNC in 200 µl of RPMI 1640 without added serum. Cultures were pulsed with 0.5 µCi ^{3}H-thymidine on day 2 and harvested on day 3. Results are expressed as a stimulation index (SI) calculated as follows:

$$SI = \frac{\text{cpm experimental (responder + irr. stimulator)}}{\text{cpm control (responder + irr. responder)}}$$

RESULTS AND DISCUSSION

Previously we have presented evidence that only two MHC haplotypes are present among all domestic inbred strains of Syrian hamsters (7). Incompatibility at the MHC equivalent, Hm-1, elicits
acute skin graft rejection, mixed lymphocyte reactivity, and graft-
vs-host reactivity, without the concomitant production of alloantibodies (See Table 1). The apparent restricted polymorphism at Hm-1
could easily be explained by the limited gene pool from which the
classical inbred strains were derived, i.e., three littermates
trapped in 1930 (16). To test this hypothesis we obtained a new
source of wild Syrian hamsters, trapped in 1970 (14).

We were able to detect strong mutual cellular alloimmune reactions between the classical inbred and the recently-wild strains, as
evidenced by acute skin graft rejection and graft-vs-host reactions
(13). These preliminary studies suggested that this new source of
hamsters expressed additional strong histocompatibility determinants,
possibly encoded by the hamster MHC equivalent, Hm-1.

An analysis of T cell-mediated alloreactions was carried out by
use of the mixed lymphocyte reaction assay. Reciprocal MLR's using
both the classical inbred and recently wild strains were performed
and representative results are presented in Table 2. The classical
inbred strains gave strong MLR's when tested against the recently-
wild lines: MIT, TX, and UT2, with stimulation indices in the range
of 6.1 to 38.4. Recently-wild lines also responded reciprocally to
the classical inbred strains, with stimulation indices in the range
of 3.8 to 12.1, suggesting that the recently-wild lines express unique
Hm-1 haplotypes.

Table 1. Characterization of Hm-1 Among Classical Inbred Strains

Haplotype	MLR[1]	GvHR[2]	SGR[3]	Ab[4]	Strains
a	+	+	+	−	MHA, LSH, PD4, LVG
b	+	+	+	−	CB

[1]Positive MLR = stimulation index of 3.0 or more.

[2]Positive GvHR = Graft-vs-host reaction as measured in the popliteal
lymph node hypertrophy assay. Positive reactions were assigned when
a hypertrophy index of 5.0 or more was obtained.

[3]Positive SGR = skin graft rejection with a median survival time of
less than 21 days.

[4]Positive Ab = induction of alloantibody responses.

Table 2. Mixed Lymphocyte Reactions Between Recently-Wild and
          Classical Inbred Strains

Responder	Stimulator	Stimulation Index
MHA	TX	38.4
TX	MHA	5.9
MHA	MIT	20.9
MIT	MHA	3.8
CB	UT2	6.1
UT2	CB	12.1

Results from complete checkerboard MLR combinations suggested
that at least four new MLR-defined phenotypes were present among the
recently-wild lines (Table 3). Moreover, this new catch of hamsters
produced progeny expressing MLR phenotypes quite similar, if not
identical, to the Hm-1^a haplotype expressed in the classical inbred
strain, MHA. Apparently, the UT1 and DFW strains express this Hm-1^a
haplotype. Genetic studies revealed that only a single genetic locus
encodes for the allodeterminants responsible for induction of strong
MLR in the Syrian hamster, suggesting that the six MLR haplotypes
listed in Table 3 represent alleles at a single locus.

Utilizing several different combinations of inbred and recently-
wild lines, we were able to generate 13 putative alloantisera. The
results of the direct cytotoxic reactions of several of these antisera are shown in Table 4. All of the antisera were cytotoxic, ex-

Table 3. Model for MLR Disparity

Strain	Haplotype
MHA, LSH, PD4, UT1, DFW	a
CB(ZO)	b
MIT	c
TX, GS	d
UT2	e
SYR	f

Table 4. Cytotoxic Activity of Hamster Alloantisera

Antisera	Reciprocal of 50% cytotoxic titer with target[1] cells					
	MHA	CB	MIT	TX	UT2	SYR
MHA anti-MIT	0	0	>32	0	>32	4w
MHA anti-UT1/UT2	0	0	>32	8w	>32	>32
MHA anti-TX	0	0	0	>32	0	>32
CB anti-MHA	0	0	0	0	0	0

[1]Symbol "w" with a number indicates that less than 95% (but more than 50%) cells were killed at a 1:2 dilution of antiserum.

cept CB anti-MHA, and we have previously shown that this inbred/ anti-inbred combination fails to produce cytotoxic antibodies (4).

In summary, the classical inbred strains MHA and CB were both capable of producing cytotoxic antibodies following immunization with the recently-wild semi-inbred lines MIT, TX, UT2, and SYR. Often, when an antiserum was prepared against one of the recently-wild lines, the antiserum was also cytotoxic for cells derived from several other recently-wild lines, suggesting that the new lines share some antigenic specificities. None of the antisera produced by inbred strains in response to recently-wild lines reacted with cells from any of the classical inbred lines.

The recently-wild lines, MIT, SYR, TX and UT2, were capable of producing cytotoxic antibodies following immunization with classical inbred strains, MHA and CB. When an antiserum was made against MHA or CB, it reacted equally well with cells from all the classical inbred strains: MHA, CB, LSH, and PD4. Some of the antisera reacted with cells from a few of the recently-wild lines, suggesting that these antisera detect specificities shared between these two different groups of animals.

Absorption analyses were performed on selected antisera to determine the complexity of these sera. MIT anti-MHA reacted strongly with several different strains. Absorption with UT2 removed activity for UT2 but left activity for MHA and CB (Table 5). Absorption with MHA or CB removed all cytotoxic activity. These data suggest that this antiserum contains at least two antibodies: one antibody detects a specificity shared by UT2, MHA, and CB; another antibody detects a specificity shared only by MHA and CB. Moreover, the MIT strain does not produce antibodies that can distinguish between the Hm-1^a and Hm-1^b allodeterminants, suggesting that these two haplotypes are truly serologically indistinguishable.

Table 5.   Absorption Analysis of Hamster Alloantisera: Differences
           Between Classical Inbred Strains

| | | Cytotoxicity with target cells[1] | | |
Antisera	Absorbed by	MHA	CB	UT2
MIT anti–MHA	---	+	+	+
	MHA	0	0	0
	CB	0	0	0
	UT2	+	+	0

[1]Cytotoxicity: + = greater than 90% lysis at a 1:16 dilution of
                  antiserum.
              0 = no lysis at a 1:2 dilution of antiserum.

       The antiserum MHA anti–UT reacts strongly with several recently-
wild lines. Absorption with UT2 or SYR removes all reactivity. Absorption with MIT leaves reactivity for UT2 and SYR (Table 6). These
data suggest that this antiserum contains at least two antibodies:
one antibody recognizes a specificity shared by UT2, SYR, and MIT;
the second antibody recognizes a specificity present only in UT2 and
SYR.

       The new catch of recently-wild Syrian hamsters therefore allows
the definition of new histocompatibility determinants, some of which
induce T cell proliferation as measured by MLR, while others elicit
the production of cytotoxic alloantibodies. To determine whether

Table 6.   Absorption Analysis of Hamster Alloantisera: Differences
           Between Recently-Wild Strains

| | | Cytotoxicity with target cells[1] | | |
Antiserum	Absorbed by	MIT	UT2	SYR
MHA anti–UT1/UT2	--	+	+	+
	UT2	0	0	0
	SYR	0	0	0
	MIT	0	+	+

[1]Cytotoxicity: + = greater than 90% lysis at a 1:16 dilution of
                  antiserum.
              0 = no lysis at a 1:2 dilution of antiserum.

these determinants are encoded by genes at identical, closely linked, or unlinked loci, we performed genetic linkage studies. To summarize, we found evidence in two studies for linkage of genetic loci that encode for determinants that induce both MLR and alloantibody (UT2 and SYR strains); in all other strains, however, no evidence for linkage of MLR and alloantibody elicitation could be detected. These genetic linkage studies indicate that some of the antisera produced by the inbred MHA strain in response to histocompatibility antigens of some wild lines (MHA anti-UT and MHA anti-SYR) contain antibodies that react with determinants encoded by loci identical or closely linked to the loci encoding for the strong MLR determinants. Other antisera (MHA anti-MIT and MHA anti-TX) fail to recognize determinants encoded by loci linked to the MLR loci. Since we presume that the strong MLR determinants are encoded by the hamster MHC equivalent, we propose that MHA anti-UT and MHA anti-SYR recognize hamster MHC determinants and that MHA anti-MIT and MHA anti-TX predominantly recognize non-MHC determinants.

The results summarized in this report document the vigorous allo-immune responses obtained between the classical inbred and recently-wild hamsters. The fact that, using a new source of hamsters, we could easily detect a high titer of cytotoxic antibodies suggests that our previous attempts to raise alloantisera failed primarily be-

Table 7. Characterization of Hm-1 as Defined by Alloreactions Among the Classical Inbred and Recently-Wild Strains

Haplotype	MLR[1]	Cytotoxic[2] antibody	SGR[3]	Strains
a	+	−	+	MHA, LSH, PD4, LVG, UT1, DFW
b	+	−	+	CB (ZO)
c	+	−	n.d.[4]	MIT
d	+	−	+	TX,GS
e	+	+	+	UT2
f	+	+	n.d.	SYR

[1]Positive MLR = stimulation index of 3.0 or more when tested with all other haplotypes.

[2]Positive cytotoxic antibody = induction of alloantibody which reacts with a determinant genetically linked to the MLR locus.

[3]Positive skin graft rejection = induction of acute SGR genetically linked with the MLR locus.

[4]n.d. = not done.

cause the classical inbred strains do not express sufficient immunogenetic disparity that is required for the induction of alloantibody
body formation. Further, since hamster inbred strains are capable of
producing cytotoxic antibodies, it is highly unlikely that the hamster B cell repertoire is deficient for clones of alloreactive cells.
These results, however, do not resolve the dilemma that strong cellular alloreactivity between strains MHA and CB is not matched by strong
(or even detectable) alloantibody responses.

Previous studies (4) using xenoantisera (rabbit anti-hamster and
rat anti-hamster) suggested that all the available inbred strains of
hamsters expressed very similar if not identical MHC Class I and possibly Class II determinants, as detected serologically. Using several
different alloantisera, we were unable to distinguish serologically
between the alloantigens encoded by the $Hm-1^a$ and $Hm-1^b$ haplotypes,
suggesting that the two inbred derived haplotypes induce reciprocal
T cell proliferation without the subsequent induction of alloantibody
production. The most likely explanation for this limited immunogenetic disparity between the two inbred Hm-1 haplotypes is that they
represent minor variants at either Class I or Class II MHC loci.

The antisera produced by the inbred strains in response to the
recently-wild lines were extremely useful. Data obtained using these
sera indicate that the recently-wild lines are polymorphic for serologically detectable histocompatibility determinants. Genetic linkage
studies indicate that at least two of the MLR defined haplotypes can
be defined serologically, and we believe that these antisera contain
antibodies that recognize determinants encoded by the hamster MHC
equivalent, Hm-1.

Table 7 lists the number of possible different Hm-1 haplotypes
present among the two separate populations of hamsters. Six unique
haplotypes have been tentatively assigned to various inbred and recently-wild lines. All haplotypes can be defined using mixed lymphocyte reactions and skin graft rejection. Presently, only two haplotypes can be defined serologically, $Hm-1^e$ and $Hm-1^f$. This is unusual,
since most other species exhibit extensive serologically detectable
polymorphism at the MHC (12,17).

In an attempt to further characterize the hamster MHC, we are
currently producing congenic lines containing the wild- and inbred-
derived haplotypes, by selecting for MLR reactivity. Preliminary
biochemical evidence suggests that the antisera directed at UT2 (the
$Hm-1^e$ haplotype) detects cell surface molecules reminiscent of murine
Class II, or Ia-like, determinants. Our data suggest that Syrian hamsters possess a polymorphic MHC, Hm-1, but the extent of polymorphism
appears to be limited in comparison with other species in that:
1. only two of six haplotypes are serologically detectable; and 2.
the alloantigenic variation at Hm-1 is limited to Class II-like determinants.

ACKNOWLEDGMENTS

    We wish to thank Ms. Glenda Schroeder and Jalynn Graves for ex-
cellent technical assistance. This work was supported in part by
U.S.P.H.S. grants RR01133 and CA09082.

REFERENCES

1. Billingham, R.E.; Hildemann, W.H.   Proc R Soc Lond [Biol] 148
    (1958) 216.
2. Duncan, W.R.; Streilein, J.W.   Transplantation 25 (1978a) 12.
3. Streilein, J.W.; Billingham, R.E.   J Exp Med 132 (1970) 168.
4. Duncan, W.R.; Streilein, J.W.   J Immunol 118 (1977) 832.
5. Palm, J. et al.   J Hered 58 (1967) 40.
6. Billingham, R.E. et al.   Reconstr Surg Traumatol 34 (1967) 329.
7. Duncan, W.R.; Streilein, J.W.   Transplantation 25 (1978b) 17.
8. Klein, J.   Adv Immunol 26 (1978) 55.
9. McKenzie, I.F.C. et al.   Immunogenetics 3 (1976) 241.
10. Nabholz, M.H. et al.   Immunogenetics 1 (1975) 457.
11. Shreffler, D.C.; David, C.S.   Adv Immunol 29 (1975) 125.
12. Klein, J.   Science 203 (1979) 516.
13. Streilein, J.W.; Duncan, W.R.   Immunogenetics 9 (1979) 563.
14. Murphy, M.R.   Am Zool 11 (1971) 632.
15. Klein, J. et al.   Immunogenetics 2 (1975) 141.
16. Yerganian, G.   Prog Exp Tumor Res 16 (1972) 2.
17. Duncan, W.R. et al.   Immunogenetics 9 (1979) 263.

IgE-DEPENDENT RELEASE OF INFLAMMATORY MEDIATORS FROM HAMSTER MAST

CELLS IN VITRO

Timothy J. Sullivan, David A. Hart, and J. Wayne Streilein

Departments of Internal Medicine, Microbiology, and
Cell Biology
University of Texas Health Science Center at Dallas,
Dallas, TX   75235

INTRODUCTION

The release of mediators from mast cells is an essential step in immediate hypersensitivity reactions and also appears to play a significant role in delayed hypersensitivity and some forms of complement mediated reactions (1). Mediator release from rat or human mast cells can be provoked by antigen-IgE interactions on the surface of cells, by C3a or C5a anaphylatoxins, by bradykinin, by basic lysosomal proteins from neutrophils, by certain lymphokines and by a variety of other molecules (1-4). Preformed molecules such as histamine and newly formed molecules such as slow reacting substance-A (SRS-A) and prostaglandin D_2 (PGD_2) are released which exert potent regulatory influences on tissue function in areas of mast cell secretion. In addition to roles in the effector arms of immune and non-specific inflammation, recent evidence indicates that mast cell mediators may exert important regulatory influences on the evolution of immune responses (5). While the precise roles of mast cells in these immunologic events are not entirely clear, it seems likely that important roles will be delineated in several areas of immune function.

Surprisingly little is known about the nature and functions of hamster mast cells. There have been reports, however, that mast cells are abundant in the tissues of hamsters and that they appear in the serosal fluid of the peritoneal cavity (6-9). Hamster mast cells have been found to release histamine upon exposure to bacterial endotoxin (6), concanavalin A or phytohemagglutinin (7), compound 48/80 (8), basic lysosomal proteins and other cationic proteins (9), and a variety of other chemical stimuli. No clear evidence of an IgE system or responsiveness to anaphylatoxins or lymphokines has been reported.

33

The purpose of the present study was to examine serosal mast cells from MHA-strain Syrian hamsters for evidence of an IgE system and IgE-activatable secretory processes. Mast cells purified to near homogeneity released up to 77% of their preformed histamine after stimulation with anti-immunoglobulin antisera. Direct evidence was obtained that immunoglobulin with characteristics of IgE binds to the surface of hamster mast cell. These studies indicate that Syrian hamsters do have an IgE system and that IgE-ligand interactions can lead to marked degrees of mediator release from hamster mast cells.

MATERIALS AND METHODS

Goat antiserum against the rat IgE myeloma protein IR-162 was prepared and characterized as described in a separate report (10). Rabbit anti-hamster IgG was obtained from Miles Laboratories. All the other reagents were obtained from previously described sources (11-13).

Adult male and female MHA-strain Syrian hamsters were anesthetized with ether, exsanguinated by decapitation, and the thoracic and abdominal cavities were opened. Cells were harvested and processed in a medium containing 140mM sodium chloride, 4mM potassium chloride, 1mM sodium phosphate, 1mM calcium chloride, 5.6mM dextrose, 2mM piperazine-N,N'-Bis (α-ethane sulfonic acid), 0.1% (w/v) bovine serum albumin, and heparin 1 U/ml (pH 6.80). The mast cell medium was prepared fresh daily by taking a concentrated stock solution of salts and glucose and adding heparin, bovine albumin and calcium chloride and then diluting to volume with distilled water. The pH was adjusted to 6.80 with 5N sodium hydroxide. The abdominal and thoracic cavities were flooded with 14 ml of medium and then the trunks of the animals were massaged 100 times. Medium containing suspended cells was recovered by aspiration with a capillary pipet and placed in polypropylene test tubes. Mast cells in mixed serosal cell preparations were counted after staining with toluidine blue dye (14).

The pooled cell suspension was centrifuged at 50 x g for seven minutes. The medium was decanted and the cell pellet was resuspended in medium at a concentration of 6 million cells/ml. We purified the mast cells by layering the mixed cells over a 32% bovine serum albumin density gradient as described for the purification of rat mast cells (11). Two milliliters of cell suspension were layered over 4 ml of bovine albumin in medium in 50-ml polycarbonate centrifuge tubes. Cells were allowed to settle for 20 minutes and then were centrifuged at 450 x g for 20 minutes. The cells retained at the interface were aspirated and discarded. The interface was washed twice with 2 ml of medium. Mast cells contained in the bovine albumin were recovered by diluting the albumin with 40 ml of medium, sedimenting the mast cells at 50 x g for 10 minutes and then washing the cells twice with medium. The cells were then resuspended, counted, and diluted to the desired concentrations in medium.

Mast cells (10^5) in 0.09 ml of medium were added to 12 x 75-mm polypropylene tubes containing 0.01 ml of a solution of secretory agonist or medium alone as a control. All experiments were performed in triplicate. Incubations were carried out at 37°C without agitation after initial mixing. At the end of incubation periods, 0.4 ml of medium were added to each tube and the cells were sedimented at 1400 x g for two minutes at room temperature. Supernatant solutions were obtained by decantation, frozen, and stored at -80°C for histamine assay.

Histamine was determined by the radioenzymatic method previously described (15). Total histamine was determined on cell samples that had been boiled for three minutes.

The methods used to label the surface of mast cells with ^{125}I by use of lactoperoxidase, to lyse the cells with NP-40, to purify molecules with lentil lactin affinity chromatography, to preclear, to precipitate, and to analyze immunoprecipitates by SDS-polyacrylamide gel electrophoresis have been described in detail (13). Briefly, 20 million purified mast cells were suspended in phosphate buffered saline (PBS) and labeled with ^{125}I with lactoperoxidase and hydrogen peroxide. After cells were washed with ice cold PBS, the cell membranes were solubilized with 0.5% NP-40. After centrifugation, the supernatant was dialyzed and then subjected to lentil lectin column chromatography. After elution from lentil lectin with alpha methyl D-mannoside, immunoprecipitations were performed with rabbit anti-hamster immunoglobulin antisera, goat anti-rat IgE antisera, and rabbit anti-hamster IgM, and normal MHA, rabbit and goat sera as controls. The resulting immunoprecipitates were subjected to SDS-polyacrylamide gel electrophoresis and the resulting fractions were analyzed by gamma scintillation count.

RESULTS

Characterization of the Hamster Serosal Mast Cells

The total number of cells recovered by lavage of the thoracic and peritoneal cavities of 16 hamsters averaged 6.14 ($\pm$ 2.3) million per hamster. The cells were macrophages (58.6 $\pm$ 5.2%), lymphocytes (23.0 $\pm$ 3.2%), mast cells (17.9 $\pm$ 6.8%), and neutrophils (0.6 $\pm$ 0.3%). In a total of 35 animals, an average of 1.46 $\pm$ 0.3 million mast cells were present per animal, 20.8 $\pm$ 1.8% pure. The range of the number of mast cells was from 1.2 to 4.3 million cells per animal. The range in percent of mast cells in these preparations was from 14.1% to 43.0%. The thoracic cavity contributed 25.7 $\pm$ 4.3% of the total mast cells. These unpurified cell preparations contained 28.3 $\pm$ 5.7 pg histamine per mast cell. Viability as assessed by trypan blue dye exclusion was 98.4 $\pm$ 1.7%.

Table 1.   Mediator Release from Isolated Hamster Mast Cells

Addition[1]	Histamine released[2] (%)
Medium	5.1 ± 0.3
A-23187 (0.5 µg/ml)	54.2 ± 3.0
(0.1 µg/ml)	20.7 ± 4.4
Concanavalin A (1 µg/ml)	45.4 ± 6.4
(0.1 µg/ml)	31.1 ± 2.6
Compound 48/80 (1 µg/ml)	8.4 ± 3.4

[1]Mast cells (10^5) were incubated with the indicated concentrations of stimuli in 0.10 ml of medium for 15 minutes at 37°C as described in Methods.

[2]The amount of histamine released is expressed as the mean ± S.E.M. of results in three experiments.

Purification of the mast cells according to the scheme presented in the methods section of this paper resulted in preparations which were 98.6 ± 1.1% pure mast cells. The remaining cells in the preparation were macrophages, by morphologic criteria. These purified cells were 97.2 ± 0.8% viable. Of the mast cells applied to the gradients for purification, 77.0 ± 6.3% were recovered. The histamine content of these purified mast cells was 26.8 ± 4.3 pg/cell. Thus this purification method permitted a high degree of purification of viable cells with no significant loss of histamine during the procedure.

Mediator Release from Hamster Mast Cells

As summarized in Table 1, isolated hamster mast cells released substantial amounts of histamine in response to the calcium ionophore A23187 and to the lectin concanavalin A, with a less marked degree of release provoked by the polycationic compound 48/80. Viability of cells after 15 minutes' incubation in the presence of these releasing agents was not significantly decreased. These results confirm the ability of hamster mast cells to secrete mediators in a non-cytotoxic fashion after stimulation with diverse chemical stimuli.

If antibody is present on the surface of hamster mast cells, and if such an antibody can transmit a signal to the interior of the cell in a manner similar to that delineated for rat mast cells, then cross linking of surface immunoglobulin molecules should lead to mediator

Table 2. Reversed Anaphylaxis in Isolated Hamster Mast Cells

Addition[1]	Histamine released[2] (%)
Medium	2.7 ± 0.2
Anti-hamster Ig	
30 µg/ml	64.6 ± 5.3
10 µg/ml	69.2 ± 4.6
1 µg/ml	56.8 ± 5.0
0.1 µg/ml	25.8 ± 3.1
Anti-rat IgE	
30 µg/ml	27.1 ± 2.3
10 µg/ml	24.2 ± 3.4

[1]Mast cells (10^5) were incubated with the indicated concentration of agonists in 0.1 ml of medium for 15 minutes at 37°C.

[2]The results of three experiments are presented as the mean ± S.E.M.

release. Two approaches were taken to provoke a reversed anaphylactic reaction in hamster mast cells as an initial step toward demonstrating an IgE system in the hamster. As summarized in Table 2, incubation of isolated hamster mast cells with heteroantisera against hamster light chains and gamma chains resulted in a marked degree of mediator release. The viability of the mast cells following challenge with optimal concentrations of anti-light chain antibody was not significantly decreased. Heating of the anti-hamster light chain antibody at 56°C for 30 minutes did not change the ability of the antibody to provoke mediator release, indicating that complement activation and anaphylatoxin-mediated release were not active in the system. The second approach to provoking reversed anaphylaxis in hamster mast cells involved the use of goat anti-rat myeloma IgE antibody (Table 2). Again, non-cytotoxic release of histamine was provoked by this antiserum. Normal rabbit and normal goat sera at similar concentrations had no effect on mediator release (data not shown).

Characterization of the Molecules Bound by Antibodies Against Hamster Light and Gamma Chains and Rat Epsilon Chains

The ability of rabbit anti-hamster light chain antibodies and goat antibodies directed against rat epsilon chains to provoke non-cytotoxic mediator release from hamster mast cells strongly suggested the presence of a molecule on the surface of these mast cells which

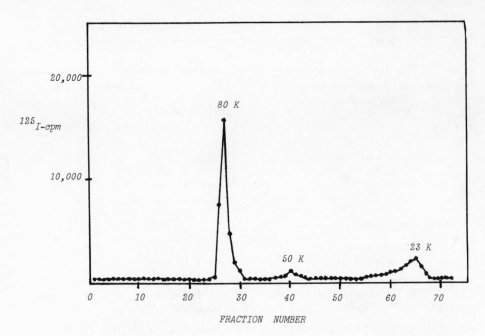

Fig. 1: Cell surface molecules immunoprecipitated from hamster mast
         cell lysates with goat anti-rat IgE. Intact mast cells were
         radioiodinated and lysed as described in Methods. Immuno-
         precipitates of mast cell lysates were analyzed by SDS-
         polyacrylamide gel electrophoresis followed by gamma scintil-
         lation counting of the gel fractions.

bore immunoglobulin light chains and expressed determinants that were
sufficiently homologous to determinants on rat IgE that cross-reactions
occurred with antibodies induced by immunization with rat IgE. In
order to obtain direct information bearing upon the nature of the
ligands bound by these two antisera, the surface of hamster mast cells
was iodinated with lactoperoxidase. Cell membranes were solubilized
with NP-40 and the materials bound by these antisera were precipitated
as described above. As depicted in Fig. 1, immunoprecipitates of
labeled hamster mast cells subjected to SDS-polyacrylamide gel electrophoresis demonstrated the presence of two dominant molecular species.
One was a molecule migrating with an apparent molecular weight of
23,000 daltons which co-migrated with authentic hamster light chains.
The second principal molecule had an apparent molecular weight of
80,000 daltons. In experiments not shown, immunoprecipitates of labeled
hamster mast cells produced by antisera against hamster light chains
gave identical gel patterns. Again, two principle molecular species
were precipitated, one 23,000 daltons and the other 80,000 daltons.
Immunoprecipitation with antisera directed against hamster μ chains

did not precipitate any detectable molecular species. Incubation of
extracts of labeled mast cells with normal goat, rabbit or hamster sera
also did not result in the precipitation of any detectable molecular
species. These results strongly suggest the presence of an immunoglobulin on the surface of hamster mast cells bearing a heavy chain with an
apparent molecular weight of 80,000 daltons, which is distinct from
that of known hamster heavy chains. A small amount of material with
an apparent molecular weight of 50,000 daltons was consistently co-
precipitated with the apparent heavy and light chains when either an
anti-light chain antibody or anti-rat epsilon antibody was used. The
nature of this molecular species has not been determined.

DISCUSSION

        The results of these experiments indicate that the Syrian ham-
ster can produce IgE antibodies which bind to mast cells and which
can trigger the release of inflammatory mediators from mast cells.
Functional evidence for the presence of immunoglobulin on the surface
of hamster mast cells was obtained by use of two very different kinds
of antibodies. Anti-immunoglobulin antisera containing anti-light
chain activity as well as anti-heavy chain activity caused a marked
release of mediators from mast cells, suggesting that immunoglobulin
was present on the surface of these carefully washed cells in a form
capable of mediating a signal to the interior of the cell. Radiolabeling and immunoprecipitation studies indicate that these anti-
immunoglobulin antisera precipitated an immunoglobulin that did not
contain the heavy chains of previously recognized hamster immunoglobulins. The 80,000-dalton molecule, which appears to represent the
heavy chain of this mast-cell-bound antibody, was distinct in size
from other hamster immunoglobulin heavy chains, with the exception of
μ chain. Potent anti-μ chain antibody did not precipitate radiolabeled materials from the surface of mast cells, suggesting that the
immunoglobulin heavy chain being detected was similar in size but did
not bear μ determinants. The ability of goat anti-rat IgE antibody
to trigger release from hamster mast cells and to precipitate an immunoglobulin containing an 80,000-dalton heavy chain is further evidence that an antibody is present on the surface of the hamster mast
cell. In addition, this result suggests that the hamster antibody has
substantial sequence homology with rat IgE antibody. While much work
remains to be done to characterize the nature of the antibody on the
surface of mast cells and to characterize the functional response of
cross-linking of such immunoglobulin molecules, the data available do
indicate that the IgE class of antibody exists in the Syrian hamster.
The epsilon heavy chain has an apparent molecular weight of 80,000
daltons. Assuming a two-heavy-chain, two-light-chain molecule, the
approximate molecular weight of this immunoglobulin would be 206,000
daltons.

The ability of goat antibodies against rat epsilon chains to cause mediator release from hamster mast cells and to precipitate an apparent immunoglobulin from the lysates of hamster mast cells suggests that there has been substantial conservation of the IgE molecule in these rodents. In support of the notion that some rodent IgE antibodies have considerable sequence homology, recent preliminary findings in our laboratory indicate that monoclonal antibodies of the IgE class from both rats and mice bind to the surface of hamster mast cells, and that when cross-linked these heterologous IgE molecules initiate secretion of histamine from hamster mast cells. Thus there is preliminary evidence that the regions of the IgE molecule which bind to mast cell receptors are very similar for the rat, mouse, and hamster. In addition, other areas of the epsilon chain accessible to immunoglobulin also have a degree of sequence homology, even though the IgE antibody is bound to surface receptors. Detailed comparative studies of mouse, rat and hamster IgE antibodies will be of considerable interest.

The 50,000-dalton peak of radioactivity appearing in SDS-polyacrylamide gels of immunoprecipitates of hamster mast cell surface immunoglobulin may represent the IgE receptor of these cells. Though the counts appearing in the 50,000-dalton peak were consistently low, this peak was consistently present. The apparent molecular weight of the possible hamster IgE receptor is similar to that reported for rat IgE receptors (16). Studies similar to these recent rat IgE receptor studies to characterize these putative receptor molecules will have to be undertaken before this issue can be resolved.

The availability of homogenous populations of viable mast cells responsive to a variety of immunologic and chemical secretory stimuli may be quite valuable as a model system for the study of immediate hypersensitivity. Syrian hamster mast cells contain a sufficient amount of histamine to permit functional studies on as few as 10,000 cells. This would permit over 100 observations to be made from the cells obtained from one animal. The availability of a variety of well-characterized inbred strains of hamsters makes this system especially attractive. While mouse mast cells are present in the peritoneal and thoracic cavities, the numbers available are quite small, severly hampering any efforts to exploit the genetic advantages available in the many inbred mouse systems. This system would be particularly valuable not only to characterize immediate hypersensitivity reactions of the hamster, but also to provide data for comparison with information already in existence bearing upon immediate hypersensitivity reactions involving rat, mouse or human mast cells. As background information bearing upon the hamster system evolves, and as more background information is accumulated bearing specifically upon hamster mast cells, this system may be of particular value as a model system with quantitative advantages over inbred strains of mice and functional advantages over the rat mast cell system. The amount of mediator release provoked by antibodies directed against mast cell surface IgE is substantially greater in the hamster than in the rat system. This could be an important advantage in experiments designed to unravel the biochemical basis of mediator release from mast cells.

The hamster mast cell system appears well-suited for studying IgE responses and antigen-induced IgE-mediated mast cell secretion. Future functional and biochemical studies of hamster IgE, of hamster mast cells and of the biochemical basis of mediator release from hamster mast cells may be of great value. In addition, it will be of considerable interest to examine the effects of complement anaphylatoxins in the hamster mast cell system and to examine the role of mast cells in delayed hypersensitivity reactions in hamster systems. In vitro studies of hamster mast cells can be coupled to in vivo functional and pharmacologic experiments which may yield considerable new insight into the role of mast cells in immune events in the hamster.

REFERENCES

1.   Sullivan, T.J.; Parker, C.W. Am J Pathol 85 (1976) 437.
2.   Johnson, A.R. et al. Immunology 28 (1975) 1067.
3.   Johnson, A.R.; Erdos, E.G. Proc Soc Exp Biol Med 142 (1973) 1252.
4.   Seegers, W.; Janoff, A. J Exp Med 124 (1966) 833.
5.   Plaut, M. J Allergy Clin Immunol 63 (1979) 371.
6.   Hook, W.A. et al. Infect Immun 2 (1970) 462.
7.   Hook, W.A. et al. Infect Immun 9 (1974) 903.
8.   Boreus, L.O. Acta Physiol Scand 49 (1960) 251.
9.   Keller, R. Int Arch Allergy 34 (1968) 139.
10. Sullivan, T.J. et al. J Immunol 117 (1976) 713.
11. Sullivan, T.J. et al. J Immunol 114 (1975) 1473.
12. Marquardt, D.L. et al. J Immunol 120 (1978) 871.
13. Eidels, L. et al. Mol Immunol 16 (1979) 541.
14. Bray, R.E.; Arsdel, P.P. Proc Soc Exp Biol Med 106 (1961) 255.
15. Snyder, S.H. et al. J Pharmacol Exp Ther 153 (1966) 544.
16. Kulczycki, A. Jr. et al. J Biol Chem 254 (1979) 3194.

INDUCTION AND REGULATION OF CONTACT HYPERSENSITIVITY IN SYRIAN HAMSTERS

J. Wayne Streilein, Pamela Witte, Kim Burnham and
Paul R. Bergstresser

Departments of Cell Biology and Internal Medicine
The University of Texas Health Science Center at Dallas
Dallas, TX   75235

INTRODUCTION

Syrian hamsters were introduced into experimental biology more than 50 years ago when it was found that they were particularly useful for the study of certain parasitic diseases (1). Within a relatively short period of time, their usefulness as experimental subjects was extended into several seemingly unrelated fields. They came to be used extensively for the study of experimental neoplasms (2), virus infections (3), and transplantation immunology (4). After the first 20 years of experience, the hamster came to be regarded as a relatively unique experimental subject because of certain putative aberrations: 1. hamsters reject skin allografts poorly or not at all (4); 2. hamsters are unusually susceptible to induction of tumors with a variety of oncogenic agents (2); 3. hamsters are highly susceptible to infection with viruses from many different species (3). Over the last two decades immunologists have learned that rejection of allografts, resistance to viral infection, and resistance to tumor induction are properties of the immune response that are presided over by the thymus and its cellular progeny. Because of the paramount role played by the thymus-dependent system in these various immune reactivities, it seemed reasonable to question the nature and extent of thymic function in the Syrian hamster. Surprisingly little is known about the T-cell system in this species. It was discovered more than 15 years ago that the ontogenetic maturation of the thymus as studied histologically is delayed (5). Evidence in support of this idea includes the facts that: 1. induction of neonatal transplantation tolerance can be achieved in hamsters up to a week following birth (4); 2. seeding of peripheral lymphoid organs with lymphocytes labeled intrathymically is delayed following birth compared to mice and rats (6); and 3. thymectomy performed as late as four weeks after birth results in a progressive wasting syndrome in hamsters resembling that following neonatal thymectomy in mice and rats (5,7). More recently, it has been found that hamsters fail to regulate certain alloimmune reactions thought to be governed by functional subsets of T lymphocytes in mice and other species. For example, hamsters fail to suppress graft-versus-host reactions in vivo following specific alloimmunization (8), and they do not develop suppressor cells in mixed lymphocyte cultures designed to delineate a putative allogeneic T-cell suppressor (9). In response to alloimmunization in vivo or in vitro, hamster lymphoid cells fail to assume significant cytotoxic activity as measured in vitro (10). Moreover, there is evidence that hamsters fail to develop cytotoxic T cells in response to acute virus infection (11).

In an effort to define more fully the nature and extent of the hamster T-cell system, we have developed a model of contact hypersensitivity in this species (12) based on the model developed successfully in mice over the past decade. The study of contact hypersensitivity in mice has permitted definitive description of participation of $Ly1^{+}23^{-}$ T lymphocytes in the mediation of contact hypersensitivity (13). Moreover, these studies have allowed the examination of populations of T-suppressor cells that regulate contact hypersensitivity in mice. Analogous studies have been conducted in hamsters in order to describe the role of the hamster thymus in this T cell-mediated system.

MATERIALS AND METHODS

Inbred hamsters of the MHA, LSH and CB lines were used in these experiments as adults between the ages of 2 and 6 months. The MHA and LSH lines share the same MHC allele ($\underline{Hm-1}^{a}$) and differ at a few minor histocompatibility loci. They also share the same IR-BSA allele and in general give comparable immune responses to a variety of immunogens. The CB line possesses the $\underline{Hm-1}^{b}$ allele and a different IR-BSA allele from the other two strains ($\overline{14,15}$).

Spleen and lymph nodes were rendered into single-cell suspensions as described previously (12). Viable cell counts were assessed with trypan blue exclusion and cell concentrations were adjusted to appropriate levels in balanced salt solution containing 1% heat-inactivated calf serum.

Abdominal skin was shaved and painted as described elsewhere (12) with 100 μl 7% TNCB, 25 μl 0.5% DNFB, or 25 μl of 10% oxazolone on day 0 and day 1. Ears were challenged with 20 μl of 1% TNCB, 0.2% DNFB, or 1% oxazolone on day 5, and degree of swelling was measured with a micrometer at 24, 48, 72 and 96 hours thereafter as described previously (13). Swelling was expressed in 10^{-4} inches. Maximum difference between experimental and control ears of each animal was used

as the measure of specific reactivity. Positive controls were hamsters
that were sensitized in the conventional fashion through normal abdominal wall skin. Negative controls were unsensitized hamsters whose
ears were challenged with the appropriate hapten.

Sensitization through hamster cheek pouch was achieved by everting
one pouch of an anesthetized hamster on two successive days and ap-
plying the contactant directly as described above. The pouch when dry
was returned to its anatomic position.

Ultraviolet light irradiation was conducted as described previously (16). Each animal received four daily exposures of eight
minutes' duration to shaved abdominal wall skin. This dose of irradiation reduced the number of Langerhans cells in exposed epidermis to
3% of control values as measured by ATPase reactivity.

For cheek pouch grafts, pouches were excised and everted, loose
areolar tissue was removed, and 2.5 x 2.5 cm grafts were fashioned and
placed on raw dermal beds on the thoracic cage of syngeneic hamsters.
Plaster of Paris bandages were applied for eight days, then removed.
At 30 days the graft epithelium was appropriately rugous as expected
of this type of epidermal surface exposed to room air.

Protocols for inducing unresponsiveness by intravenous infusion
of soluble salts or hapten-derivatized lymphoid cells have been described elsewhere (12). Seven days after inoculation of appropriate
tolerogen, abdominal skin was shaved and painted in typical immunizing
fashion with the appropriate hapten.

Lymph node and spleen cells were harvested from skin-sensitized
donors seven days after cutaneous painting with hapten. Using one
donor equivalent per recipient, pooled lymph node and spleen cells
were inoculated intravenously into syngeneic hamsters that had received
250 R whole-body gamma irradiation 24 hours previously (Gammacell 40
Irradiator, Atomic Energy of Canada, Ltd.). One hour later the ears
of these animals were challenged with dilute solutions of the appropriate haptens.

Lymph node and spleen cells were harvested from animals exposed
to a tolerizing stimulus seven days previously. Using one donor equivalent as described above, the cells were inoculated intravenously
into lightly irradiated recipients. One hour later the abdominal
skin was shaved and painted in conventional immunizing regimen with
the appropriate hapten.

Lymphoid cells were fractionated by passage through nylon wool
columns as described (17). Cells in the eluate, and cells gently
teased from the column, were prepared separately and injected into
lightly irradiated recipients as above. One donor equivalent was

routinely used, although significant losses of cells were observed frequently after passage through the columns.

A goat anti-hamster thymocyte serum (GαHT) described previously was used to remove T cells from lymphoid suspensions (11). After treatment with serum and complement, the remaining cells were washed, counted, and inoculated into lightly irradiated recipients at a dose of one donor equivalent. Following treatment with GαHT serum, 16% of pooled lymphoid cells remained.

Rabbit anti-hamster immunoglobulin (RαHIg) was used with complement to treat lymphoid cell preparations in an effort to remove B cells. Following treatment with RαHIg, 73% of pooled lymphoid cells remained and were inoculated at one donor equivalent into lightly irradiated syngeneic recipients.

Hapten-specific antibodies in the serum of hamsters exposed to TNCB or TNP-modified syngeneic lymphoid cells was measured by a hemagglutination assay with TNP-modified hamster erythrocytes as targets. The assay was described previously (12).

EXPERIMENTS AND RESULTS

Induction of Contact Hypersensitivity

Syrian hamsters of three inbred strains, MHA, LSH and CB, were exposed on shaved abdominal skin to immunizing doses of the chemical contactants DNFB, TNCB and oxazolone. Subsequently, their ears were challenged with the immunizing (or a different) hapten in dilute concentration. The ears were measured for degree of swelling 24, 48, 72 and 96 hours later as a measure of contact hypersensitivity. The results of these studies are presented in Table 1. All three haptens successfully immunized recipient hamsters. The degree of ear swelling is roughly comparable to that achieved by similar immunizing procedures in mice, and the hypersensitivity is immunologically specific (12).

Contact hypersensitivity has been employed to examine the cellular basis of T cell-mediated immunity in mice and guinea pigs. It has been learned that, when highly reactive haptens (such as DNFB) are painted on cutaneous surfaces, they derivatize host protein components (18). The precise nature of the proteins that are derivatized is not known, but immunogenetic evidence suggests that the gene products of the major histocompatibility complex are involved. Specifically, it is known that class I (murine K/D) alloantigens and class II (Ia) determinants are essential for the promotion, and ultimately the restriction, of the cell-mediated response to hapten (19). It is assumed that haptens derivatize the histocompatibility determinants directly, but it is not known whether this is the crucial step in induction of contact hypersensitivity. Recently, it has been shown that epidermal Langerhans cells are alone among the cells of the epidermis in their ability to display cell-surface Ia antigens in mice (20), guinea pigs (21), and man (21). These curious cells of mesenchymal origin also display on their surfaces Fc and C3b receptors (22) and have been found to be effective antigen presentors in vitro to primed T lymphocytes (23). As a consequence, it has been hypothesized that Langerhans cells are the critical cells within the epidermis whose derivatization is essential to the induction of contact hypersensitivity (16).

Langerhans Cell Requirements for Induction of Contact Hypersensitivity

Hamster cheek pouch, mouse tail skin, and the cornea of all mammals have markedly reduced (or absent) concentrations of epidermal Langerhans cells (24). Experiments were designed to test whether Langerhans cell-deprived cutaneous surfaces could sustain induction of contact hypersensitivity. Companion studies in mice have been reported elsewhere (16). LSH hamsters received two daily paintings of 0.5% DNFB on one everted cheek pouch. Five days later the ears of these hamsters were challenged with 0.2% DNFB. The results, shown in Table 2, indicate that contact hypersensitivity cannot be induced through intact cheek pouch epithelium. To test whether application of DNFB to the cheek pouch permitted the animals to swallow the agent (and therefore elicited specific unresponsiveness as has been reported in guinea pigs [25]), syngeneic cheek pouch grafts were placed heterotopically on thoracic cages of LSH hamsters. Thirty days later, when

Table 1. Induction of Contact Hypersensitivity with Haptens in Inbred Hamsters

Strain	(N)	Sensitizing agent	Challenge agent	Ear swelling response (x 10^{-4} inches $\pm$ SEM)
CB	(15)	TNCB	TNCB	29 $\pm$ 5
CB	(5)	none	TNCB	8 $\pm$ 5
CB	(5)	TNCB	Oxazolone	11 $\pm$ 5
MHA	(11)	TNCB	TNCB	33 $\pm$ 3
MHA	(4)	None	TNCB	2 $\pm$ 2
LSH	(13)	DNFB	DNFB	42 $\pm$ 5
LSH	(5)	DNFB	Oxazolone	15 $\pm$ 4
LSH	(4)	Oxazolone	Oxazolone	53 $\pm$ 6
LSH	(4)	None	Oxazolone	14 $\pm$ 5

these 2.5 x 2.5 cm grafts had healed and appeared to be healthy, two
applications of 0.5% DNFB were made. When the ears of these animals
were challenged with DNFB five days later, no hypersensitivity was
seen. These data are consistent with the notion that a critical concentration of Langerhans cells is required for induction of contact
hypersensitivity. However, because the cheek pouch has no lymphatic
drainage, it was possible that no hapten had escaped systemically,
and therefore the immune system of these hamsters was never perturbed.
To answer this question more directly, advantage was taken of the observation that the numbers of histochemically normal epidermal Langerhans cells can be drastically reduced by cutaneous irradiation with
ultraviolet light (24). Accordingly, panels of LSH hamsters were
shaved on the abdomen and exposed to ultraviolet light for eight
minutes over a four-day interval (16). This treatment produced a profound reduction in ATPase-positive Langerhans cells at the treatment
site (only 4% of control density). Immediately after the last exposure, the skin was painted with 0.5% DNFB. A second application was
made 24 hours later and the animals' ears were challenged with DNFB
five days later. No evidence of induction of contact hypersensitivity
was seen (see Table 2). It was concluded that hamsters resemble mice
(and probably guinea pigs, man and other mammals) in their requirement
for a threshold density of normal Langerhans cells at cutaneous sites
through which contact hypersensitivity to reactive haptens is to be
attempted.

Role of T Lymphocytes in Contact Hypersensitivity

A major reason for developing a contact hypersensitivity model in
hamsters was to be able to investigate the putative role of T lymphocytes in the response. In mice, man, guinea pigs, rats, and other animals, it has been established that T cells mediate contact hypersensitivity reactions. Since the nature and extent of T-cell function in
hamsters has been called into question, the availability of this model
offered an excellent opportunity to study the thymus-dependent system.

A direct approach to this question involved determining whether
contact hypersensitivity could be adoptively transferred to naive hamsters with living lymphoid cells and then to determine whether the responsible cell type was a T lymphocyte. Panels of LSH hamsters were
sensitized to DNFB in the conventional manner. Seven days later, their
lymph nodes and spleens were removed, made into single-cell suspensions, pooled and inoculated intravenously (at one donor equivalent)
into lightly irradiated (250 R) syngeneic recipient hamsters. One
hour later the ears of these animals were challenged with dilute DNFB.
As the findings presented in Table 3 reveal, contact hypersensitivity
can be successfully transferred by the passage of living lymphoid
cells to syngeneic recipients.

Whether the responsible cell was of thymus-derived lineage was
examined in two ways. In the first, lymphoid cell suspensions from

Table 2. Langerhans Cell Requirements for Induction of Contact Hyper-
          sensitivity in LSH Hamsters

Site of DNFB application	(N)	Ear swelling response (% positive control)
Abdominal skin (positive control)	(6)	100
Cheek pouch	(9)	35
Body wall skin graft	(5)	97
Cheek pouch graft	(5)	37
UVL-treated skin	(5)	0
Negative control	(8)	5

Positive control = 91 ± 4 inches x 10^{-4}.

DNFB-sensitive donors were passed over nylon wool columns, a procedure
known to produce an eluate rich in T lymphocytes and poor in B lymphocytes and macrophages. In the second, a highly specific, cytotoxic
goat anti-hamster thymocyte serum was used to treat suspensions of
 lymphoid cells from DNFB-sensitized donors. These fractionated or
serum-treated cells were injected into lightly irradiated syngeneic
recipients whose ears were challenged with DNFB one hour later. Contact hypersensitivity was transferred adoptively with nylon wool non-
adherent cells, but not with cell suspensions treated with the anti-
thymocyte reagent and complement. It seems reasonable to conclude
that contact hypersensitivity is mediated in hamsters by a population
of T lymphocytes, a population that we presume to be the hamster homologue of murine Lyl^+23^-.

B Lymphocyte Activation by the Induction Regimen Used for Contact Hypersensitivity

Although T lymphocytes appear to mediate contact hypersensitivity,
activation of B lymphocytes was also considered. In mice, cutaneous
painting with hapten rarely results in measurable amounts of circulating anti-hapten antibody (26). More often, but not always, guinea
pigs painted with contactants do develop specific serum antibodies
(27). Whether antibodies are produced in response to cutaneous
painting with hapten is important in the context of regulation of contact hypersensitivity. Serum was obtained from MHA and CB hamsters
skin-painted with TNCB and assayed for anti-TNP antibodies. Virtually
every animal developed measurable titers of anti-TNP antibody. Progressively rising titers were found in sera of MHA hamsters over the
60-day observation period, whereas titers of anti-TNP antibody reached

Table 3. Adoptive Transfer of Contact Hypersensitivity: Identifica-
          tion of Responsible Lymphoid Cell

Donors of lymphoid cells	Cells used for adoptive transfer	Number of recipients	Ear swelling response (% positive control)
DNFB-immune	Pooled lymph node and spleen	(6)	100
DNFB-immune	Nylon wool adherent	(3)	58
DNFB-immune	Non-adherent	(3)	71
DNFB-immune	Goat anti-thymocyte serum	(3)	23
DNFB-immune	Normal goat serum	(3)	102
Non-immune	Pooled lymph node and spleen (positive control)	(6)	100
None	Negative control	(3)	18

a maximum after 30 days in CB hamsters, then faded away. Thus, hamsters differ from mice in the capacity of their B lymphocytes to be
activated to secretion of specific antibody following cutaneous
painting with chemical contactants. The relationship of this response
to questions about regulation of hamster contact hypersensitivity will
be considered again below.

Regulation of Contact Hypersensitivity--Induction of Unresponsiveness

     The model system of contact hypersensitivity has proven to be par-
ticularly useful in the mouse to examine the role of T-lymphocyte subsets in regulation of immune responses (28). Since the system seems
to be reproducible in hamsters, it afforded an excellent opportunity
to ask similar questions about the hamster thymus-dependent immune
system. The most dramatic expression of immunoregulation of contact
hypersensitivity in the mouse is the induction of specific unresponsiveness. The classic maneuver of inducing unresponsiveness (described
first in guinea pigs [25]) by oral feeding of the chemical contactant
has been supplanted more recently by infusion of soluble salts of reactive chemicals such as DNFB and TNCB (29). Intravenous administration of these salts to mice produces a state of specific unresponsiveness; this is revealed when IV-treated animals fail to develop contact
hypersensitivity when immunized in the conventional fashion by cutaneous painting with hapten. Comparable experiments were conducted in
hamsters. DNBS was administered IV (500 mg/kg) to adult LSH hamsters.
Seven days later these animals were painted twice at 24-hour intervals

with 0.5% DNFB. When their ears were challenged with DNFB five days later, the degree of ear swelling was virtually indistinguishable from negative controls (Table 4). Thus, unresponsiveness can be achieved in hamsters, as in mice and guinea pigs, by intravenous exposure to the soluble salt of a hapten. MHA hamsters thus rendered unresponsive to DNFB retained their capacity to become contact hypersensitive to oxazolone, a non-cross-reacting hapten, indicating that the unresponsive state was immunologically specific for the eliciting agent (12).

A second line of investigation gave similar results. Murine lymphoreticular cells, when haptenated in vitro and then injected intravenously, induce hapten-specific unresponsiveness in syngeneic recipient mice (30). To test whether this situation applies in hamsters, spleen and lymph node cells from MHA and from CB hamsters were derivatized in vitro with TNBS; then 30×10^6 haptenated cells were injected intravenously into syngeneic recipients. These animals were subjected to the sensitizing TNCB regimen seven days later. When their ears were challenged with dilute TNCB, trivial swelling was observed (Table 4).

Finally, hamsters that had been exposed to DNFB through cutaneous surfaces depleted of Langerhans cells (naturally, as in the cheek pouch, or artificially, following ultraviolet light irradiation) were painted with DNFB on normal skin in the typical immunizing regimen. These animals also failed to develop contact hypersensitivity to this hapten (Table 4). These results are particularly interesting; they

Table 4. Induction of Hapten-Specific Unresponsiveness

Primary exposure to hapten	(N)	Ear swelling response to secondary exposure (% positive control)
TNP-modified lymphoid	(4)	40 (MHA)
cells IV	(5)	50 (CB)
None (negative control)	(8)	40
DNBS IV (LSH)	(5)	16
DNFB painted on cheek pouch	(5)	15
DNFB painted on UVL treated skin	(5)	6
None (negative control)	(8)	20

Positive control = hapten painted on abdominal skin without prior exposure; ear swelling response = 100%.

indicate that Langerhans cells play an essential role in the skin by preventing the development of unresponsiveness to antigens applied cutaneously, and they suggest that the absence of a lymphatic drainage pathway from the cheek pouch does not prevent antigen from leaking into the systemic circulation, since animals treated on the cheek pouch with DNFB become profoundly unresponsive.

Adoptive Transfer of Unresponsiveness

Unresponsiveness can be achieved by two quite different mechanisms: on the one hand, deletion of specific antigen-reactive cells by exposure to antigen may rob the host of the capacity to recognize antigen subsequently--a passive process. On the other hand, antigen, when appropriately presented, may elicit an active process of suppression in which populations of regulatory cells suppress or inhibit antigen-reactive cells from responding to antigen in the conventional way--an active process. Adoptive transfer studies offer an opportunity to choose between these alternative mechanisms. LSH hamsters were rendered unresponsive to DNFB by intravenous inoculation of DNBS as above. Seven days later, lymphoid cells from these animals were inoculated into lightly irradiated (250 R) syngeneic recipients. Two hours later, the recipients received two skin paintings with 0.5% DNFB at 24-hour intervals. Ear challenge of these animals five days later revealed that unresponsiveness had been transferred (see Table 5). Similarly, lymphoid cells harvested from donor hamsters rendered unresponsive by the application of 0.5% DNFB to cutaneous surfaces deficient in Langerhans cells were also able to transfer the unresponsiveness to syngeneic recipients (Table 5). While the level of unresponsiveness achieved in these latter recipients was not profound, the ear swelling was nevertheless significantly less than that found in positive control ears.

Table 5. Adoptive Transfer of Hapten-Specific Unresponsiveness with Pooled Lymph Node and Spleen Cells

Primary exposure of donor to hapten	Number of recipients	Ear swelling response (% positive control)
DNBS IV	(12)	35
DNFB painted on cheek pouch	(6)	50
DNFB painted on UVL treated skin	(7)	67
None (negative control)	(4)	5

Positive control = normal recipients of normal lymphoid cells, then skin sensitized with DNFB; ear swelling response = 100%.

Thus, we conclude that hapten-specific unresponsiveness induced in hamsters by these several methods is mediated by an active process.

Cellular Basis of Unresponsiveness

On the assumption that regulation of unresponsiveness in hamsters would resemble that described in mice, we next employed nylon wool fractionation and treatment with anti-thymocyte serum to determine whether T cells were responsible for the transfer of hapten-specific unresponsiveness. Pooled lymph node and spleen cells from DNBS-treated MHA hamsters were passed through nylon wool columns. The non-adherent fraction, as well as cells teased from the column (adherent fraction), were transferred into lightly irradiated syngeneic recipients. In companion experiments, lymphoid cells from DNFB-unresponsive hamsters were treated with goat anti-hamster thymocyte serum before transfer into syngeneic recipients. Immediately thereafter, these panels of recipients were immunized in the conventional manner to DNFB. When their ears were challenged five days later, every panel showed evidence of profound, hapten-specific unresponsiveness (see Table 6).

Table 6. Adoptive Transfer of Hapten-Specific Unresponsiveness:
         Analysis of Responsible Cell Type

Donor of lymphoid cells	Cells used for adoptive transfer	Number of recipients	Ear swelling response (% positive control
DNFB-unresponsive	Pooled lymph node and spleen	(12)	35
DNFB-unresponsive	Nylon wool adherent	(3)	38
DNFB-unresponsive	Non-adherent	(3)	38
DNFB-unresponsive	Goat anti-thymocyte serum	(3)	19
DNFB-unresponsive	Normal goat serum	(3)	36
DNFB-unresponsive	Rabbit anti-hamster Ig	(3)	23
DNFB-unresponsive	Normal rabbit serum	(3)	60
-----	Serum from DNFB-unresponsive donors	(4)	101
None	Negative control	(8)	9

Positive control = normal recipients of normal lymphoid cells, then skin sensitized with DNFB; ear swelling response = 100%.

That is, nylon wool adherent cells (enriched for B lymphocytes and depleted of most, but not all, T lymphocytes) were able to transfer unresponsiveness; similarly, suspensions from which T cells had been selectively removed by specific antisera also transferred unresponsiveness.

We next examined the possibility that B cells were responsible
for transfer of unresponsiveness. Rabbit anti-hamster immunoglobulin
(RαHIg) serum is cytotoxic (with the aid of complement) for most, but
not all, surface Ig-bearing lymphocytes. Lymphoid cells from hamsters
rendered unresponsive to DNFB were treated with RαHIg and then injected
intravenously into syngeneic recipients. Within two hours, these animals were immunized with two skin applications of 0.5% DNFB, but when
their ears were challenged five days later, they too proved to be profoundly unresponsive (Table 6). This line of investigation is not yet
complete, and it is premature to state categorically that B cells are
not responsible for maintaining the unresponsive state. However, we
are reasonably certain that T lymphocytes are not involved in this
aspect of immunoregulation.

Antibody Production Concomitant with Induction of Unresponsiveness

Serum was harvested from hamsters that had been rendered unresponsive to TNCB by intravenous injection of TNP-modified syngeneic lymphoid cells. Unexpectedly, every serum sample contained anti-TNP antibodies, with titers indistinguishable from those induced by skin
painting with TNCB. Thus, B-cell activation (and secretion of hapten-
specific antibodies) takes place following exposure to hapten by virtually any route and presentation, irrespective of whether contact
hypersensitivity or unresponsiveness is induced. It seemed possible,
therefore, that regulation of unresponsiveness could be a function of
antibody. One experiment was designed to test this possibility. Serum
was harvested seven days after unresponsiveness had been induced in
LSH hamsters by intravenous inoculation of DNBS. One ml of serum was
administered intravenously plus 0.5 ml intraperitoneally to normal LSH
hamsters. One hour later, these animals were subjected to the conventional DNFB immunizing regimen. Challenge of their ears five days
later with dilute DNFB revealed intense swelling, comparable to that
found in animals who were immunized following administration of normal
LSH serum (Table 6). Although not every reasonable permutation of
this experiment had been tried, the data do not hold promise that regulation of hapten-specific unresponsiveness in hamsters is mediated by
antibody.

DISCUSSION

Characterization of the thymus-dependent component of hamster
immune responses has proven to be more arduous than we had originally

expected. Except for early claims that hamsters did not reject skin allografts (which, if true, would have suggested that hamsters lack thymic function completely), there has never been any question in our minds that a functioning thymus exists in this species. The diversity of functions currently thought to be assumed by the thymus and its cellular progeny in mice and other species, however, is extreme. Accurate identification of these various cellular and functional components of the T-cell system is not always easy, even in the mouse where the greatest experience has been gained. In part, our difficulties in describing the thymus system in hamsters relate to the paucity of cell-surface markers and reagents that can be used to identify various cell types. We are only now beginning to address this important issue. Our difficulties in defining the T-cell system, however, must also relate in part to differences between the T-cell system as it is currently described in the mouse and that which we are able to identify and describe in hamsters.

There is ample experimental evidence from this and other laboratories that the functional T-cell subset that in the mouse bears the $Ly1^+23^-$ surface phenotype also exists in hamsters (10,31). Even though we are unable to show that murine alloantisera specific for the Ly1 and Ly2 alloantigens cross-react on hamster lymphocytes, there are overwhelming functional data to indicate that the $Ly1^+23^-$ cell population is present. Hamster T cells participate in mixed lymphocyte reactions and graft-versus-host reactions (10,31); they are required to help B lymphocytes in the production of IgG antibody to a variety of T-dependent antigens (5,32), and now with this series of studies we report that a similar cell population exists that mediates contact hypersensitivity in hamsters. This last observation has been particularly gratifying since it establishes the presence of a T cell-mediated reaction that is unrelated to transplantation immunity. While there remain some lingering doubts about the efficacy of the putative $Ly1^+23^-$ T-cell population in hamsters (e.g., the efficiency of T-cell help provided in the switch of hamster B cells from IgM to IgG synthesis [32] has been questioned), we are satisfied that a reasonable homologue for the murine $Ly1^+23^-$ population is present and functional in hamsters.

The induction of contact sensitivity on the part of this population of T lymphocytes also appears to be conventional in hamsters. The method of sensitization by skin painting with reactive haptens is identical to that employed in mice. Moreover, a threshold density of Langerhans cells within the cutaneous surface to be painted is essential in both species. The fact that hamster B cells are also activated to make specific antibody by cutaneous painting with TNCB, whereas mouse B cells are usually not so activated, may not represent a critical species difference. It has been reported that B lymphocytes of guinea pigs may be similarly activated (27).

While induction of contact hypersensitivity may be comparable in mice and hamsters, the modalities used by each species to regulate this response are dissimilar. At the present time, it is not possible to describe in all particulars the means by which regulation of contact hypersensitivity and unresponsiveness is achieved in mice. However, the broad outlines of the control are apparent. At least three populations of T lymphocytes suppress the inductive and the effective phases of the primary response (33) (two suppressor cells with Lyl^-23^+ phenotypes and a Ts auxiliary cell with Lyl^+23^+ surface markers). Recently, evidence has been produced (33,34) that antibody regulates contact hypersensitivity. The precise mechanism and specificity through which antibody mediates control remain to be elucidated. It is currently attractive to speculate that idiotypic and anti-idiotypic antibodies regulate through an elaborate, anastomosing network. While our analysis of regulation of hamster contact hypersensitivity response is comparatively primitive and certainly naive, it nonetheless appears that this species does not use a cell of thymic origin in regulating the response; at least, we cannot detect such a cell through the adoptive transfer studies presented here.

We do not believe that this failure to find evidence of T-cell suppression is trivial or due to technical artifacts. The GαHT serum is able to deplete T cells that mediate hypersensitivity from a cellular suspension, but is unable to remove the cell that is responsible for unresponsiveness. If the latter cell is of thymic origin, then its expression of the hamster homologue of Thy-1 is markedly reduced or aberrant. It seems simpler to conclude that the responsible cell is not a T lymphocyte. This represents the second time we have looked experimentally for a suppressor-cell population by using an experimental paradigm designed optimally to demonstrate such a cell. Previously, we have failed to find evidence of suppression of allogeneic reactions in vitro and in vivo (8,9). In fact, our original reasons for considering whether hamsters produced suppressor cells in allogeneic reactions turned on clinical observations made in hamsters undergoing graft-versus-host disease. While normal lymphoid cells from parental strain donors are capable of initiating graft-versus-host disease in semiallogeneic hamster recipients disparate at the major histocompatibility complex, Hm-1, cells harvested from specifically sensitized parental strain donors are even more effective (35). This finding stands in direct contrast to what has been found with cells from specifically sensitized mice and rats; in these species, immune cells perform no better and are frequently less good at inducing GVHR against major transplantation antigens. Moreover, while refractoriness to subsequent graft-versus-host reaction can be induced in hamsters as it can in mice and rats, refractoriness does not depend upon immunoregulatory processes in hamsters (35). Instead, acute graft-versus-host disease can be reinitiated in F^1 hybrid hamsters that have recovered from graft-versus-host disease by simply providing these animals with a new source of F^1 lymphohemopoietic cells. Thus, refractoriness does not result from positive suppression but from progressive deletion of F^1 target cells.

The observations presented in this and related papers suggest that hamsters are relatively unable to use suppressor T cells to regulate their immune responses. It has been reported that hamsters also do not develop cytotoxic T cells in response to acute vaccinia virus infections (11). It is interesting to consider that both of these functions are usually ascribed to the Lyl⁻23⁺ T cell subsets in mice. Perhaps hamsters as a species have a restricted thymus defect that relates to their ability (or lack thereof) to generate cytotoxic and suppressor cells, both of which have a common cell-surface determinant. What this putative set of deficiencies has to do with unusual aspects of hamster responses to viruses and to tumors is worthy of consideration.

REFERENCES

1.   Adler, S.; Theodor, O.   Proc R Soc Lond [Biol] 108 (1931) 447.
2.   Trentin, J.   Fed Proc 37 (1978) 2084.
3.   Toolan, H.   Fed Proc 37 (1978) 2065.
4.   Billingham, R.E.   Fed Proc 37 (1978) 2024.
5.   Sherman, J. et al.   Blood 23 (1964) 375.
6.   Linna, T.J.   Blood 31 (1968) 727.
7.   Adner, M. et al.   Blood 25 (1965) 511.
8.   Lause, D.; Streilein, J.W.   Transplantation 25 (1977) 211.
9.   Lause, D.; Streilein, J.W.   Transplantation 26 (1978) 80.
10. Duncan, W.; Streilein, J.W.   J Immunol 118 (1977) 832.
11. Nelles, M.; Streilein, J.W.   Immunogenetics (1980) in press.
12. Streilein, J.W.   J Immunol 124 (1980) 577.
13. Benacerraf, B.; Unanue, E.R.   Textbook of Immunology.   Williams and Wilkins, Baltimore (1979).
14. Duncan, W.; Streilein, J.W.   Transplantation 25 (1978) 12.
15. Duncan, W.; Streilein, J.W.   Transplantation 25 (1978) 17.
16. Toews, G. et al.   J Immunol 124 (1980) 445.
17. Julius, M. et al.   Eur J Immunol 3 (1973) 654.
18. Macher, E.; Chase, M.   J Exp Med 129 (1969) 103.
19. Vadas, M. et al.   Immunogenetics 4 (1977) 137.
20. Rowden, R. et al.   Immunogenetics 7 (1978) 465.
21. Stingl, G. et al.   J Immunol 120 (1978) 570.
22. Stingl, G. et al.   Nature 268 (1977) 245.
23. Stingl, G. et al.   J Invest Dermatol 71 (1978) 59.
24. Bergstresser, P. et al.   J Invest Dermatol 74 (1980) 77.
25. Chase, M.   Proc Soc Exp Biol Med 61 (1946) 257.
26. Scott, D.; Long, C.   J Exp Med 144 (1976) 1369.
27. Polak, L. et al.   Immunology 25 (1973) 451.
28. Miller, S. et al.   J Exp Med 147 (1978) 788.
29. Phanuphak, P. et al.   J Immunol 112 (1974) 115.
30. Miller, S.; Claman, H.   J Immunol 117 (1976) 1519.
31. Singh, S.; Tevethia, S.   Proc Soc Exp Biol Med 142 (1973) 433.
32. Streilein, J.W. et al.   Transplant Proc 9 (1977) 1229.
33. Sy, M-S. et al.   J Exp Med 149 (1979) 1197.
34. Sy, M-S. et al.   J Exp Med 151 (1980) 896.
35. Streilein, J.W.   J Exp Med 135 (1972) 567.

ALLERGIC CONTACT DERMATITIS IN THE HAMSTER AND IN OTHER RODENTS

Henry C. Maguire, Jr.

Division of Dermatology
Hahnemann Medical College
230 North Broad Street
Philadelphia, PA   19102

INTRODUCTION

The first, and for a long time the only, experimental animal for the study of allergic contact dermatitis (ACD) was the guinea pig (1). Thus the basic studies that related sensitization potential to the ability of a low molecular weight allergen to couple to protein, that established the requirement for viable lymphoid cells (not sera) for the passive transfer of hypersensitivity to simple chemical allergens, and that demonstrated the induction of a specific immunological unresponsiveness to contact allergens, were done in the guinea pig (2,3, 4,5). Indeed, the guinea pig still remains the animal of choice for the identification of contact allergens of man (6,7). In 1968, the technique of measuring increased ear thickness as a way of assessing induced inflammation by contact allergens in the mouse was introduced (8); in contrast to the guinea pig, inflammatory skin reactions on the flank of the mouse are difficult to evaluate since these reactions lack both erythema and easily defined induration. The ear thickness technique recently has been extended to studies of allergic contact dermatitis in the hamster (9,10) and we are using the same methodology to evaluate ACD hypersensitivity in rats (11). This report examines ACD in the hamster and relates it to ACD in other species.

MATERIALS AND METHODS

Hamsters purchased from Lakeview Laboratories, Waltham, Mass., were housed four or five to a cage on wood shavings in a light-cycled, temperature-controlled room. They were maintained on Purina Chow and had unlimited access to acidified water (pH about 3). Females were used throughout; they were about 10 weeks old at the beginning of an experiment. Fighting sometimes was a problem, particularly with the

LVG and LHC strains. PD-4 hamsters were the least bellicose. The
health of the animals was excellent; unintended losses did not occur.
The following reagents were purchased from commercial sources: oxazolone (4-ethoxymethylene-2-phenyl oxazolone)(BDH Chemicals Ltd., Poole,
England); DNCB (1-chloro-2,4-dinitrobenzene), DNFB (1-fluoro-2,4-
dinitrobenzene), and $DNBSO_3$ (1-sulfonate-2,4-dinitrobenzene) (Eastman
Chemicals, Rochester, N.Y.); cyclophosphamide (Cy) (Sigma, St. Louis,
Mo.); complete Freund's adjuvant (CFA) (Difco Laboratories, Detroit,
Mich.). Hamsters were sensitized by a high concentration of allergen
applied to a clipped area on one flank; challenge was made with a
dilute, relatively non-irritating concentration of allergen applied
to the dorsal aspect of a normal ear. Induced inflammation was assessed by measuring the ear before and at different times after the
challenge application of allergen using an engineer's micrometer
bearing a rachet (8). In some experiments, hamsters were sensitized
to allergens by the split-adjuvant technique described previously (12).
Briefly, CFA was injected intradermally at multiple sites. Twenty-four
hours later, allergen was inoculated directly into these sites.

RESULTS AND DISCUSSION

    In the guinea pig, the application of allergen to skin sites pre-
viously injected with complete Freund's adjuvant (CFA) results in a
considerable intensification, by the adjuvant, of the induced hypersensitivity (12). The same sort of intensification by CFA of the induction of delayed-type hypersensitivity (DTH) to low molecular weight
contact allergens can be obtained in hamsters. The result of a typical experiment is shown in Fig. 1. The induced DTH was recognizable
as specific inflammation in the challenge sites at 24 and 48 hours but
not at four hours. CFA preparation of the sensitization sites resulted in a marked increase in the resultant sensitivity. We have
also had similar findings with contact allergens and CFA in the rat
(11). Our attempts to date to boost the acquisition of DTH to simple
chemicals with CFA in the same way in mice have been totally unsuccessful, for unknown reasons. Although the mechanism whereby CFA height-
ens the acquisition of DTH is not well understood, our studies in
guinea pigs have led us to conclude that, in immunopotentiation of
DTH, the site of action of CFA is in the lymph nodes draining the site
of sensitization (13).

    Numerous studies have established that the alkylating agent Cy is
a potent immunosuppressive drug in humans as well as in a variety of
experimental animals. Not only suppression of the primary antibody
response but induction of specific immunological tolerance has been
produced in several rodent species when Cy is given at the same time
as primary immunization (14,15). In the area of cellular hypersensitivity, Cy is used to inhibit T-cell reactions such as allograft rejection and the graft-versus-host reaction. Some years ago, during
studies of the effect of Cy on allergic contact dermatitis in the

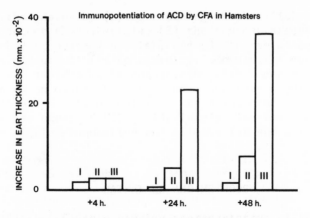

Fig. 1:   Immunopotentiation of ACD by CFA in hamsters. Two groups
           of LVG female hamsters were sensitized to oxazolone by the
           application of 0.02 ml of 5% oxazolone in acetone to a
           clipped site on the left flank on day 0 and day 1. Animals
           of one group had their sensitization site injected in two
           areas with 0.1 ml of complete Freund's adjuvant one hour
           before the first application of sensitizer. All hamsters
           as well as a toxicity control group were challenged on the
           ear on day 7 by the application of 1% oxazolone contained
           in a solvent consisting of one part corn oil and four parts
           acetone. The average reaction, as indicated by increase in
           ear thickness, for each group at four hours, 24 hours and
           48 hours is shown.
           Group I: Toxicity control; Group II: Sensitization without
           CFA; Group III: Sensitization with CFA.

guinea pig, we came upon the seemingly paradoxical finding that pretreatment of guinea pigs with Cy potentiated rather than suppressed
the acquisition of ACD to strong contact allergens (16). In a typical experiment, guinea pigs were pretreated with Cy and sensitized to
DNCB (Fig. 2). The sensitizing stimulus, which was modest, resulted
in most animals of the control group showing weak contact reactions
24 hours after challenge; the sites were negative at 48 and 72 hours.
In contrast, guinea pigs pretreated with Cy prior to sensitization
with DNCB developed much more intense challenge reactions which persisted to 72 hours and beyond. This result has been confirmed and extended to other animal species and to a variety of antigens including
purified foreign proteins, sheep red blood cells, bacteria, parasites
and fungi as well as allogeneic cells (17-22). Indeed, Cy has been
shown to immunopotentiate the acquisition of delayed-type hypersensitivity to syngeneic tissue, e.g., to testicular tissue in mice (23). F
Further, we have found that in man, the non-specific suppression of
delayed-type hypersensitivity that is associated with advanced malig-

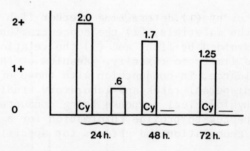

Fig. 2:   Guinea Pig sensitization using CY. Hartley female guinea
          pigs weighing approximately 400 g were injected with Cy (10
          mg/kg IP) on days 0,1,2,3 and 4. On day 4 this group, as
          well as a positive control group, were sensitized on the
          flank by the application of 0.5 mg DNCB in acetone. On day
          14 the guinea pigs of both groups were challenged with 0.1%
          DNCB in acetone on the opposite flank. The intensity of
          the challenge reactions were scored at 24, 48 and 72 hours.
          The mean intensity of the reactions at each time point in
          each group are shown.

nancy can be reversed by immunopotentiation with Cy (24). In addition
to man and the guinea pig, we have studied immunopotentiation by Cy
of ACD in hamsters, rats and mice; Cy immunopotentiation is readily
obtained in these species. In a typical experiment in hamsters, LVG
females were injected on day -3 with Cy and then sensitized to DNCB,
in parallel with a positive control group, on day 0. Both groups, as
well as a toxicity control group, were challenged with DNCB eight days
later. The readings at 24 and 48 hours are shown in Fig. 3; Cy substantially increased the induced ACD. In the mouse, not only does Cy
regularly heighten the acquisition of ACD in normal mice, but Cy immu-
nopotentiates as easily in mice rendered B-cell deficient by treatment
from birth with a goat antiserum against mouse IgM (25). Mice so
treated are considered B-cell deficient on the bases that: their sera
lack detectable mouse immunoglobulin and contain circulating goat
anti-mouse IgM; their spleens lack cells containing surface immunoglobulin by immunofluorescence; and their spleen cells fail to give
a mitogenic response above background to stimulation by the B-cell
mitogen LPS but react normally to the T-cell mitogen Con A. Such
mice fail to produce detectable serum antibody when immunized with
sheep red blood cells or DNP-KLH. The target of Cy immunopotentiation in the mouse appears to be a population of T suppressor cells
that would otherwise damp the challenge response. It is likely that
the inhibition of a similar population of T suppressor cells accounts
for Cy immunopotentiation in the other rodent species, guinea pig,
hamster, and rat, and perhaps in man as well, although direct evidence
is lacking.

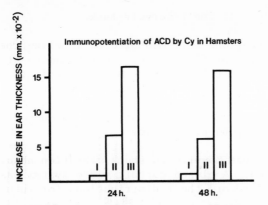

Fig. 3:   Immunopotentiation of ACD by CY in hamsters. Two groups of
           LVG hamsters were contact sensitized by the application of
           0.02 ml of 10% DNCB in acetone in the morning and again in
           the afternoon to a clipped site on the flank on day 0.
           Three days earlier the hamsters of one group had received
           Cy, 150 mg/kg, IP. Both groups as well as a toxicity group
           were challenged on the ear on day 8 by the application of
           0.015 ml of 1% DNCB in a solvent consisting of one part
           corn oil and four parts acetone.
           Group I: Toxicity controls; Group II: Sensitization without
           Cy; Group III: Cy then sensitization.

        More than 50 years ago it was noted in man and in the guinea pig
that immunological tolerance to a low molecular weight skin sensitizer
(neoarsphenamine) could readily be induced by the intravenous or in-
tracardiac injection of allergen prior to sensitization (26,4). In
the case of guinea pigs, mice, rats, and hamsters, pretreatment with
parenteral DNBSO$_3$ (about 750 mg/kg) consistently induces specific unresponsiveness to subsequent attempts to engender sensitivity with
DNFB (or DNCB); such tolerant animals are as readily sensitized to
oxazolone as are normal animals of the same species. The results of
a typical experiment in which immunological tolerance was induced with
DNBSO$_3$ in hamsters are shown in Fig. 4. Tolerance can be induced as
well with lymphoid cells that have been haptenized in vitro by reaction with DNFB (10). Analysis of the mouse model indicates that tolerogen generates a population of T suppressor cells (27).   A similar
induction of T suppressor cells by parenteral DNBSO$_3$ is likely, but
has not yet been established experimentally, in the hamster, rat, and
guinea pig.

        The "flare reaction," which is a specific reactivation of old ACD
test sites by systemic allergen, has been demonstrated by others in
the guinea pig, and recently by ourselves in mice, rats, and hamsters
(28,11). The flare reaction is specific in that it can be produced,

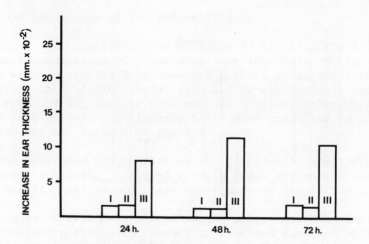

Fig. 4:   Immunologic tolerance induced by DNBSO₃ in hamsters. On
day 0 two groups of female LVG hamsters were putatively sensitized by two applications, four hours apart, of 0.02 ml of
1% DNFB in a solvent consisting of four parts acetone and
one part corn oil. Seven days previously, one group of hamsters had received IP 750 mg/kg of DNBSO₃. On day 7 both
groups as well as a toxicity control group were challenged
on the ear with 0.015 ml of 0.4% DNFB in the acetone-corn
oil solvent. The average reactions at 24, 48 and 72 hours
for each group are shown.
Group I: Toxicity controls; Group II: DNBSO₃, DNFB sensitization; Group III: DNFB sensitization alone.

for example, by parenteral DNBSO₃ if the rodent has been sensitized
previously and challenged with DNFB (or DNCB), but not in animals sensitized and challenged with an unrelated sensitizer such as oxazolone.
Indeed, in a doubly sensitized mouse, intravenous DNBSO₃ causes swelling of the DNFB-challenged ear but not of the oxazolone-challenged
ear. We have demonstrated the flare reaction in B-cell depleted mice
(28). This finding, together with the specificity of the flare reaction, implies that parenteral allergen reacts with a population of
antigen-reactive T cells remaining in the old challenge site, thereby
eliciting a local inflammatory reaction. The observation gives functional evidence for the selective sequestering of a subpopulation of
T cells that reacts specifically with allergen at the site of challenge tests. The selective pooling of antigen-reactive cells at challenge sites has been difficult to demonstrate anatomically (29,30).
The results of a typical experiment demonstrating the flare reaction
in hamsters is shown in Fig. 5.

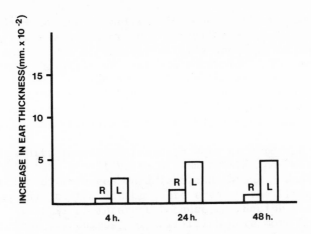

Fig. 5:   Flare reaction induced by $DNBSO_3$ in hamsters. A group of
           five female LVG hamsters were sensitized on days 0 and 1 by
           the application of 0.015 ml of 1% DNFB in a solvent consis-
           ting of four parts acetone and one part corn oil to a clipped
           area on the right flank. Challenge was made on day 7 to the
           left ear with 0.015 ml of 0.4% DNFB in the same solvent. On
           day 34 the hamsters were injected IP with $DNBSO_3$, 750 mg/kg.
           Baseline and subsequent measurements of the previously chal-
           lenged left (L) ear and the normal right (R) ear were made.
           The average increase in thickness at 4, 24 and 48 hours is
           shown.

     In summary, we have studied the generation and expression of ACD
in the hamster, guinea pig, mouse and rat. The general principles
appear to be similar in all four species. The application to the skin
of a high concentration of a strong sensitizer, such as DNFB or oxazolone, induces sensitization in four to five days. Intensification of
the acquisition of sensitivity may be obtained by means of CFA or Cy;
in the guinea pig, a synergism is obtained when the two immunopoten-
tiators are used together (Maguire & Cipriano, unpublished). How CFA
immunopotentiation works is unclear. The mechanism of Cy immunopotentiation in the mouse, and probably in the other three species, involves the inhibition by Cy of T regulator cells. The flare reaction
is readily demonstrable in all four rodent species and has been seen
clinically in man. There appears to be an activation by parenteral
allergen of a specific population of antigen-reactive T cells in the
old challenge site. The flare phenomenon provides functional evidence
for the selective localization of antigen-reactive T cells in challenge sites. The similarity of the expressions of ACD in the guinea
pig, mouse, hamster and rat suggests a similarity of the mechanisms
regulating ACD in these species.

ACKNOWLEDGMENTS

NIH grants AI 13337 and CA-14043.

The invaluable technical assistance of Ms. Barbara Pfeiffer in putting
together this manuscript is gratefully acknowledged.

REFERENCES

1. Chase, M.W. Harvey Lectures, Series 61, pp. 169-203 (1965-1966)
    Academic Press (1967).
2. Landsteiner, K.; Jacob, J. J Exp Med 61 (1935) 643.
3. Landsteiner, K.; Chase, M.W. Proc Soc Exp Biol Med 49 (1942) 688.
4. Sulzberger, M.B. Arch Dermatol Syph 20 (1929) 669.
5. Chase, M.W. Proc Soc Exp Biol Med 61 (1946) 257.
6. Magnusson, B.; Kligman, A.M. Allergic Contact Dermatitis in the
    Guinea Pig; Identification of Contact Allergens. Charles C.
    Thomas, Springfield, Ill. (1970).
7. Maguire, H.C. Jr. Animal Models in Dermatology, ed. Maibach.
    Churchill-Livingston, New York (1975) 67.
8. Asherson, G.L.; Ptak, W. Immunology 15 (1968) 405.
9. Magure, H.C., Jr. Fed Proc 38 (1979) 1173 (Abst #4996).
10. Streilein, J. W. et al. J. Immunol 124 (1980) 577.
11. Jaffee, B.; Maguire, H.C. Jr. Allergic Contact Dermatitis in the
    Rat (in preparation).
12. Maguire, H.C. Jr.; Chase, M.W. J Exp Med 135 (1972) 357.
13. Maguire, H.C. Jr. Immunol Commun 1 (1972) 239.
14. Maguire, H.C. Jr.; Maibach, H.I. J Allergy 32 (1961) 406.
15. Santos, G.W. Fed Proc 26 (1967) 907.
16. Maguire, H.C. Jr.; Ettore, V.L. J Invest Dermatol 48 (1967) 39.
17. Hunziger, N. Dermatologica 135 (1968) 187.
18. Turk, J.L. et al. Immunology 23 (1972) 493.
19. Lagrange, P.W. et al. J Exp Med 139 (1974) 1529.
20. Easmon, C.S.F.; Glynn, A.A. Immunology 33 (1977) 767.
21. Finerty, J.H. Fed Proc 34 (1975) 1025 (Abst. #4568).
22. Kerckhaert, J.A.M. et al. J Immunol 113 (1974) 180.
23. Yoshida, S. et al. Clin Exp Immunol 38 (1979) 211.
24. Maguire, H.C. Jr. et al. Proc Am Assoc Cancer Res 21 (1980) 203
    (Abst. #814).
25. Maguire, H.C. Jr. et al. Immunology 37 (1979) 367.
26. Frei, W. Klin Wochenschr 7 (1928) 539.
27. Claman, H.N.; Moorhead, J.W. Contemp Top Immunobiol 5 (1976) 211.
28. Maguire, H.C. Jr.; Weidanz, W.P. Clin Res 28 (1980) 574A.
29. Turk, J.L. Immunology 5 (1962) 478.
30. Kay, K.; Rieke, W.O. Science 139 (1963) 487.

SECTION II

MOLECULAR IMMUNOLOGY

Chairpersons:

David A. Hart

J. Donald Capra

about 0.033 there was a brief period of avoidance closely followed by a period of complete rejection of the dosed chamber. Note that the fish continued to sample the dosed chamber as indicated by continued brief crossings of the partition. The fish continued to reject the dosed chamber until the waste concentration in the second chamber reached the avoidance level (0.017%).

A second example of an avoidance response is shown in Fig. 4. In this case, five juvenile spot were exposed to the Squibb waste. The fish moved freely between the two test chambers during the control period, spending about half of the time on each side. Response to injection of waste was almost immediate. The fish continued to move between the chambers without perceptible change in number of crossings. However, behavior in other respects changed sharply as the fish remained in the rear of the chamber, diving frequently and nosing at the downstream screen.

During the first hour of the test period, time spent in the dosed chamber was actually increased over the control period. However, as waste concentration reached 0.012 the fish moved out of the dosed chamber and continued to reject the area of higher concentration until the avoidance level was exceeded in both

Fig. 4. Behavioral responses of juvenile spot Leiostomus xanthurus to a composite pharmaceutical and petrochemical waste. Five fish. August 30, 1975.

IMMUNOCHEMICAL CHARACTERIZATION OF SYRIAN HAMSTER MAJOR

HISTOCOMPATIBILITY COMPLEX HOMOLOGUES

J. Theodore Phillips, J. Wayne Streilein, Diane A. Proia,
and William R. Duncan

Departments of Cell Biology and Internal Medicine
The University of Texas Health Science Center at Dallas
Dallas, TX   75235

INTRODUCTION

The genes within the chromosomal segment known as the major histocompatibility complex (MHC) encode products that enable immunologic
communication among cells and promote self-versus-nonself recognition--
capabilities considered vital to every mammalian species (1). Gener-
alizations of the mechanisms involved in MHC function are derived from
studies performed in various animal models (1,2). Historically, the
Syrian hamster has been considered unique with regard to certain MHC-
mediated phenomena. Abnormal structure and/or expression of hamster
MHC products have been suggested to account for certain of these features (3-5). To investigate these alternatives, cell-surface molecules putatively homologous to MHC products of other species have been
identified and immunochemically characterized in the Syrian hamster
(6-8). The possible relationships between these homologues and newly
defined hamster cell-surface alloantigens are considered in this study.

MATERIALS AND METHODS

Mouse anti-H-2 alloantisera utilized in this study were obtained
from the Transplantation Branch, NIAID, National Institutes of Health,
and Dr. J. Klein, Max Planck Institut fur Biologie, Tubingen, FRG.
The potential reactivities of these sera are shown in Table 1.

The methods of hamster alloantisera production and detection of
hamster cell-surface determinants by immunoprecipitation from radiolabeled antigen preparations have been described in detail (6-8).
Non-equilibrium pH gradient electrophoresis (pH 3-10) was performed
as described (12).

Table 1. Potential Reactivities of Murine Antisera Used in this Study[1,2]

Code	Recipient	Donor	K	A	B	J	E	C	S	G	D	Qa-1	Qa-2	Qa-3	Tla	Known specificities
					(I)											
K304	(A.BY X B10.AKM)F_1		b	b	b	b	b	b	b	b	b	b	a	a	c	
		B10.A	k	k	k	k	k	d	d	d	d	a	a	a	a	H-2.4, 40, 41 (Klein et al. 1976)[10]
NIH anti-D^d	(A.SW X B10.AKM)F_1		s	s	s	s	s	s	s	s	s	b	a	a	b	
		A.TH	s	s	s	s	s	s	s	s	d	a	a	a	a	H-2.43
K595	(B10 X R107)F_1		b	b	b	b	b	b	b	?	d	b	a	a	b	
		B10.A(5R)	b	b	b	k	k	d	d	d	d	a	?	?	a	Ia.7 (Wakeland and Klein 1979)[11]
NIH anti-Ia.7	B10 X HTI)F_1		b	b	b	b	b	b	b	?	d	b	a	a	b	
		B10.A(5R)	b	b	b	k	k	d	d	d	d	a	?	a	a	Ia.7 (possibly Ia.22)[3]

(I = A, B, J, E, C)

[1] Potential reactivities are enclosed; dotted enclosures indicate incomplete data.

[2] Haplotype designations are according to Klein et al. 1978 (9).

[3] NIH Catalog of Mouse Alloantisera.

The two-stage microcytotoxicity test was performed essentially as described (13). Antiserum absorptions were performed as previously described (7,8).

RESULTS

Criteria have been suggested (1) by which MHC products of diverse species may be categorized. Class I (e.g., HLA-A,B,C; H-2K,D) products are the classical major transplantation antigens responsible for allograft rejection and non-transplantation antigen recognition by specific T cells. Class II (e.g., HLA-D, DR; H-2Ia) products also may influence allograft rejection, but more generally promote immunologic collaboration among subsets of functionally diverse lymphocytes. Class I and II products exhibit remarkably conserved molecular structures throughout mammalian evolution. This property has enabled the detection of class I and II molecules in several species by suitably cross-reactive antisera (14-17).

Class I Homologues

A survey of murine anti-class I alloantisera has identified two antisera that cross-react with determinants expressed by hamster lymphoid cells. These antisera (K304 and NIH anti-D^d; see Table 1) detect the murine H-2D^d class I product. Various hamster lymphoid cell types were tested in an in vitro cytotoxicity assay with these antisera and a representative summary of results is shown in Table 2. The cross-reactive determinants detected by cytotoxicity assay are expressed on 70% or more of each hamster lymphoid cell type tested (except bone marrow), which is consistent with the expected ubiquitous distribution of class I determinants (1,2,18).

Table 2. Summary of NIH Anti-D^d Reactivity Against Various Hamster Lymphoid Tissues

Cell type	Maximum cytotoxicity[1]	Reciprocal of titer at 50% maximum cytotoxicity
GD36 B-cell lymphoma	70%	4
Lymph node	85%	8
Spleen	80%	4
Thymus	80%	8
Bone marrow	20%	4

[1]Complement (C') cytotoxicity controls are subtracted and did not exceed 10% for any of the tested cell types.

Table 3.   Absorption of Anti-H-2D[d] Alloantiserum by Hamster Cells

	Absorption with:[1]		
	Erythrocytes	Lymph node cells	Fibroblasts
% Reduction:[2]	0	30	40

[1]Cells from MHA hamsters.

[2]Calculated by comparison to activity of appropriately diluted anti-D[d] tested on radiolabeled H-2D[d] antigen preparations.

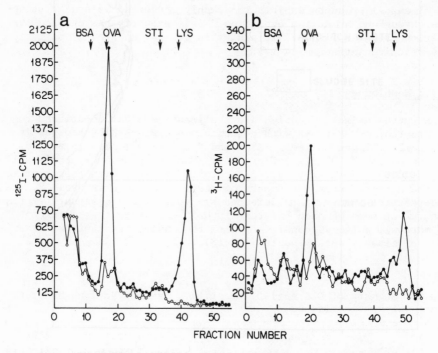

Fig. 1a, b: SDS-PAGE of radiolabeled antigens from MHA lymph node
cells detected by rabbit anti-human β_2-microglobulin.
(a) Lectin-purified extracts from 10^8 ^{125}I-labeled cells
were reacted with anti-β_2M (●) or normal rabbit serum (O).
(b) Lectin-purified extracts from 2.5 x 10^6 ^{3}H-leucine
labeled cells were reacted with anti-β_2M (●) or rabbit
anti-hamster IgG (O).   Immunoprecipitates were analyzed
on 13% reduced gels.   Molecular weight markers included
bovine serum albumin (BSA; 68K), ovalbumin (OVA; 45K),
soybean trypsin inhibitor (STI; 20.1K) and lysozyme
(LYS; 14.3K).

To examine whether the murine anti-D^d cross-reaction with hamster determinants was due to serologically-shared structures rather than a non-specific interaction, aliquots of murine anti-D^d antisera were absorbed with equal volumes of hamster erythrocytes, lymph node cells or fibroblasts, and then tested for their capacity to immunoprecipitate H-2D^d molecules from radiolabeled murine lymphoid cell preparations (Table 3). Absorption with hamster erythrocytes did not appear to reduce specifically anti-D^d activity. Absorption with either hamster lymph node cells or fibroblasts, in comparison, reduced by similar amounts the capacity of anti-D^d antisera to immunoprecipitate the H-2D^d product. Determinants expressed on hamster lymphoid cells and fibroblasts must therefore display significant serologic homology with murine H-2D^d class I products.

Attempts to immunoprecipitate anti-D^d reactive determinants directly from radiolabeled hamster preparations have been unsuccessful, perhaps because of the low affinity of the cross-reacting antibodies. When a cross-reacting rabbit anti-human β_2-microglobulin antiserum was used, however, a 43,000-dalton cell-surface glycoprotein (p43) and 12,000-dalton putative hamster β_2-microglobulin (p12) have been co-immunoprecipitated from hamster lymph node cell preparations (6; Fig. 1). By implication from similar studies in other species (19-22), hamster p43 likely represents a family of MHC-associated molecules, including MHC class I products, which are characteristically non-covalently associated with β_2-microglobulin.

These studies show that hamsters express cell-surface products that are serologically and structurally homologous to class I MHC products of other species. These products are also distributed among a variety of hamster tissues, compatible with the ubiquitous tissue distribution characteristic of MHC class I products.

Class II Homologues

Murine alloantisera directed against H-2 Ia^k products (Table 1) have been reported to cross-react with MHC class II homologues expressed on rat (15,16), miniature swine (17), and human (23, 24) lymphoid cells. When tested on various hamster lymphoid cell types, murine anti-Ia^k was found to cross-react with determinants present on 20% to 90% of each cell type (Table 4). GD36 (B cell) lymphoma cells were most readily killed by murine anti-Ia^k, hamster bone marrow cells were least readily killed. Absorption-immunoprecipitation experiments similar to those previously described concerning hamster class I homologues were performed next to test the specificity of the apparent cross-reaction of murine anti-Ia^k with hamster cell-surface determinants. Aliquots of murine anti-Ia^k were absorbed with equal volumes of either hamster erythrocytes, lymph node cells or fibroblasts and tested for their capacity to immunoprecipitate Ia^k products from radiolabeled murine lymphoid cell preparations (Table 5). In contrast to

Table 4. Summary of Anti-Ia^k Reactivity Against Various Hamster
Lymphoid Tissues

Cell type	Maximum cytotoxicity[1]	Reciprocal of titer at 50% maximum cytotoxicity
GD36 B-cell lymphoma	93%	16
Lymph node	85%	16
Spleen	80%	32
Thymus	55%	8
Bone marrow	20%	4

[1]Complement (C') cytotoxicity controls are subtracted and did not
exceed 10% for any of the tested cell types.

hamster class I homologues, class II homologues were found to be absent
from both hamster erythrocytes and fibroblasts, but are expressed by
lymph node cells. In addition, absorption with hamster thymocytes or
GD36 lymphoma cells showed a reduction of anti-Ia^k activity similar to
that observed after absorption with lymph node cells. Therefore, cell-
surface structures serologically homologous to murine Ia^k MHC class II
products are expressed by some, but not all, hamster somatic cells.
This somewhat limited tissue distribution of these determinants is characteristic of MHC class II products (1,2,18).

Immunoprecipitation of ^{3}H-leucine labeled hamster lymph node
cell preparations with murine anti-Ia^k yields two molecular populations of 39,000 and 29,000 daltons (7; Fig. 2). These molecules
show no tendency towards covalent association with each other or with
other molecules; preliminary data, however, suggest that the 39- and
29-kD species may exist as a non-covalently bound complex which is disrupted under standard conditions of analysis (Phillips, unpublished
data). With regard to radiolabeling characteristics, lactoperoxidase-

Table 5. Absorption of Anti-H-2Ia^k Alloantiserum by Hamster Cells

	Absorption with:[1]				
	Erythrocytes	Lymph node cells	Fibroblasts	Thymocytes	GD36
% Reduction:[2]	0	40	0	20	35

[1]All cells, except GD36 lymphoma, from MHA hamsters.

[2]Calculated by comparison to activity of appropriately diluted anti-
Ia^k tested on radiolabeled H-2Ia^k antigen preparations.

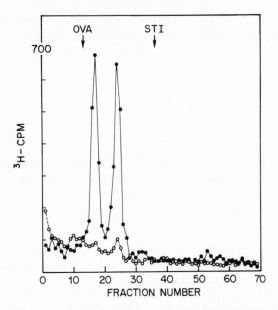

Fig. 2: SDS-PAGE of ^{3}H-leucine-labeled MHA hamster lymph node cells
immunoprecipitated with murine anti-Ia^k (K595). Lectin-
purified extracts from 2 x 10[7] cells were reacted with anti-
Ia^k (●) or anti-D^d (K304; 0) and analyzed on 15% reduced gels.

catalyzed iodination appears to label only the 29-kD component (7).
This property has also been demonstrated for mouse and guinea pig MHC
class II products (25).

Therefore, we have described hamster cell-surface molecules with
serologic and structural homology to MHC class II products. Hamster
class II homologues appear to be distributed among a variety of lymphoid tissues including thymocytes. Hamster erythrocytes and fibroblasts, as expected, do not express detectable amounts of these determinants.

Hamster Cell-Surface Alloantigens

Recent studies from this laboratory have demonstrated serologically-detectable alloantigenic differences among recently wild hamsters and classically inbred strains (6,26). The serologic typing of
these alloantisera is reviewed elsewhere in this volume (27). The
structural characteristics of all hamster alloantigens thus far identified are exemplified by the prototypic molecules identified by the
alloantiserum, MIT anti-MHA (6;Fig. 3). In each case in which immuno-

Table 6. Detection of Hamster Alloantigens p39/p29 in Various Strains[1]

	MIT anti-MHA	TX anti-MHA	SYR anti-MHA	CB anti-MIT	MHA anti-UT	CB anti-UT	CB anti-GS
MHA	+	+	+	−	−	−	−
UT	+		+	+	+	+	
TX	−	−		+		+	+
MIT	−		+	+			

[1]Radiolabeled lymph node cell preparations from each strain were immunoprecipitated with each alloantiserum; + denotes the detection of p39/p29 components.

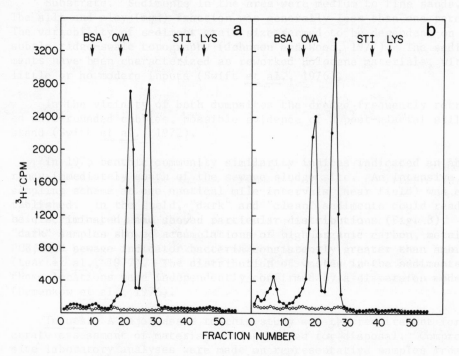

Fig. 3a, b: SDS-PAGE of alloantigens from ^{3}H-leucine-labeled MHA lymph node cells. Lectin-purified extracts from 2.5 x 10[7] cells were reacted with MIT anti-MHA (O) or normal MIT serum (●) and the immunoprecipitates were analyzed on 13% reduced (a) or unreduced (b) gels.

precipitable material has been analyzed (Table 6), hamster alloantisera are found to react only with populations of cell-surface glycoproteins with MWs of 39,000 (p39) and 29,000 (p29). Preliminary studies
indicate that p39 and p29 components may form a labile non-covalently
bound complex similar to that described for hamster class II homologues.
In contrast to the class II homologues, however, the p39/p29 alloantigens identified by MIT anti-MHA (and TX anti-MHA) are both well-labeled
by lactoperoxidase-catalyzed radioiodination (6).

By immunoprecipitation and cytotoxicity analyses, alloantigens
p39 and p29 are expressed by a variety of hamster lymphoid tissues,
but are absent from fibroblasts (Table 7). Alloantiserum MIT anti-
MHA, however, does detect determinants expressed by MHA erythrocytes.
These determinants probably represent a separate class of alloantigens,
since erythrocyte-absorbed MIT anti-MHA retains activity comparable to
the unabsorbed serum tested on various hamster lymphoid cell types
(not shown). This tissue distribution is generally comparable to that
of the similarly-sized hamster class II products defined by cross-
reactive murine anti-Ia^k (cf. Table 7). Thus, hamster alloantisera
define cell-surface antigens, which by structure and tissue distribution appear to resemble MHC class II rather than class I molecules.
Significantly, no evidence of class I allotypic variation has yet been
detected in this species.

Table 7. Tissue Distribution of p39/p29 Alloantigens and MHC Class
          II Homologues[1]

	MHA						
	Lymph node	Thymus	Spleen	Bone marrow	1° fibro- blast	MHST fi- broblast	GD36 lymphoma
MIT anti-MHA	+	+	+	+	−	−	+
TX anti- MHA	+	+	+	+	−		
Murine anti-Ia^k	+	+	+	+		−	+

[1]Derived from immunoprecipitation and cytotoxicity data.

Relationships Between Hamster Cell-Surface Alloantigens and Class II
Products

The apparent similarities of cell-surface products detected by
hamster alloantisera and cross-reactive murine anti-Ia^k pertain to
their nominal molecular weights and tissue distributions. Additional
experiments designed to test the relationship between antigens recognized by separate antisera involve "preclearing" the antigen preparation with one antiserum and then testing the remaining fraction with
a second antiserum. Pretreatment of an ^{125}I-labeled MHA antigen preparation with MIT anti-MHA has been found not to affect the precipitation of the 29-kD component by murine anti-Ia^k (Phillips, unpublished
results). This observation suggests that hamster alloantigens detected by MIT anti-MHA are non-identical to the similarly-sized and
distributed hamster class II products detected by murine anti-Ia^k.
The relatively weak reactivity of the anti-Ia^k reagent, however, prevented complete analysis of reciprocal preclearing.

Non-equilibrium pH gradient electrophoresis (NEPHGE) has proven
useful in separating cell-surface molecules on the basis of native
charge (12,28). MIT anti-MHA alloantigens and anti-Ia^k reactive components were examined by this method (Fig. 4). In both instances a
relatively non-complex pattern was obtained, consisting of two or
three major components. Additional studies (not shown), combining
isoelectric focusing and SDS-PAGE, have identified the highly acidic
component as the 39-kD entity and the relatively basic component as
the 29-kD entity. NEPHGE analysis of these components on a common gel
(Fig. 5) shows at least four separate major peaks, thus confirming
their nonoverlapping identities. Thus, at least two distinct populations of 39- and 29-kD cell-surface components are identified by these
studies. One population is homologous to murine MHA class II products
by size, labeling characteristics, tissue distribution and serologic
cross-reaction; another similar, yet distinct, population represents
the first alloantigens described immunochemically in this species.

Relationships Between Hamster Cell-Surface Alloantigens and Hm-1

To assess the linkage relationships between loci encoding p39/p29
alloantigens and the hamster MHC-equivalent, Hm-1, experiments were
performed with partially congenic hamster strains derived by repeated
backcrosses to the MHA background. In each backcross generation, progeny expressing allogeneic Hm-1 determinants were identified by the capacity of lymphocytes from these animals to act as stimulators in mixed
lymphocyte reactions (MLRs) with MHA (Hm-1^a) lymphocytes as responders
(3,26,27). Backcross progeny that were incapable of stimulating MHA
lymphocytes in MLR were presumed to bear the Hm-1^a homozygous genotype.
Antigen preparations derived from MLR stimulator (+) and non-stimula-
tor (-) progeny were then reacted with hamster alloantisera to determine the expression of p39/p29 alloantigens by these phenotypes (Table

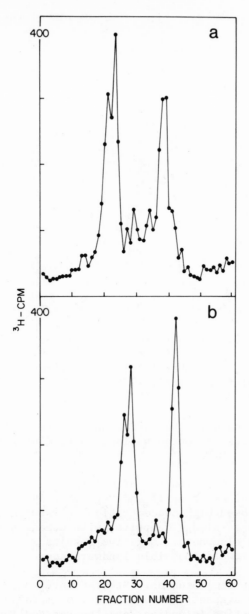

Fig. 4a, b: NEPHGE analysis of immunoprecipitates obtained from ^{3}H-leucine-labeled MHA glycoprotein fractions. 2 x 10[7] cell-equivalents were reacted with (a) murine anti-Ia[k] (K595) or (b) 5 x 10[6] cell-equivalents were reacted with MIT anti-MHA and analyzed as described in Materials and Methods. The acidic end is to the right; the basic end to the left.

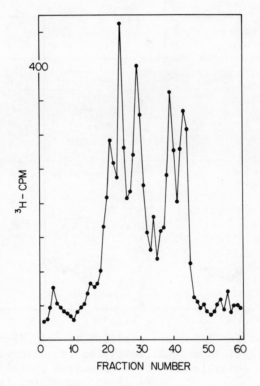

Fig. 5: NEPHGE analysis of a mixture of the immunoprecipitates shown
         in Fig. 4a and b.

8). Alloantiserum MIT anti-MHA immunoprecipitates p39/p29 alloantigens from MLR$^+$ and MLR$^-$ progeny of both [(MHA X UT) X MHA] N_6 and
[(MHA X TX) X MHA] N_5 backcrosses. This observation demonstrates the
expected detection of p39/p29 alloantigens encoded by a portion of
the MHA genome expressed in each of these partially congenic combinations. Alloantiserum CB anti-UT, however, reacts only with antigen
preparations derived from MLR$^+$ [MHA X UT) X MHA] N_6 progeny. This
finding strongly implies the linkage of loci governing the expression
of UT p39/p29 alloantigens and loci defining Hm-1. The failure of CB
anti-UT to immunoprecipitate cross-reactive TX p39/p29 alloantigens
from the MLR$^+$ [(MHA X TX) X MHA] N_5 antigen preparation implies that
the loci encoding these alloantigens have been successfully removed
by repeated backcrosses and selection of the TX Hm-1 haplotype. Therefore, TX p39/p29 alloantigens which cross-react with CB anti-UT must
not be encoded by loci linked to Hm-1. The data suggest that CB anti-
UT detects two categories of p39/p29 alloantigens: those that are encoded by loci linked to Hm-1 and those that are not.

DISCUSSION

MHC class I and II products demonstrate characteristic immunochemical properties that are apparently well-conserved throughout evolution (1,29,30). By criteria of molecular sizes, chemical properties,
tissue distributions and interspecies serological cross-reactions with
homologous MHC products, likely candidates for hamster MHC class I
and II products have been identified. Hamster cell-surface molecules
(p39/p29) detected by all known cytotoxic hamster alloantisera are
remarkably similar to the previously designated hamster class II homologues. Logically, p39/p29 alloantigens probably also represent hamster class II MHC products, even though in at least one instance, p39/
p29 and anti-Ia^k reactive hamster molecules are non-identical (Fig.
5). Despite apparent class II polymorphism, however, hamster MHC
class I homologues do not appear to express serologically detectable
allotypic variation. The closest known parallel to this uncommon situation is the series of serologically-silent H-2K^b class I mutations
in the mouse (31).

The functional MHC-equivalent of the Syrian hamster, Hm-1, encodes alloantigens responsible for acute skin graft rejection (SGR),
MLR and graft-versus-host reactions (GVHR) among inbred and recently
wild hamster strains (4,26,27). Allogeneic MLRs serve as a convenient
phenotypic marker for Hm-1 since the hamster MLR is known to be controlled by a single locus (or tightly linked loci) closely linked to
other loci governing SGR and GVHR. Although non-MHC loci capable of
promoting MLR do exist in other species, in no instance have these
loci been associated with acute SGR and GVHR (1,2,18). The association of loci controlling SGR, MLR, and GVHR therefore appears to be a
unique characteristic of the MHC in general (1).

Within the MHC, class II (and occasionally class I) products mediate the MLR (1,2,18). Class II-like hamster p39/p29 alloantigens
are therefore expected to be encoded by loci closely linked to Hm-1.
Genetic analysis has demonstrated this proposed association in the
case of UT p39/p29 alloantigens detected by CB anti-UT. This observation provides additional strong evidence that p39/p29 hamster alloantigens may represent typical class II MHC products. The apparent expression of anti-Ia^k reactive molecules by many, if not all, hamster
strains has precluded the formal demonstration of their proposed relationship to Hm-1.

Additional genetic analysis has, however, raised the possibility
that more complex relationships may exist between loci encoding p39/
p29 and Hm-1 alloantigens. In particular, TX p39/p29 alloantigens
appear to be encoded by loci unlinked to Hm-1. This conclusion is
also supported by recent serologic and MLR-typing analysis of certain
partially congenic hamster strains (27).

Table 8. Genetic Relationships Between Hamster Cell-Surface
Alloantigens and Hm-1

	[(MHA X UT) X MHA] N_6[1]			
	MLR$^-$	[2]MLR$^+$	MHA	UT
MIT anti-MHA	[3]+	+	+	+
CB anti-UT	−	+	−	+

	[(MHA X TX) X MHA] N_5[1]			
	MLR$^-$	MLR$^+$	MHA	TX
MIT anti-MHA	+	+	+	−
CB anti-UT	−	−	−	+

[1]Segregant populations.

[2]Cells from these animals stimulated MHA lymphocytes to respond in
mixed lymphocyte cultures.

[3]+ indicates immunoprecipitation of p39/p29; − indicates that no
immunoprecipitable components were detected.

Several hypotheses may be advanced to explain this unexpected observation: 1. During the process of backcrossing, intra-Hm-1 recombi-
nation occurred and resulted in the separation of certain TX p39/p29
loci from the intact TX Hm-1 haplotype. Although plausible, this explanation is unlikely, because the linkage relationships between several Hm-1 haplotypes and loci encoding serologically-detectable alloantigens are established and are apparently not due to random genetic
events (27). 2. Some hamster haplotypes (e.g., TX) may exhibit relatively loose linkage among the component loci of Hm-1. This may be
secondary to a deficient regulator locus (T locus?) or may simply reflect a natural genetic state for this species. 3. Alloantigens p39/
p29 represent class II homologues some of which are naturally associated with Hm-1, others of which are naturally associated with class
II loci scattered throughout the genome. In many species, immune response (Ir) genes may be MHC-linked, but also are known to occur
throughout the genome (1,2,18). Numerous theories have suggested that
class II and Ir loci are one and the same, and that the Ir gene product
is therefore a class II alloantigen (1,2,18). According to this model,
certain hamster p39/p29 alloantigens might represent non-Hm-1-associ-
ated Ir gene products. 4. Alloantigens p39/p29 consist of a family
of molecules sharing only grossly similar immunochemical characteristics; thus, only a subset is MHC-related, and the remainder have no
further discernible relationship to class II or any other MHC-related
product. This unlikely hypothesis would require a preponderance of
chemically similar cell-surface alloantigens encoded by loci which
bear no obvious evolutionary relationship to each other.

Of these four hypotheses, the second and third alternatives seem to be the most tenable. Neither theory, however, is without its difficulties: all currently described MHCs are composed of tightly linked loci, and the nature of the Ir gene product still remains conjectural. Nonetheless, the existence of class II-like alloantigens outside of the MHC domain is clearly without precedent. This observation, along with the continued lack of evidence of serologically detectable hamster class I polymorphism, implies that certain immunogenetic features may be unique to Syrian hamsters. Further analysis of these issues awaits the development of additional congenic strains and specific alloantisera. At present, there is strong evidence that class I and II MHC homologues are expressed by the Syrian hamster and that certain serologically-detectable hamster alloantigens are Hm-1-encoded class II products. This view is compatible with the generalized features of the mammalian MHC. Other facets of hamster MHC structure and organization may, however, be atypical.

SUMMARY

Based primarily on studies in mice and man, the organization and gene-product structures of the mammalian major histocompatibility complex (MHC) are thought to be extensively conserved. However, attempts to generalize from the specific observations of other species to Syrian hamsters have not been completely successful. Previous studies in hamsters have suggested abnormal structure, expression, and/or function of the putative hamster MHC and its products. Characterization of hamster MHC gene-products is therefore of interest.

This study concerns the identification and characterization of hamster cell-surface glycoproteins homologous to MHC products of man and mouse. Utilizing radioimmunoprecipitation and serologic techniques, these molecules have been characterized with regard to molecular weight, tissue distribution and immunochemical homology to human and murine class I and II MHC products. In addition, alloantisera raised between histoincompatible hamster strains have been similarly used to identify cell-surface alloantigens of this species. The alloantisera detect cell-surrace hamster molecules with immunochemical properties and tissue distribution resembling MHC class II rather than class I products. Thus, in contrast to other species, hamsters appear not to express extensively polymorphic major transplantation antigens of the class I type. Some hamster alloantigens are apparently homologues of Ia determinants since their genes are linked to Hm-1. However, other alloantigens with similar molecular weights are seemingly encoded by genes unlinked to the hamster MHC. These data support the hypothesis that the hamster MHC contains genes which encode for molecular products similar to those described in man and mouse, but that the organization and/or expression of these genes may be atypical.

ACKNOWLEDGMENTS

This work was supported in part by USPHS Grants AI-10678, RR01133 and CA-09082. We gratefully acknowledge excellent preparation of the manuscript by Ms. Sara Howard.

REFERENCES

1. Götze, D., ed. The Major Histocompatibility System in Man and Animals. Springer-Verlag (1977).
2. Klein, J. Biology of the Mouse Histocompatibility-2 Complex. Springer-Verlag (1975).
3. Duncan, W.R.; Streilein, J.W. Transplantation 25 (1978) 12.
4. Duncan, W.R.; Streilein, J.W. Transplantation 25 (1978) 17.
5. Duncan, W.R.; Streilein, J.W. J Immunol 118 (1977) 832.
6. Phillips, J.T. et al. Immunogenetics 7 (1978) 445.
7. Phillips, J.T. et al. Immunogenetics 9 (1979) 477.
8. Phillips, J.T. Dissertation, University of Texas Health Science Center at Dallas (1979).
9. Klein, J. et al. Immunogenetics 6 (1978) 489.
10. Klein, J. et al. Transplantation 22 (1976) 572.
11. Wakeland, E.K.; Klein, J. Immunogenetics 8 (1979) 27.
12. O'Farrell, P.Z. et al. Cell 12 (1977) 1133.
13. Klein, J. et al. Immunogenetics 2 (1975) 141.
14. Smilek, D.E. et al. J Exp Med 151 (1980) 1139.
15. Shinohara, N. et al. J Immunol 121 (1978) 637.
16. Blankenhorn, E.P. et al. Eur J Immunol 10 (1980) 145.
17. Lunney, J.K.; Sachs, D.H. J Immunol 122 (1979) 623.
18. Snell, G.D. et al. Histocompatibility. Academic Press (1976).
19. Vitetta, E.S. et al. J Exp Med 144 (1976) 179.
20. Michaelson, J. et al. J Exp Med 145 (1977) 1066.
21. Schwartz, B.D. et al. J Immunol 121 (1978) 835.
22. Grey, M.H. et al. J Exp Med 138 (1973) 1608.
23. Delovitch, T.L.; Falk, J.A. Immunogenetics 8 (1979) 405.
24. Lunney, J.K. et al. Scand J Immunol 10 (1979) 403.
25. Schwartz, B.D. et al. J Immunol 120 (1978) 671.
26. Streilein, J.W.; Duncan, W.R. Immunogenetics 9 (1979) 563.
27. Duncan, W.R.; Streilein, J.W. This volume.
28. Jones, P.P. et al. J Exp Med 148 (1978) 925.
29. Maizels, R.M. et al. Immunogenetics 7 (1978) 425.
30. Cook, R.G. et al. In: Current Trends in Histocompatibility. Plenum Press (1979).
31. Klein, J. Adv Immunol 26 (1978) 56.

ADDENDUM

Studies on tissue expression of hamster alloantigens by the technique of immunoprecipitation have recently been extended to include two other major tissue types: macrophages and epidermal cells.

In the former case, peritoneal exudate cells were induced by thioglycollate, harvested and allowed to adhere to plastic surfaces. They
were then washed free of non-adherent cells, and cultured for 48 hours
at 37°C under conditions in which metabolic labeling with ^{3}H-leucine
occurred. Lysates were prepared from the adherent cells and analyzed, after appropriate immunoprecipitation, with SDS-PAGE. Epidermal cells were prepared from hamster cheek pouch skin by trypsiniza-
tion to produce a single cell suspension. The monodisperse cells
were then cultured for 48 hours under conditions that allowed metabolic labeling with ^{3}H-leucine. Lysates were prepared from cells harvested at the end of the culture interval, immunoprecipitated and
analyzed by SDS-PAGE. MIT anti-MHA antiserum identified p29 and p39
on the surfaces of hamster macrophages (plastic-adherent peritoneal
exudate cells), a finding in agreement with the hypothesis that these
molecules are hamster homologues of murine Ia antigens. However, the
same antiserum failed to immunoprecipitate any molecules from the
surfaces of hamster epidermal cells. This finding is also consistent
with the idea that this reagent identifies only class II-like molecules. It further implies that class II molecules are not present on
hamster epidermal cells, a realization that has recently emerged from
study of murine skin. The failure to find class II molecules by this
method on cheek pouch cells has another implication: we have recently
shown that the frequency of Langerhans cells within hamster cheek
pouch epidermis is much lower than in normal body wall skin, although
they are clearly identifiable. Since Langerhans cells would be expected to express hamster Ia-antigen homologues, it is important to
note that Ia-like antigens were not detected on cultured epidermal
cell preparations. We must presume that Langerhans cells are deleted
by the culturing maneuver from the epidermal cell preparations.

IMMUNOGLOBULINS ON THE SURFACE OF HAMSTER LYMPHOCYTES

Claire P. Robles, Richard L. Proia, David A. Hart and
Leon Eidels

Department of Microbiology, The University of Texas Health
Science Center at Dallas, Dallas, TX   75235

INTRODUCTION

Cell surface immunoglobulin (Ig) is important as an antigen specific receptor on B lymphocytes. It is distributed in a clonotypic
fashion and may also function in the antigen-dependent triggering of
B lymphocytes. In most species, the predominant isotypes of cell surface Ig are 7-8S membrane IgM (mIgM) and IgD (mIgD). Evidence from
experiments with mouse lymphoid cells indicates that the class of Ig
present on the B cell can determine whether a cell is triggered or
tolerized after exposure to specific antigen (reviewed in 1,2). Onto-
genic development of cell surface Ig in the murine system begins with
the appearance of mIgM-bearing cells and is followed by cells expressing both mIgM and mIgD. Immature murine B lymphocytes display predominantly mIgM at the cell surface and constitute a population of lymphocytes that are readily tolerized. In contrast, mature B cells express
both mIgM and mIgD on their surface. Exposure of these mature cells
to antigen leads to subsequent proliferation and differentiation to
antibody secretion. Furthermore, removal of mIgD from the surface of
these mature lymphocytes (by treatment with papain or capping by specific antisera) results in a population of cells that becomes preferentially tolerized by antigen (2). Thus, the two classes of surface
Ig, mIgM and mIgD, appear to regulate the response of B lymphocytes
to antigen presentation.

In several species, including man and mouse, cell surface Ig has
been well characterized. Less is known, however, about these important molecules in the hamster. Immunofluorescence studies have been
reported, indicating that subpopulations of hamster splenocytes express
IgM (25%), IgG (6%), and IgA (5%) (3). Whereas recent evidence suggests hamsters have serum IgE (4), IgD in the hamster has not been

identified. Since the serum concentration of IgD in other species is
low, it seemed reasonable to use cell surface immunoglobulins, of
which IgD is a major constituent in many species, to look for hamster
IgD. This report relates data which, together with previous investigations (5), indicate that two Ig isotypes are predominant on the cell
surface of hamster lymphoid cells. One of these isotypes is mIgM and
the other is a likely candidate for the hamster equivalent of membrane
IgD.

MATERIALS AND METHODS

Female MHA or CB hamsters, 1 to 6 months old, were obtained from
Charles River Laboratories. Radiolabeling of cells, immunoprecipitations and sodium dodecyl sulfate (SDS)-polyacrylamide gel electrophoresis (PAGE) were carried out as previously described (5). Briefly,
single-cell suspensions of the lymph nodes from unimmunized hamsters
were prepared. These cells (1×10^8), in 1 ml of phosphate buffered
saline (PBS) (0.01M sodium phosphate, 0.15M NaCl, pH 7.2), were iodinated by the lactoperoxidase method (6) utilizing carrier-free ^{125}I
(Amersham-Searle Corp). Radiolabeled cells were washed and lysed in
2 ml of 0.5% NP-40 in Tris buffered saline (TBS) (0.01M Tris-HCl, 0.15M
NaCl, pH 7.4). Where indicated, protease inhibitors (0.5 mg soybean
trypsin inhibitor/ml, 1mM iodoacetamide, 100 μM $ZnCl_2$, and 0.2 mg pheny-
lmethylsulfonylfluoride/ml) were added to the lysing buffer. Nuclei
were pelleted by centrifugation and the resulting supernatant dialyzed
against TBS for three hours at $4^\circ C$. The radiolabeled glycoprotein
fraction, containing all of the cell surface Ig, was obtained by lentil lectin affinity chromatography (7).

A rabbit anti-hamster IgM (μ chain) (RαHμ) was prepared using purified hamster serum IgM as the immunizing agent. In order to obtain
hamster IgM, serum was collected from MHA and CB female hamsters, immunized four days earlier with sheep RBC to increase IgM titers. The
serum was centrifuged ($10^5 \times g$, two hours, $2^\circ C$) to remove aggregates
and lipoproteins. The clarified serum was subjected to gel filtration
with Sephacryl G-300 (Pharmacia). The column was developed in a descending fashion with PBS as the buffer and the ascending portion of
the highest molecular weight peak was pooled. This fraction was then
subjected to affinity chromatography on rabbit anti-hamster Ig-Sepha-
rose (prepared by the cyanogen bromide-activation method [8]). The adsorbed protein was eluted with 3.5M $MgCl_2$ and was shown to be pure IgM
by SDS-PAGE analysis. Electrophoresis of 100 μg of the unreduced purified IgM showed only one band (1×10^6 daltons), and two bands (80,000
and 23,000 daltons) when the samples were reduced. No contaminating
bands were detected by Coomasie blue staining. Unreduced and reduced
MOPC 104E (Bionetics) were used as molecular weight markers. The purified hamster IgM did not react with an antiserum to $alpha_2$ macroglobulin (Dr. J. Stein-Streilein, University of Texas Health Science Center
at Dallas) when analyzed by double diffusion in gels. This latter

result indicated that the purified protein did not contain alpha$_2$ macroglobulin, the major high molecular weight serum component which
could have co-purified with the IgM.

New Zealand white rabbits were immunized with 75 µg of the purified IgM in Freund's complete adjuvant (Difco) and then boosted twice
more at three-week intervals in Freund's incomplete adjuvant (Difco).
Light chain specificity was removed from the resulting immune serum by
affinity chromatography on hamster IgG-Sepharose (hamster IgG prepared
as described [9]). The non-adherent fraction was analyzed by double
diffusion in gels and was shown to have activity against IgM but not
IgG. When the antiserum was reacted with ^{125}I-labeled normal hamster
serum, IgM was specifically precipitated.

For detection of cell-surface Ig, aliquots of the ^{125}I-labeled
glycoprotein fraction from lymphoid cells were incubated with the prepared RαHµ and various other immunoglobulin reagents. These reagents
included normal rabbit IgG (NRIg) (9), rabbit anti-hamster IgG (heavy
and light chain specificities, Cappel Laboratories) (RαHIg), rabbit
anti-mouse IgM (µ chains) (RαMµ) and rabbit anti-mouse IgD (δ chain)
(Dr. E. Vitetta, UTHSCD), rabbit anti-hamster IgA (α chain) (Dr. P.
Kelly, N.Y.U. Dental Center). The antigen-antibody complexes formed
during incubation with the RαHµ and other reagents were precipitated
with Protein A-bearing Staphylococcus aureus. Immune precipitates were
washed in TBS-NP-40 (0.1%)-BSA (0.1 mg/ml) and solubilized by boiling
in SDS (1%)-Tris-HCl (0.1M)-Urea (8M) (pH 8.4). The insoluble S. aureus
was collected by centrifugation. When 2-mercaptoethanol (2-ME) was
added, to a 1.2M final concentration, to reduce disulfide bonds, samples were analyzed by SDS-7.5% PAGE. For analyzing unreduced samples,
SDS-5% polyacrylamide gels were used. Internal molecular weight
markers of reduced and unreduced ^{3}H-mouse IgM (HP-76 plasmacytoma,
Dr. M. Sawyer, UTHSCD) and ^{3}H-hamster IgG (GD-36 lymphoma) were included in each sample. After development of the gels for 14 to 16
hours at 5 mA/gel for unreduced samples, or 7 mA/gel for reduced samples, the gels were fractionated and analyzed for radioactivity. Internal markers were analyzed as described (5). For purposes of determining the polypeptide composition of unreduced molecules, the radiolabeled protein peaks were extracted from the 5% gels, pooled and lyophilized. After the pooled samples were reconstituted, and reduced
with 2-ME, they were applied to SDS-7.5% polyacrylamide gels and electrophoresed.

RESULTS AND DISCUSSION

Hamster lymph node cells were surface radiolabeled, lysed with
NP-40 and fractionated on a lentil lectin-Sepharose column. Aliquots
of the ^{125}I-glycoprotein fraction were immunoprecipitated with RαHIg,
RαMµ, or NRIg. The immune precipitates were analyzed on SDS-PAGE under
reducing conditions. As might be expected with a reagent possessing

light chain specificity, the RαHIg precipitated more than one class
of heavy chain. Two species of heavy chains, 84,000 dalton and 68,000
dalton, were consistently precipitated along with light chains of
23,000 daltons. The major cell-surface heavy chain was the 84,000
dalton species, somewhat heavier than the μ chain of murine IgM myeloma HP-76 (80,000 daltons), and the less prominent peak was electrophoretically distinct from the gamma chain of GD-36 (52,000 daltons),
with a mobility corresponding to a molecular weight of 68,000. The
cross-reactive RαMμ reagent was able to precipitate material that contained the 84,000 dalton heavy chain as well as the light chain, but
not material containing the 68,000 dalton chain (Table 1). The maximum amount of the 84,000 dalton chain detected by use of increasing
concentrations of the cross-reactive reagent, however, was always approximately 40% to 60% of that detected using the RαHIg. All three
peaks of radioactivity (heavy and light chains) were absent in the
NRIg control immune precipitate.

     To determine whether the cross-reactive RαMμ reagent was less ef-
fective than the RαHIg because of affinity considerations,glycoprotein
fractions of ^{125}I-labeled lymph node cells were precleared with the
RαMμ reagent using two sequential rounds of precipitation. The resulting supernatants were divided and treated with either RαMμ or
RαHIg. Essentially no radioactivity was detected by additional treatment with the RαMμ reagent, indicating that molecules recognized by
this antiserum had been successfully depleted. The RαHIg reagent, however, was still able to recognize additional material containing the
84,000 dalton molecules which were not reactive with the RαMμ reagent.
Approximately 40% to 60% of the 84,000 dalton peak that was present
before the preclearing was precipitated by the polyvalent RαHIg, but
not by the cross-reactive μ chain-specific reagent. Thus, the RαMμ
reagent appears to recognize a subpopulation of the molecules containing the 84,000 dalton heavy chain.

     When glycoprotein fractions of cell lysates were analyzed with a
rabbit anti-hamster IgA (α chain) reagent or a rabbit anti-mouse IgD
(δ chain) reagent, no radioactive peaks were detected by SDS-PAGE.
Therefore, the antigenic identity of molecules containing the 68,000
dalton heavy chains could not be ascertained.

     To determine the apparent molecular weights of the precipitated
molecules in their unreduced form, aliquots of the glycoprotein fraction were precipitated as before, with RαHIg and RαMμ, and analyzed by
SDS-5% PAGE. Three peaks of radioactivity were observed using the
RαHIg reagent. These corresponded to molecular weights of 220,000,
170,000, and 110,000. When the unreduced radiolabeled proteins were
extracted from the gels, reduced with 2-ME and analyzed on SDS-7.5%
polyacrylamide gels, the results listed in Table 1 were obtained. The
220,000 dalton peak consisted of 84,000 dalton heavy chains and 23,000
dalton light chains. This was also the case with the 110,000 dalton
molecule. The 170,000 dalton peak, on the other hand, gave rise to

Table 1. Polypeptide Chain Composition

| Antiserum | Apparent mol. wt. $(\times 10^{-3})$[1] | | Structure |
	Unreduced	Reduced	
RαHIg[2]	220	84 + 23	
RαMμ[3]	220	84 + 23	$\mu_2 L_2$
RαMμ			
then RαHIg	220	84 + 23	$(84_2 L_2)$
RαHIg	170	68 + 23	$(68_2 L_2)$
RαMμ	110	84 + 23	μ–L
RαMμ			
then RαHIg	110	84 + 23	84–L

[1]Apparent mol. wt. were determined on SDS 5%–PAGE and on SDS-7.5% PAGE for unreduced and reduced molecules, respectively (see Materials and Methods).

[2]RαHIg = rabbit anti-hamster IgG (heavy and light chains).

[3]RαMμ = rabbit anti-mouse IgM (μ chain).

the 68,000 dalton heavy chain as well as light chains. By use of a pre-clearing protocol similar to that described earlier, it was found that only a subpopulation of the 220,000 dalton and 110,000 dalton molecular weight classes, which contain the 84,000 dalton chain, were recognized by the cross-reactive RαMμ antiserum. The percentage of the subpopulation recognized by the RαMμ reagent was similar to what was found earlier in the reduced system (40% to 60%).

Therefore, at least some of the 220,000 dalton molecules represent intact mIgM, and they are composed of two heavy (84,000 daltons) and two light (23,000 daltons) chains. The 110,000 dalton molecule appears to be, at least in part, half-molecules of mIgM. Such half-molecules of surface immunoglobulin have been reported in the mouse (10). The 170,000 dalton immunoglobulin also appears to consist of two heavy (68,000 dalton) and two light chains (Table 1).

The inability of the RαMμ reagent to recognize a subpopulation of the 84,000 dalton molecules that is recognized by the RαHIg reagent could have at least two explanations. First, it is possible that two distinct isotypes have heavy chains falling into the same 84,000 dalton molecular weight class. It is reasonable to suggest this because both in the human (11) and in the rat (12,13), the delta chain of cell-surface IgD co-electrophoreses with the μ chain of mIgM under conditions similar to those described here. Therefore, if the 84,000 dalton molecules consist of two types of heavy chains, it would be conceivable that the heavy chain, not cross-reactive with the RαMμ reagent, is hamster mIgD. An alternative explanation is that the antiserum against mouse μ chains (RαMμ) cross-reacts with only a subpopulation of hamster

Table 2.   Identification of 84,000 Dalton Heavy Chain

Antiserum	Precleared with RαMμ	Per cent ^{125}I-cpm at 84,000 dalton[1]
RαHIg[2]	−	100
	+	43
RαHμ[3]	−	109[5]
	+	43
RαMμ[4]	−	54[5]
	+	16

[1][125]I-cpm relative to RαHIg (100%).

[2]RαHIg = rabbit anti-hamster IgG (heavy and light chains).

[3]RαHμ = rabbit anti-hamster IgM (μ chain).

[4]RαMμ = rabbit anti-mouse IgM (μ chain).

[5]Average of three experiments.

mIgM. This would mean that the subpopulation not recognized by the RαMμ reagent (approximately 40% to 60%) differs antigenically from the mIgM that is precipitated.

A rabbit anti-hamster IgM (RαHμ) was prepared, to distinguish between the two possibilities discussed above. The RαHμ reagent was generated against hamster serum IgM and rendered specific for the μ heavy chain. When added to the glycoprotein fraction of ^{125}I labeled cell lysates, the RαHμ reagent immunoprecipitated 220,000 dalton molecules that could be shown to consist of 84,000 dalton heavy chains and 23,000 dalton light chains. The antiserum did not recognize molecules containing the 68,000 dalton heavy chains. The RαHμ reagent, made against serum IgM, should react with all of the mIgM present on the cell surface regardless of antigenic differences, provided these differences were represented in the serum IgM. Again, a preclearing experiment was performed, in which sequential rounds of the RαMμ reagent were used to deplete the lysate of all molecules recognized by that reagent.   The resulting supernatant was divided and one aliquot was treated with the RαMμ reagent, showing that the RαMμ reactivity had been almost completely removed as expected because of the prior depletion.   More importantly, when RαHIg, or RαHμ, was used on the remaining supernatant, either reagent was still able to precipitate the remaining molecules (approximately 40%) containing the 84,000 dalton heavy chain (Table 2). Treatment with the RαHIg continued to precipitate the 68,000 dalton molecule under these conditions. Therefore, both the anti-IgM reagent made against the hamster (RαHμ), and the polyclonal RαHIg, precipitate the same population of immunoglobulins

containing the 84,000 dalton polypeptide. These results strongly suggest that all of the 84,000 dalton heavy chains belong to the IgM class
of immunoglobulin.

An unresolved issue concerns the fact that the RαMμ reagent was
unable to recognize a portion of the hamster mIgM. Complete removal
of all mIgM precipitated by this reagent leaves behind some 40% to 60%
of the total mIgM available to the polyclonal RαHIg reagent. A possible explanation for this observation is that there are two subclasses of hamster IgM, both expressed on the cell surface, and that
RαMμ recognizes only one of them. It is unlikely, however, that an
antiserum against mouse IgM would fail to recognize shared determinants between subclasses within the hamster, since the antiserum recognizes determinants shared between the mouse and hamster species.
Another consideration is that the RαMμ reagent used was generated
against a myeloma IgM containing lambda light chains (MOPC 104E). Residual anti-light chain activity would not be detected in cell lysates
of mice, since this species has 95% kappa chains (14). The ratio of
kappa to lambda chains in the immunoglobulins of the hamster is not
known. If the hamster should resemble the human species, in which
there are approximately equal amounts of kappa and lambda chains (15),
then possible residual anti-lambda activity, and not specificity for
μ-chain determinants, might account for the hamster mIgM precipitated.
The RαMμ reagent, however, did not react with the molecules containing
the 68,000 dalton heavy chains, which also should have been precipitated in the hamster by virtue of such anti-lambda activity.

The identity of the 68,000 dalton heavy chain is still unresolved.
As previously mentioned, this heavy chain appears to have a mobility
on SDS-PAGE that is slower than the hamster gamma chain (52,000 daltons), and appears not to react with an anti-hamster IgA reagent. An
anti-mouse IgD reagent also failed to precipitate a 68,000 dalton
heavy chain, but this could be due to an inability of the reagent to
cross-react with the hamster IgD. Interestingly, cell-surface delta
chains from mouse IgD have an apparent molecular weight (16) that is
similar to that found for the unidentified hamster cell-surface molecule (ie. 68,000 daltons). Consistent with the known proteolytic lability of mIgD in the mouse (17) are the earlier investigations (5),
utilizing hamster lymph node cells, that proved the molecules containing the 68,000 dalton heavy chains to be susceptible to proteolytic
digestion by papain under conditions that did not degrade mIgM. In
the mouse, the ratio of δ to μ in cell-surface Ig approaches 1.0 in
adult animals (1,2), whereas in adult hamsters the 68,000:μ ratio had
been reported to be much lower (5). In recent experiments, however,
when a mixture of protease inhibitors (soybean trypsin inhibitor, iodoacetamide, zinc chloride and phenylmethylsulfonylfluoride) were included in the lysing and immunoprecipitation protocols, the 68,000
dalton:μ ratio of hamster cell-surface Ig became remarkably similar
to that described for the δ:μ ratio in adult mice. Thus, in the presence of protease inhibitors the 68,000 dalton:μ ratio rose from an

average of 0.36 to 0.92. These results further demonstrate the proteolytic lability of the unidentified 68,000 dalton molecule, and suggest it to be present in a ratio with IgM that is similar to the $\delta:\mu$
ratio found in the mouse.

The data presented in this report indicate that there are two
major classes of mIg on the surface of hamster lymphoid cells. By
use of a reagent prepared specifically against the μ chain of hamster
IgM, it has been demonstrated that the class of immunoglobulin containing the large heavy chain (84,000) is mIgM. The identity of the other
class containing 68,000 dalton heavy chains is not known, since none
of the antisera utilized thus far have reacted specifically with those
molecules. However, this as yet unidentified class seems a likely candidate for hamster mIgD because of its many similarities to murine
cell-surface IgD. Further studies on the appearance and relative abun-
dance of these isotypes during ontogeny may yield additional insights
into the development of immune responsiveness in hamsters.

REFERENCES

1.   Moller, G. Immunol Rev 37 (1977) 3.
2.   Vitetta, E.S., et al. Biological Basis of Immunodeficiency,
      ed. Gelfand and Dosch. (1980) 189.
3.   Coe, J.E.; Green, I. J Natl Cancer Inst 54 (1975) 269.
4.   Sullivan, T. et al. This volume.
5.   Eidels, L. et al. Molec Immunol 16 (1979) 541.
6.   Haustein, D. J Immunol Meth 7 (1975) 25.
7.   Hayman, M.; Crumpton, M.J. Biochem Biophys Res Commun 47 (1972)
      923.
8.   Cuatrecasas, P. J Biol Chem 245 (1970) 359.
9.   Hart, D.A. Infect Immun 11 (1975) 742.
10.   Eidels, L. J Immunol 123 (1979) 846.
11.   Finkleman, F.D. et al. J Immunol 116 (1976) 1173.
12.   Ruddick, J.H.; Leslie, G.A. J Immunol 118 (1977) 1025.
13.   Golding, H. et al. J Immunol 123 (1979) 2751.
14.   McIntire, K.R.; Potter, M. J Natl Cancer Inst 33 (1964) 631.
15.   Fahey, J.L.; Solomon, A. J Exp Med 117 (1963) 81.
16.   Melcher, U. et al. J Exp Med 140 (1974) 1427.
17.   Vitetta, E.S.; Uhr, J.W. J Immunol 117 (1976) 1579.

COMPARATIVE IMMUNOLOGY OF OLD WORLD HAMSTERS -- CRICETINAE

John E. Coe

Department of Health and Human Services, Public Health
Service, National Institutes of Health, National Institute
of Allergy and Infectious Diseases, Laboratory of Persistant
Viral Diseases, Rocky Mountain Laboratory
Hamilton, MT 59840

Previous work in our laboratory has centered on the immunoglobulins (Ig) and immune response of the Syrian hamster. Various other
hamster species are becoming available (1), however, and will be
useful as models in medical research. The question arises whether
these hamsters have Ig's comparable to and antigenically cross-reactive
with those described in the Syrian hamster, so that antisera to previously characterized serum proteins of Syrian hamsters would be useful in studies with non-Syrian hamsters. In addition, the degree of
identity of the various Ig classes in these other species would provide some idea of their relative taxonomic distance from Syrian hamsters. To answer these questions sera fromheterologous non-Syrian hamsters were tested on simple gel diffusion for precipitin reactions
with rabbit antisera specific for Syrian hamster IgG_1, IgG_2, IgA, and
IgM (2). The hamsters also were evaluated for the presence of an interesting sex-limited serum protein called Female Protein (FP) (3).
In the diffusion analysis, the antisera were reacted with the heterologous hamster sera and an adjacent well contained homologous Syrian
hamster sera so that the heterologous protein could be evaluated for
its antigenic identity (+ = fusion reaction) or antigenic deficiency
($+_s$ = spur formation) with the homologous interaction. The results are
shown in Table 1. In regard to Ig, all the hamster species tested contained serum IgG_1, IgG_2, IgA and IgM, which cross reacted with antisera specific for that Ig in Syrian hamsters. The degree of cross-
reactivity, however, varied among the groups and complete identity
(fusion reaction) was found only with serum from "wild" Syrian hamsters. Closely related Mesocricetus hamsters, such as Kurdistan and
Rumanian, contained antigenically identical serum IgG_1, IgA and IgM,
whereas IgG_2 was deficient, that is, it lacked some antigens found in

Table 1. Hamster Serologic Taxonomy

Hamster	IgG$_2$	IgG$_1$	IgA	IgM	FP	
					F	M
Mesocricetus auratus[1]	+	+	+	+	+	0
Syrian domestic						
Syrian wild	+	+	+	+	+[2]	0
Mesocricetus brandti	$+_s$	+	+	+	+[2]	0
Kurdistan						
Mesocricetus newtoni	$+_s$	+	+	+	?	?
Rumanian						
Cricetulus migratorius	$+_s$	$+_s$	$+_s$	+	0	0
Armenian						
Cricetulus griseus	$+_s$	$+_s$	$+_s$	$+_s$	0	0
Chinese						
Cricetus cricetus	$+_s$	$+_s$	$+_s$	$+_s$	0	0
European						
Phodopus songorus	$+_s$	$+_s$	$+_s$	$+_s$	0	0
Dzungarian						

[1]Homologous reference species.

[2]Electrophoretic variants.

+ = reaction of identity; $+_s$ = spur reaction compared to homologous.
Syrian wild - descendants from those captured by Dr. Murphy in 1971 (obtained from Maureen Connelly, MIT, Cambridge, Mass.).
Kurdistan - from Dr. Murphy, NIH, Bethesda, Md.
Rumanian - lyophilized sera kindly provided by Dr. Raicu, Bucharest, Rumania.
Armenian - from H.J. Gagnon, Boston, Mass.
Chinese - from Chickline Co., Vineland, N.J.
European - from Dr. Thomas Cameron, NCI, NIH, Bethesda, Md.
Dzungarian - from Dr. M. Murphy, NIH, Bethesda, Md.

Syrian hamster IgG$_2$. Examination of hamsters representing another genus, Cricetulus, showed that Armenian hamsters had antigenically deficient IgG$_2$, IgG$_1$ and IgA (only IgM was identical), whereas the Chinese hamster was antigenically deficient in all four Ig classes. This suggested that the Chinese hamster was taxonomically the more distant from Syrian hamsters. The other hamsters representing the genus

Cricetus (European) and Phodopus (Dzungarian) were also nonidentical in all four Ig classes, and from a serological standpoint also are distant relatives to Syrian hamsters. Previous studies comparing antigenic variability of IgG_1, IgG_2 and IgM among 15 species of Peromyscus (4) showed a different rate of variation among the Ig classes (IgG_2 > IgG_1 > IgM), suggesting that the IgG_2-Fc gene has evolved more rapidly than IgG_1-Fc gene, etc. The spectrum of hamsters examined in the present study was quite limited, but the results were consistent with greatest variation in IgG_2 and least variation in IgM. Whereas similar Ig-Fc-gene products were detectable in all hamsters, the FP gene appears to have evolved independently within a Mesocricetus ancestor and been preserved so that an antigenically identical Female Protein was detected in only Syrian and Kurdistan hamsters. The status of FP in Rumanian hamsters, another member of Mesocricetus, is unknown at present. Some FP gene alleles do exist, however, since an electrophoretic polymorphism of FP has been detected in some strains of wild Syrian hamsters and also appears to be present among individual Kurdistan hamsters.

Although antisera specific for Syrian hamster Ig do cross react with serum Ig from Chinese, European and Dzungarian hamsters, the reaction was so poor that such antisera would have only limited use in these species, unless a sensitive assay system was utilized. For example, Fig. 1 shows an immunoelectrophoretic pattern (IEP) of Syrian and Chinese hamster sera reacted in both homologous and heterologous fashion with rabbit antisera against whole Syrian and Chinese hamster serum. The IgG_1-IgG_2 cross-reactions appear erratic and inconclusive. The electrophoresed hamster sera were obtained from animals immunized to hen egg albumin (HEA); the bottom portion of Fig. 1 shows the HEA-^{131}I autoradiograph of the same IEP. The IgG_1-IgG_2 precipitin line fusions were seen clearly after autoradiography amplification. In addition, note that the Chinese hamster IgM was detected on IEP (arrow) and autoradiograph only with heterologous anti-Syrian hamster, which had a good titer of anti-IgM. The autoradiograph also shows that IgG_2 was electrophoretically comparable in the two species, whereas IgG_1 was electrophoretically faster in Chinese than in Syrian hamsters. Consequently, Chinese hamster IgG_1 actually can be isolated from IgG_2 by Pevikon or DEAE (in contrast to Syrian IgG_1), (2), and we have used such preparations for production of specific antisera to IgG_1 and IgG_2. Fig. 2 shows the pattern of these Chinese hamster Ig's when developed with specific anti-Chinese hamster IgG_1 and IgG_2, and the more anodal extent of the IgG_1 vs. IgG_2 migration can be visualized.

Although the Chinese hamster was antigenically distant (by Ig analysis) from the Syrian hamster, it was similar, in fact superior, to the Syrian hamster in its propensity to produce an IgG_1 antibody response without detectable IgG_2 antibody production. Table 2 shows the results of IgG_1-IgG_2 antibody production as detected by radioimmunoelectrophoresing at intervals after various immunization schemes.

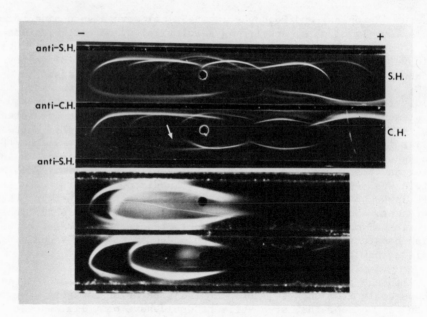

Fig. 1:   Immunoelectrophoresis (top) and respective HEA-^{131}I auto-
          radiograph (bottom) of HEA-immune Syrian hamster (SH) and
          Chinese hamster (CH) sera when developed with both rabbit
          anti-whole SH or CH serum. The heterologous-homologous
          IgG$_1$-IgG$_2$ precipitin reactions can be seen more clearly in
          the autoradiograph below. CH IgM was detected on IEP (arrow)
          and autoradiograph only with heterologous anti-SH. Note,
          the similar electrophoretic mobility of CH and SH IgG$_2$,
          whereas IgG$_1$ of CH is slightly faster than IgG$_1$ of SH.

The 7S Ig antibody response of the animals was grouped according to
extent of IgG response, i.e., number of hamsters with IgG$_1$ antibody
alone (G$_1$) vs. those with both IgG$_1$ + IgG$_2$ antibody (G$_{1+2}$). No instance was found of IgG$_2$ antibody alone. Chinese hamsters inoculated
with HEA in saline (subcutaneously, intraperitoneally or footpad) produced anti-HEA only in the IgG$_1$ class (Table 2). Even after eight
sequential injections of HEA saline, sera from all 10 animals contained IgG$_1$ antibody without detectable IgG$_2$ anti-HEA. For example,
Fig. 3 shows an IEP of day 28 serum from a Chinese hamster injected
thrice (day 0, 14, 21) with 500 µg HEA-saline; in the respective autoradiograph (below), HEA-^{131}I was bound only in the IgG$_1$-precipitin
line of the IEP (arrow). A similar response was found in Syrian hamsters in which a concomitant IgG$_2$ unresponsiveness to HEA was shown
to be present in IgG$_1$-responding hamsters after repeated inoculations
of HEA saline (5, 6). Syrian hamsters, however, did produce IgG$_2$
anti-HEA after 5 µg HEA injected in incomplete Freund's adjuvant (IF)

Table 2. IgG_1-IgG_2 Antibody Response in Chinese Hamsters[1]

Inoculum	No. animals	Day after primary inoculation									
		7		14		21		35		100	
		G_1	G_{1+2}	G_1	G_{1+2}	G_1	G_{1+2}	G_1	G_{1+2}	G_1	G_{1+2}
500 γ HEA Saline	10	–		0[2]	0↓	2	0↓↓	10	0↓↓↓↓↓	10	0
5 γ HEA IF	10	0	0	10	0	6	4	3	7	4	6
500 γ HEA IF	10	5	3	3	7	2	8	1	9	1	9
5 γ HEA CF	9	0	0	2	7	0	9	1	8	1	8
500 γ BSA Maalox	4	1	0	4	0	4	0	4	0	4	0

↓   Repeat challenge with primary inoculum.

[1] Anti-HEA and anti-BSA detected in IgG_1 and IgG_2 by radioimmunoelectrophoresis in which ^{131}I-labeled antigen was added to developed/washed immunoelectrophoretic patterns of test sera and specific binding in the IgG_1 + IgG_2 precipitin lines was detected by autoradiography.

[2] Number of animals with specific antibody in either IgG_1 alone (G_1) vs. those with both IgG_1 + IgG_2 (G_{1+2}).

No instance of IgG_2 without IgG_1 anti-HEA/BSA observed.

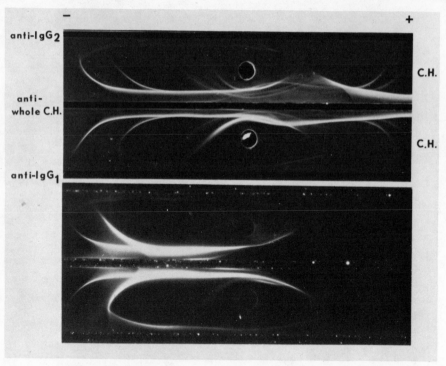

Fig. 2:   Immunoelectrophoresis (top) and HEA-^{131}I autoradiograph
          (below) of HEA immune Chinese hamster (CH) when developed
          with rabbit antisera specific for CH IgG$_1$ and IgG$_2$. Note
          that IgG$_1$ migrates more toward the anode than IgG$_2$, per-
          mitting IgG$_1$ isolation from IgG$_2$.

(5), whereas in Chinese hamsters, IgG$_1$ anti-HEA appeared first (Table
2, day 14 sera, all 10 animals with only IgG$_1$ anti-HEA), and a significant number of animals did not have IgG$_2$ anti-HEA during the course of
the experiments. Even after 500 µg HEA-IF or 5 µg HEA complete Freund's
(CF), some Chinese hamsters did not produce IgG$_2$ anti-HEA, although
all were producing IgG$_1$ anti-HEA. Limited observations for IgG antibody production with another antigen (bovine serum albumin, BSA) also
showed an exclusive IgG$_1$ response (Table 2). This IgG$_1$ and IgG$_2$ differential antibody response in Syrian and Chinese hamsters suggests
that a specific antigen processing step or an Ig class specific suppressor cell may be a ubiquitous phenomenon in hamsters.

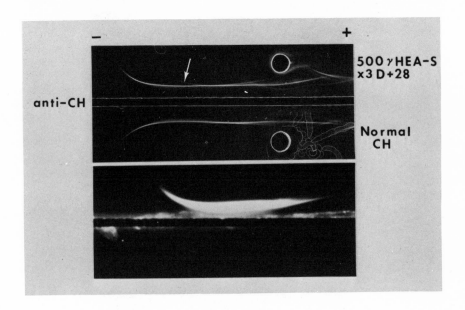

Fig. 3:   Radioimmunoelectrophoresis of sera obtained from Chinese
           hamster on day 28 after three inoculations of HEA-saline
           and developed with rabbit anti-whole Chinese hamster (CH).
           Note HEA-^{131}I binding was present only in the IgG$_1$ precipi-
           tin line (arrow).

REFERENCES

1.   Yerganian, G. Prog Exp Tumor Res 16 (1972) 2.
2.   Coe, J.E. Fed Proc 37 (1978) 2030.
3.   Coe, J.E. Proc Natl Acad Sci 74 (1977) 730.
4.   Coe, J.E. J Immunol 106 (1971) 34.
5.   Coe, J.E. Immunology 21 (1971) 175.
6.   Portis, J.L.; Coe, J.E. J Immunol 115 (1975) 693.

HEMOLYTIC COMPLEMENT AND ITS COMPONENTS IN SYRIAN HAMSTERS: A STUDY

OF FIVE STRAINS UNINFECTED AND INFECTED WITH BRUGIA PAHANGI

Ota Barta, Priscilla P. Oyekan, John B. Malone and
Thomas R. Klei

Department of Veterinary Microbiology and Parasitology
School of Veterinary Medicine, Louisiana State University
Baton Rouge, LA   70803

INTRODUCTION

Few studies have been done on the hamster complement system (C).
Our previous study showed that sensitized sheep erythrocytes were the
best target cells for the hemolytic action of hamster C. The reaction
proceeded best at pH 7.3, at an ionic strength of 0.147 and in the
presence of 1mM Mg^{2+} and 0.3mM Ca^{2+} (1). All nine C components were
tested in hamsters by use of commercially prepared cellular intermediates of sensitized sheep erythrocytes and guinea pig (C1, C8 and C9)
and human C components (C2, C3, C4, C5-7) (1). Successful testing of
hamster total C, C1, C4, and C2 has been reported (2). Other workers
(3) reporting on C6 deficiency in unspecified strains of Syrian hamsters found a correlation of this deficiency with a high incidence of
proliferative enteritis.

In our study, the levels of total C and C components were determined in one outbred (LVG) and four inbred (MHA, LHC, PD4, and CB)
strains of Syrian hamster (Mesocricetus auratus), and the effect of
Brugia pahangi infections of four- to five-month duration on total C
and C component levels was studied.

MATERIALS AND METHODS

Five strains of Syrian hamsters were included in the study: One
outbred strain, LVG, with agouti coloring, and four inbred strains:
MHA, white; PD4, white; LHC, buff; and CB, agouti coloring. All hamsters were purchased at 6 weeks of age (Charles River Breeding Laboratories, Inc., Wilmington, Mass.) and housed in neoprene plastic cages,
three to five hamsters per cage.

NaCl-barbital buffer, pH 7.3, ionic strength 0.147 (4) was used as diluent for total C testing, as recommended (1). Glucose-NaCl-barbital buffer, pH 7.3, ionic strength 0.075, containing 0.1% gelatin, was used for testing C components as recommended by the producer of cellular intermediates and C components (Cordis Laboratories,Miami, Fla.).

Erythrocytes for testing total C were collected in Alsever's solution by venipuncture from a single donor sheep. After four or more days of aging, the cells were washed three times in 0.15M NaCl solution and resuspended to 1×10^8 erythrocytes/ml in NaCl-barbital buffer. The concentration of cells was determined from photometric measurement at 412 nm.

Erythrocyte-antibody-complement component (EAC) cellular intermediates EAC1gp, EAC4gp, and EAC14gp were purchased from a commercial source (Cordis Laboratories) and treated before use as recommended by the producer. The cellular intermediates were used at a final concentration of 1×10^8 EAC/ml.

A commercially produced hemolysin (BBL, Division of Becton-Dickinson and Co., Cockeysville, Md.) was used to sensitize erythrocytes to form erythrocyte-antibody complexes (EA) for total C testing. The optimal dose of hemolysin was determined by checkerboard titrations with various dilutions of hemolysin on one side and various concentrations of hemolytic C on the other side. The optimal concentration of hemolysin was the greatest dilution that detected the smallest concentration of guinea pig and hamster serum C.

Purified C components of guinea pig origin were purchased lyophilized from a commercial source (Cordis Laboratories). They were reconstituted with distilled water to 1000 units/ml, and 0.2-ml aliquots were frozen immediately on dry-ice-methanol and stored at -72°C until used. They were used at over 100 units/ml in testing individual C components.

Hamster serum samples tested for C activity were pools of sera from four to five animals of the same strain and experimental group. The sera were harvested one hour after blood collection from the orbital sinus. The pooled serum samples were stored at -72°C until tested.

Total C testing was done at optimal conditions as described earlier (1), using 1×10^8 sheep erythrocytes/ml sensitized with an optimal dose of rabbit antibodies. NaCl-barbital buffer (1) was used as diluent. The titration was done in microtiter plates: to the diluted serum samples a mixture of sheep erythrocytes and an optimal dose of hemolysin was added, and the total volume was brought up to 0.125 ml (= 5 drops) with NaCl-barbital buffer. The plates were shaken thoroughly on Microshaker (Cooke Engineering, Alexandria, Va.) once before

and twice during the incubation. The plates were incubated floating
on water at 37°C for 60 minutes. After incubation, the plates were
centrifuged at 800 x g for two minutes, and the degree of lysis was
determined from the volume of sedimented erythrocytes and from the
color of the supernatant fluid to the nearest 10% of lysis by comparing with standards.

All results are expressed in CH^{50} units/ml of serum. One CH^{50}
unit/ml gives lysis of 50% of 1 x 10^8 EA.

C components were tested using microtiter plate procedures recommended by the producer of cellular intermediates and C components
(Cordis Laboratories). All components not in question were supplied

Table 1:   Scheme of C Components Testing

Component tested	Cellular intermediate used	Purified C components added and incubation used
C1	EAC4	30°C, 20'; C2, 30°C, 10'; C-0.04M EDTA-GBB, 37°C, 60'[1]
C4	EAC1	30°C, 20'; C2, 30°C, 10'; C-0.04M EDTA-GBB, 37°C, 60'
C2	EAC1,4	30°C, t-max+1 min[2]; C-0.04M EDTA-GBB, 37°C, 60'
C3	EAC1,4	C2,5,6,7, 30°C, 30'; C8,9, 37°C, 60'
C5	EAC1,4	C2,3,6,7, 30°C, 30'; C8,9, 37°C, 60'
C6	EAC1,4	C2,3,5,7, 30°C, 30'; C8,9, 37°C, 60'
C7	EAC1,4	C2,3,5,6, 30°C, 30'; C8,9 37°C, 60'
C8[3]	EAC1,4	C2, t-max+1 min; C3,5,6,7, 30°C, 30'; C9, 37°C, 45'
C9[3]	EAC1,4	C2, t-max+1 min; C3,5,6,7, 30°C, 30'; C8, 37°C, 45'

[1]C-0.04M EDTA-GBB, a reagent prepared by diluting guinea pig complement 1:12.5 in glucose-barbital buffer lacking Mg and Ca, but containing 0.04M sodium EDTA.

[2]t-max, an optimal time for binding of C2 to EAC1,4 cells; it is given
by the producer of EAC1,4 cells.

[3]Because EAC1-7gp cells were not available, a modification of the procedure for testing C8 and C9 was made as given in the table.

in an excess of 100 CH^{50} units/ml. The results were evaluated as in
total C testing.

    For Brugia pahangi infection, age-matched groups of seven ham-
sters of each strain were infected by subcutaneous injections of 185
to 200 infective larvae of the filarid nematode B. pahangi at 13 to
16 weeks of age by methods described previously (5).

RESULTS

    Total C. The serum pools of the inbred MHA and LHC hamsters had
the highest content of C (260 and 230 CH^{50} units, respectively). The

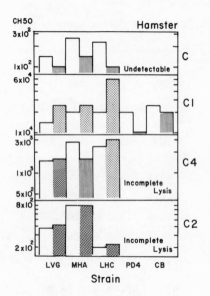

Fig. 1:   Total complement (C) concentration and levels of early-acting
           components of the complement system (C1, C4, and C2) in the
           sera of five strains of Syrian hamsters. Results given in
           CH^{50} units per ml of serum and 1 x 10^8 target erythrocytes.
           Concentrations in control groups are represented by open col-
           umns, concentrations in Brugia pahangi-infected animals by
           darkened columns: dotted columns, if levels higher than in
           controls; gray, if same levels as in controls; striped, if
           levels lower than in controls. Samples were pools of four
           to five serum aliquots from different animals.

outbred strain LVG had a lower level of C (160),and the inbred strains
PD4 and CB had no detectable C in their sera. The CH^{50} units in the
sera from infected MHA, LHC and LVG animals were below those of the
uninfected controls (140, 100, and 100, respectively) perhaps because
of utilization of C during the infection.

        C1. The C1 levels were within a narrow range from 14,000 to
25,000 CH^{50} units in all hamster strains. The pool of sera from infected animals of the LHC strain had a three-times greater concentration of C1 than the uninfected animals. Infected animals of the PD4
strain had one half of the C1 levels of uninfected animals. In the remaining strains, the C1 levels showed less difference between infected
and uninfected animals. In both strains with undetectable total C activity, the C1 levels in infected animals were higher, and in the
other three strains lower, than the levels of the uninfected controls
(Fig. 1). Our results in this study were below the 89,000 CH^{50} units
of C1 reported for hamster serum (2), but were similar to our previous
results (1).

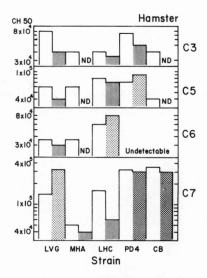

Fig. 2:   C3, C5, C6, and C7 components of the complement system in
          the sera of five strains of hamsters in control (open col-
          umns) and Brugia pahangi-infected (darkened columns) ani-
          mals in CH^{50} units. (See legend to Fig. 1 and text for de-
          tails.)

C4. The concentrations of C4, which reacts in the C activation sequence after C1 and before C2, were higher in the strains with detectable total C levels (2,000 to 2,800 CH^{50} units) than in the strains with undetectable total C activity. In these strains, the end-point was not possible to establish with confidence in fresh serum, because complete lysis was not detectable in any well, and many wells had lysis around 50% (Fig. 1). The infected LHC hamsters had more C4, and the LVG and MHA strains less, than did the uninfected animals. The C4 levels compare well with 3,500 units reported for hamster sera (2), but were higher than titers determined with human C2 in our previous work (1). The strain differences in C4 levels may indicate either that the PD4 and CB strains have inherited lower levels of C4, or that they have inhibitory factor(s) in their sera that interfere with C4 testing.

C2. Serum concentrations of C2 varied considerably by strains, but the concentrations were not affected by infection with B. pahangi. The highest levels of C2 were in the MHA strain (640 units), followed by the LVG (380 units) and the LHC strains (200 units) (Fig. 1). This compares well with the reported 310 CH^{50} of C2 (2), and 800 CH^{50} reported in our previous work (1). C2 titers were apparently lower, but could not be established with certainty in the PD4 and CB strains for the same reasons as with C4 titers. The intensity of lysis at the lower dilutions, however, increased after a prediluted serum stood for three hours in ice water, indicating that a labile serum factor might cause inhibition of the reaction in samples tested immediately after thawing. Additional studies on the latter effect have not yet been completed.

C3. There were relatively small differences in C3 concentration among the various strains tested (40,000 to 80,000 units) (Fig. 2). Although there were insufficient samples to test infected animal sera

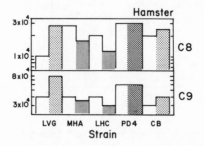

Fig. 3:   C8 and C9 components of the complement system in the sera of five strains of hamsters in control (open columns) and Brugia pahangi-infected (darkened columns) animals in CH^{50} units. (See legend to Fig. 1 and text for details.)

in two strains, all of the samples from infected animals of the other
three strains had C3 levels below that of uninfected hamsters (34,000
to 50,000 units). These levels are higher than those reported in our
previous work (6,400), when human C5 through C9 were used for C3
testing (1), indicating that guinea pig C5 has better compatibility
with hamster C3 than does human C5.

C5. No substantial differences were detected in C5 levels between the different strains or between infected and uninfected animals (40,000 and 90,000 units) (Fig. 2). These C5 levels are higher
than those reported previously (3,200) when human C3 through C9 components were used for detection (1).

C6. The level of C6 varied among inbred strains. The PD4 and CB
strains had undetectable C6, which may be the main reason for the undetectable total C activity in their sera. A similar reported C6 deficiency, not associated with any detectable C inhibitory activity,
was inherited by over 50% of the offspring (3). The C6 concentrations
in other strains tested in the present study varied between 3,000 and
8,000 units and were unaffected by B. pahangi infection. This result
compares well with 16,000 units reported in our previous paper (1).

C7. C7 levels varied considerably with the strain tested. The
highest levels were in the PD4 and CB strains, which were lacking in
C6 (300,000 and 350,000 units); the lowest C7 concentration was in the
MHA strain (50,000 units). The effect of infection varied considerably with the strains tested and had no specific pattern. All three
terminal C components in the PD4 and CB hamsters were practically unaffected by infection.

C8 and C9. Both C8 and C9 serum concentrations varied only
slightly with the strain and with infection (Fig. 3). The titers for
C8 ranged from 10,000 through 28,000 units and for C9 from 30,000 to
80,000. The concentrations of 16,000 units were reported earlier for
C8 and C9 tested with human C9 and C8, respectively (1).

Correlation of C levels and health. Of 80 animals purchased,
nine died four to seven months after purchase. Of the nine that died,
four died after the blood collection for this study; five were not
sampled. Six of the dead animals were infected with B. pahangi, and
three were uninfected. Most died of spontaneous enteritis with chronic
weight loss. The strain distribution of the dead animals was four CB,
two PD4, two MHA and one LVG. There was no apparent correlation between the C levels and the general health of the various strains of
hamsters. The CB and PD4 strains, however, which are deficient in
C6, and the MHA strain, with a low level of C7, constituted a majority
of the dead animals. The relatively high and stable C7 through C9
levels in sera from the PD4 and CB hamsters were probably caused by
blockage of their utilization due to the absence of C6. All the
tested groups of B. pahangi-infected hamsters had moderately decreased

total C and C3 levels. Previous studies (Klei, Crowell and Barta, unpublished observations) of individual, sequentially obtained sera from an outbred strain of hamsters (Sprague-Dawley) infected with the filarid nematode Dipetalonema viteae did not show significant differences in the levels of total C or C2, C3, and C4 between the infected and control animals during a 120-day infection period. In the experiments reported here, pools of sera were used and only a single bleeding at a fixed time post-infection was examined.

SUMMARY

Complement profiles were tested in outbred (LVG) Syrian hamsters (Mesocricetus auratus) and compared to the MHA, LHC, PD4, and CB inbred strains. The total C and C component concentrations in the sera varied among the strains and were in the following ranges in untreated animals (in CH^{50} units per ml): total C, 140-260 (undetectable in PD4 and CB); C1, 14,000-25,000; C2, 200-800 (except PD4 and CB); C3, 40,000-80,000; C4, 2,000-2,800 (except PD4 and CB); C5, 40,000-80,000; C6, 3,600-6,000 (undetectable in PD4 and CB); C7, 50,000-350,000; C8, 10,000-30,000; C9, 30,000-60,000. The PD4 and CB strains had undetectable total C and C6, and their exact C2 and C4 levels could not be determined, but were lower than in the other strains. The MHA strain had the highest total C levels, but had significantly lower (1/3 or less) C7 levels than the other strains of hamsters. Infection of hamsters with the filarid nematode Brugia pahangi for four to five months produced moderate decreases in the total C and C3 levels, but varied changes in other C components. Six infected and three uninfected animals died during the experiment from spontaneous enteritis and weight loss.

ACKNOWLEDGMENTS

This work was supported in part by the NIH Biomedical Research Development Grant RR 09087.

REFERENCES

1. Barta, O.; Klei, T.R. Dev Comp Immunol 2 (1978) 519.
2. Hook, W.A. et al. J Immunol 105 (1970) 268.
3. Yang, S.Y. et al. Fed Proc 33 (1974) 795 (Abstr.).
4. Mayer, M.M. In: Experimental Immunochemistry, ed. Kabat and Mayer, 2nd ed. Charles C. Thomas, Springfield, Ill. (1961) 149.
5. Malone, J.B.; Thompson, P.E. Exp Parasitol 38 (1975) 279.

ISOLATION AND CHARACTERIZATION OF HAMSTER ALPHA$_2$ MACROGLOBULIN

Joan Stein-Streilein and David A. Hart

Department of Microbiology, University of Texas Health
Science Center at Dallas, Dallas, TX 75235

INTRODUCTION

Previous reports from our laboratory have described conditions
for culturing hamster lymphocytes with mitogens in the absence of
serum (1). This finding allowed us to investigate the possibility
that a humoral factor or serum components may affect the in vitro activity of different cell populations. We have reported that a specific inhibitor of lipopolysaccharide (LPS) stimulation of MHA spleen
and lymph node cells and of dextran sulfate (DxS) stimulation of
spleen cells is present in normal isologous serum (1). This component
does not affect Con A stimulation or mixed lymphocyte reactivity and,
therefore, appears to be specific for a particular subpopulation of
lymphoid cells (B lymphocytes). We now report that the high molecular
weight inhibitor of serum or plasma is alpha$_2$ macroglobulin (α2M).

MATERIALS AND METHODS

Female MHA hamsters (Charles River, N.Y.) weighing 80-120g were
used for the source of serum, plasma and lymphocytes. New Zealand
white female rabbits were purchased from Sunny Acres Rabbitry (Tyler,
Tex.) and used for raising antisera.

Lymphoid cells were harvested from spleens of exsanguinated hamsters. Single cell suspensions were made by gently tapping the tissue
through a sterilized stainless steel screen with frequent washing with
a balanced salt solution (BSS). Cells were washed and counted by the
trypan blue exclusion technique.

Serum and plasma fractions containing $alpha_2$ macroglobulin (α2M) were tested in a bioassay for their ability to inhibit LPS stimulation of hamster splenocytes in microcultures. Microcultures contained 10^6 viable cells in 0.2 ml protein-free RPMI 1640 and were performed in round-bottom microtiter plates (Cooke Engineering). Fractions of serum or plasma containing α2M were added to the culture one hour before the mitogens. Concanavalin A (Con A) was obtained from Sigma Chemical Company. Optimum dose for microculture was 0.4 µg/0.2 ml. Lipopoly-saccharide W (LPS) was obtained from Escherichia coli 055 B5 or from Salmonella typhosa 0907 (Difco Laboratories). Optimum dose was 10 µg/0.2 ml. Cells were cultured for 72 hours at 37°C and 10% CO_2. Tritiated thymidine (^{3}H-TdR), 0.1 µCi/culture, was added 24 hours before cells were harvested on glass fiber filters and radioactivity counted in a Beckman scintillation counter.

Polyacrylamide disc gel electrophoresis in the presence of SDS (SDS-PAGE) was performed as described (2). Gels were developed with 0.1M Na_3PO_4, pH 7.2 and 0.1% SDS. Radiolabelled, crosslinked bovine serum albumin (3) and dansylated, crosslinked immunoglobulin light chains (4) were used as internal molecular weight standards (gifts from Drs. R. Proia and R. Fulton, respectively).

For immunoelectrophoresis, serum and protein samples were placed in wells cut in nobel agar (1.5%) slides. Slides (3 x 1 in.) were run for 90 minutes at 15 mA/slide in veronal buffer (pH 8.6). At termina-tion of the run, the center trough was removed and antisera added as indicated in the text. Proteins were allowed to diffuse through the gel overnight at 22°C in a moisture chamber.

The IgG fraction of anti-hamster α2M was obtained by published methods (5). IgG was precipitated from serum with 18% Na_2SO_4 and the precipitate was dialysed against 0.02M sodium phosphate, pH 6.9. The IgG fraction was further purified by anion exchange chromatography on DEAE cellulose (6).

Sepharose 4B-Cl was activated with CNBr. In brief: CNBr (15 g/ 75 ml and H_2O) was added to washed Sepharose (150 ml packed beads) with stirring and the pH of the suspension was monitored by a pH meter. The pH of the Sepharose-CNBr mixture was immediately raised to pH 11-11.5 by addition of 10M NaOH and was maintained at this pH for 10 min-utes. The CNBr-activated Sepharose was washed on a Büchner funnel with 1.5 liter of 0.1M $NaHCO_3$, pH 9.0, and left damp. An equal volume of rabbit anti-hamster α2M (IgG fraction - 2 mg/ml) was mixed with the washed CNBr-Sepharose and stirred for 18 hours at 4°C. After coupling, the conjugated Sepharose was washed with 1.0 liter of 1.0M Tris-HCl, pH 8.0, in order to block remaining activated sites on the gel. The Sepharose conjugate was stored at 4°C in PBS containing 0.02% NaN_3.

RESULTS

Hamster α2M was prepared by two methods. The first involved biochemical purification by conventional protein purification methods.
The second method utilized affinity chromatography of plasma on Sepha-
rose-rabbit anti-hamster α2M columns.

Whole blood was removed by cardiac puncture. The blood was
allowed to clot for one hour at 23°C and then stored at 4°C overnight.
The resulting serum fraction was heated at 56° for 30 minutes, then
cooled and dialysed against phosphate buffered saline (PBS, pH 7.2)
overnight at 4°C. The dialyzed serum was sterilized by passage through
a 0.45 micrometer Millipore filter. Serum was clarified by centrifugation at 10^5 x g for two hours at 5°C in a Beckman L5-75 centrifuge.
Clarified serum was removed from the center of the tube, leaving
behind the upper layer containing lipid and lipoproteins and the
pellet containing cell debris and aggregated proteins.

Aliquots (10 ml) of clarified MHA serum were applied to a Sepharose 6B column (5 x 140 cm) equilibrated with PBS. The column was developed in a descending manner at a rate of 24 ml/hour. Six-milli-
liter fractions were collected and the optical density at 280 nm was
determined for each fraction. Fractions containing the large molecular weight molecules were pooled and concentrated to the starting
volume by Amicon diaflo ultrafiltration (Amicon, Lexington, Mass.)
using a PM 10 filter (Pool A, Fig. 1).

Pevikon (C-870, Mercer Chemical Corp., N.Y.) was washed with de-
ionizrd water three times. The matrix was made to the consistency of
wet sand with barbitol buffer, pH 8.6. A block, 18 x 18 x ¼ cm, was
poured and the origin cut 13 cm from the left edge of the block.
Serum fractions (Pool A) from the column fractionation containing α2M
and other large molecular weight molecules were added to the origin.
The block was developed at 4°C for 19 hours at 400 volts or 100 mA.

Protein migration was monitored by staining the pattern of protein absorbed to a strip of filter paper. The most anodal area of
Pevikon containing protein was collected and the protein was obtained
by washing with PBS. Any remaining Pevikon was removed by centrifugation in a Sorvall RC-5 at 48,200 x g for 30 minutes. The PBS washes
were concentrated by diaflo ultrafiltration to the original sample
volume. Protein migration was also monitored by electrophoresis on
cellular acetate (Fig. 2).

Protein fractions, isolated by gel filtration and zonal electrophoresis, were separated further by ion exchange chromatography utilizing DEAE-cellulose. The sample was applied in 0.02M sodium phosphate at pH 7.2 and the column was developed with a 0.02M-0.2M sodium
phosphate gradient and a pH gradient of 7.2 to 4.5. One major peak
of protein was eluted between pH 6.8 and 6.2. These fractions were

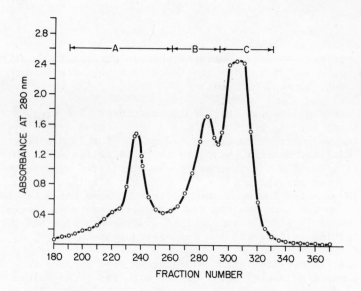

Fig. 1:   Fractionation of clarified MHA serum on Sepharose 6B. Normal
clarified serum, 15 to 25 ml, was applied to a column of
Sepharose 6B (5 x 140 cm) equilibrated with PBS. The column
was developed at a rate of 24 ml/hour at 22°C.   Fractions,
6 ml, were collected and the optical density at 280 nm was
determined.   Fractions from the areas indicated A,B, and C
were pooled, concentrated to original serum volume applied
to the column, and dialyzed against PBS.

pooled and tested for purity by SDS-PAGE analysis and immunoreactivity
with rabbit anti-hamster Ig.   The isolated molecules were homogeneous
by SDS-PAGE with a MW of 725,000 and a subunit MW of 185,000.   These
results are analogous to α2M isolated from other species (7,8).   The
isolated α2M did not react with anti-hamster Ig by double diffusion
in gel analysis.

     At each purification step the ability of various serum fractions
to suppress the LPS stimulation of hamster splenocyte cultures was
monitored.   Serum fractions able to suppress LPS stimulation co-purified with fractions that retained reactivity to antisera against hamster α2M.

     The highly purified α2M eluted from the DEAE-cellulose columns
was used to raise a monospecific α2M antisera in rabbits.   A New
Zealand white rabbit was immunized in its hind foot pads with 200 μg
of DEAE-cellulose purified α2M in complete Freund's adjuvant (CFA).
The animals were boosted four times every two weeks.

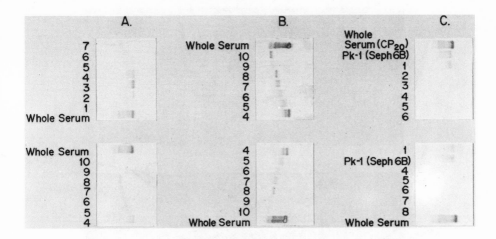

Fig. 2: Cellulose acetate analysis of fractions from zonal electrophoresis of hamster serum or Sepharose 6B fraction A (peak
1). Aliquots of clarified serum or Sepharose 6B fraction A
(peak 1) were subjected to zonal electrophoresis on a Pevikon
matrix for 19 hours at 4°C. The eluted proteins were analyzed
by cellulose acetate electrophoresis. The proteins were electrophoresed for 15 minutes in a Beckman microzone cell and
then stained with Ponceau S. Panels A and B: Separation of
normal hamster serum. Panel C: Separation of Sepharose 6B
fraction A (peak 1).

Blood was taken from the marginal ear vein prior to each antigenic challenge. Sera from the bleedings were checked for precipitating antibodies against the immunizing α2M preparation and whole
hamster serum, using immunoelectrophoresis techniques (Fig. 3). Antisera to the purified α2M precipitated a single band from both the immunizing antigen and normal hamster serum (Fig. 3).

Normal hamster serum or heparinized plasma (2 to 6 ml) containing
soybean trypsin inhibitor (SBTI, 10 μg/ml) and diisopropylfluoro-
phosphate (DFP, 1 mM) was applied to a rabbit anti-hamster α2M affinity column and allowed to incubate at room temperature for one hour.
Nonadherent proteins were washed from the column with 10 volumes of
PBS. Adherent protein (α2M) was eluted with 0.1M glycine-HCl, Ph 2.5.
One-milliliter fractions were collected and immediately neutralized
to pH 7.2 with 1N NaOH to prevent dissociation of the molecule. Fractions were monitored for protein at 280 nm utilizing a Zeiss PM Q3
spectrophotometer. Fractions were pooled and concentrated against
PBS by vacuum dialysis.

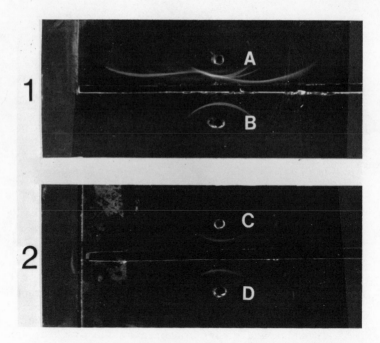

Fig. 3:   Immunoelectrophoretic analysis of α2M. Normal hamster serum
          (A,C) or DEAE-cellulose purified α2M (B,D) were electropho-
          resed as described in Materials and Methods. Panel 1: De-
          veloped with rabbit anti-hamster serum. Panel 2: Developed
          with rabbit anti-hamster α2M.

          Various preparations of serum α2M, or affinity purified α2M,
were assayed for their ability to suppress LPS stimulation of hamster
splenocytes. As indicated in Table I, as little as 300 ng was suppressive to LPS stimulation. This concentration of α2M had little or
no effect on Con A stimulation. In some experiments, where α2M partially suppressed Con A stimulation, the suppression could be overcome by increasing the Con A concentration. This effect is probably
due to the fact that Con A binds to glycoproteins such as α2M. In
contrast, increasing the LPS concentration did not overcome suppression by α2M.

DISCUSSION

          Since it was observed (9) that alpha-globulin fractions from rat
plasma prolonged graft survival, and was reported that alpha globulin
from whole human plasma caused significant prolongation of skin allo-

Table 1.   Effect of Affinity-Purified α2M on Mitogen Stimulation of
            Hamster Spleen Cells

Experiment	Control (cpm ^{3}H-TdR)[2]	Percent of control μg α2M[1]		
		0.075	0.30	7.5
unstimulated	1560	70	65	75
LPS	16240	65	25	25
Con A	47040	95	78	75

[1]α2M was added 1 hour before mitogen.

[2]CPM, counts per minute.

grafts in mice across a strong H-2 barrier (10), a number of laboratories have demonstrated immunosuppressive activities associated with
various fractions of serum (11). Most of these suppressive molecules
are of small molecular weight and appear to preferentially suppress
T-cell responses rather than B-cell responses.

Unlike most of the immunosuppressive alpha globulins isolated
from human serum, a factor, present in normal serum, has been characterized (12) that is associated with the alpha$_2$ macroglobulin fraction. Whether this active molecule is a low molecular weight entity
reversibly bound to alpha$_2$ macroglobulin, is alpha$_2$ macroglobulin with
protease inhibitor activity, or is an independent macroglobulin, remains unresolved.

The alpha globulin we isolated from hamster serum was identified
as alpha$_2$ macroglobulin because of its size and subunit composition
(7,8), its mobility in an electric field, and its capacity to inhibit
proteases by entrapment (13). Unlike the immunosuppressive α-globu-
lins reported by others, the suppressive effects of hamster α2M are
on B cells rather than T cells. This is evidenced by the fact that
affinity purified α2M suppresses LPS stimulation but not Con A stimulation of hamster spleen cells. It has been suggested, but not proven
(14), that the ability of α2M to suppress is related to its protease
inhibitor capacity. Evidence accumulated in recent years has implicated the involvement of proteolytic events during lymphocyte activation (15-19). These findings strengthen the hypothesis that α2M suppresses activation by virtue of its ability to inhibit proteases.

An alternative mechanism for suppression has been suggested,
however, by the very mechanism whereby alpha$_2$ macroglobulin interacts
with proteases and clears them through the reticuloendothelial system
(7,13). In brief, α2M interacts only with the catalytic forms of en-
dopeptidases, and all proteases probably react with the same site on
the α2M. Protease binding to α2M is believed to be an irreversible

process that involves limited proteolytic cleavage of the α2M but does not appear to involve inhibition of the active site of the enzyme. The interaction of a protease with α2M then results in conformational changes in the α2M. The conformational change results in the enzyme becoming entrapped within the complex. This α2M-protease complex is removed rapidly from the circulation by cells of the reticuloendothelial system. A receptor has been described on macrophages that binds both native and complexed forms of the molecule (20). The complex, however, binds with higher affinity, and it has been reported that internalization of the complex is mediated through coated pits (21, 22), a mechanism associated with hormones, LDL and nutrient internalization (23).

Because of its large molecular weight, the biological activity of α2M was generally believed to be associated with extracellular events. While this large molecule can be internalized by receptor-mediated endocytosis in macrophages (20), as well as cells such as fibroblasts (24), it is possible that it could also modulate intracellular events of the B lymphocytes. Earlier reports on fluorescence microscopy have demonstrated that an antigenic form of α2M is on B lymphocytes (25). It is not clear, however, whether it is the native α2M located in the membrane, or the complex form, associated with a receptor on the membrane. Not only does complex formation and uptake change the possible site of biological action, but it also offers an alternative mechanism of action. The suppression may not be caused by the native α2M, the protease inhibitor, but may be mediated through the α2M-protease complexes (26).

The affinity-purified α2M used in the present study is theoretically native α2M. While precautions were taken to insure this result, such as immediately adding protease inhibitors to the heparinized blood and rapidly purifying the α2M by affinity chromatography, the possibility remains that complex formation occurred during the isolation of the molecule. Our current investigations are directed toward separating and identifying these two forms of the molecule in order to delineate whether it is the α2M (protease inhibitor) or the α2M (complex) that suppresses B-cell activation of hamster lymphocytes by LPS.

ACKNOWLEDGMENTS

        The authors thank Nanette Broyles for her technical assistance and Daisi Marcoulides for typing the manuscript. This work was supported in part by Public Health Grants CA-24444 and CA-26842 from the National Institutes of Health.

REFERENCES

1.   Streilein, J.S.; Hart, D.A.   Infect Immun 14 (1976) 463.
2.   Shapiro, A. et al.   Biochem Biophys Res Commun 28 (1967) 815.
3.   Proia, R.L. et al.   Proc Natl Acad Sci USA 76 (1979) 685.
4.   Fulton, R.   Ph.D. Thesis, Univ Texas Health Sci Center at
     Dallas (1980).
5.   Kekwick, R.A.   Biochem J 34 (1940) 1248.
6.   Levy, H.B.; Sober, H.A.   Proc Soc Exp Biol Med 103 (1960) 250.
7.   Starkey, P.M.; Barrett, A.J.   In: Proteinases in Mammalian
     Cells and Tissues, ed. Barret.   North Holland, Amsterdam (1977)
     633.
8.   James, K.   Trends Biochem Sci Feb (1980) 43.
9.   Kamrin, B.B.   Proc Soc Exp Biol Med 100 (1959) 58.
10. Cooperband, S. et al.   Science 159 (1968) 1243.
11. Cooperband, S. et al.   Transplant Proc 111 (1976) 225.
12. Ford, W.H. et al.   Clin Exp Immunol 15 (1973) 1969.
13. Barrett, A.; Starkey, P.   Biochem J 133 (1973) 709.
14. Stein-Streilein, J.; Hart, D.A.   Fed Proc 37 (1978) 2042.
15. Streilein, J.   Ph.D. Thesis, Univ Texas Health Sci Center at
     Dallas (1976).
16. Stein-Streilein, J.; Hart, D.A.   Cell Immunol (1980) in press.
17. Vischer, T.L.   Immunology 36 (1979) 811.
18. Hart, D.A.; Stein-Streilein, J.   This volume.
19. Gisler, R.H. et al.   J Immunol 116 (1976) 1354.
20. Kaplan, J.; Nielsen, M.   J Biochem 254 (1979) 7323.
21. Maxfield, F.R. et al.   Cell 14 (1978) 805.
22. Maxfield, F.R. et al.   Nature 277 (1979) 661.
23. Goldstein, J. et al.   Nature 279 (1979) 679.
24. Van Leuven, F. et al.   J Biol Chem 254 (1979) 5155.
25. McCormick, J.N. et al.   Nature [New Biol] 246 (1973) 78.
26. Hubbard, W.J.   Cell Immunol 39 (1978) 388.

SECTION III

EFFECTOR CELLS IN VIRAL AND TUMOR IMMUNITY

Chairpersons:

Joan Stein-Streilein

John J. Trentin

FUNCTIONAL ANALYSIS OF LYMPHOID CELL SUBPOPULATIONS INVOLVED

IN REJECTION OF TUMORS INDUCED BY SIMIAN VIRUS 40

John W. Blasecki

Stine Laboratory
E.I. du Pont de Nemours and Co.
Newark, DE   19711

INTRODUCTION

Lymphoid cell surface differentiation antigens of the hamster, in contrast to those of the mouse, are not well defined, and there is little information on the functional delineation and analysis of hamster lymphocyte subpopulations. More work in this direction will be of great importance in adding to our understanding of the hamster immune system and in further developing the hamster as a useful animal model for immunologic and other studies.

Murine T lymphocytes reportedly contain subsets that differ in their responsiveness to Concanavalin A (Con A) and phytohemagglutinin (PHA)(1). Those cells that responded primarily to Con A had a relatively reduced density of surface theta determinants, and cytotoxic effector cells appeared to be contained within this T cell subset. More recently it was shown that only Ly-1,2,3[+] T cells bound PHA, and this T-cell subset lacked helper or suppressor effector function (2). While these results raise serious doubts as to the validity of using mitogen responsiveness as a measure of overall T cell function, they do suggest that mitogens may be useful probes for delineating functional lymphocyte subsets. In recent studies of cellular responses to mitogens and alloantigens, we obtained some intriguing results with respect to differential responses of hamster lymphocytes to mitogens as a function of exposure to irradiation and became interested in whether these differential responses correlated with any cellular immune functions in a DNA virus (SV40)-induced tumor system. This paper presents some of the results of our experiments.

MATERIALS AND METHODS

Inbred MHA/ssLAK and CB/ssLAK hamsters were obtained from Charles
River-Lakeview, Newfield, N.J.   Inbred BALB/c mice were obtained from
Texas Inbred Mouse Co., Houston, Tex.

Tumor cell lines used were:

MHA/ssLAK origin: MHST (SV40-transformed)
                    MHDB (Dimethylbenz(α)anthracene-transformed)
CB/ssLAK origin :   CBSV (SV40-transformed)
                    CBDB (Dimethylbenz(α)anthracene-transformed)
BALB/c origin   :   VLM-S and MKS (SV40-transformed)
                    BMC (3-methylcholanthrene-transformed)

All tumor cells were grown as described elsewhere (3,4).

The direct transplantation rejection (3,5), tumor cell neutralization (3), and macrophage migration inhibition (6) assays used to
detect specific cellular immunity to SV40 tumor-specific transplantation antigen (TSTA) have been described in detail. The preparation and
characterization of anti-hamster T cell serum (7,8), the methods for
thymectomy, lethal irradiation and bone marrow reconstitution (3), and
the purification of hamster T lymphocytes on nylon wool columns (8)
have been described recently, as have the techniques for mitogen stimulation of hamster lymphocytes (8,9) and the generation of specifically-
sensitized T cells using antigen-pulsed macrophages (10,11). In vitro
sensitization of hamster or mouse lymphoid cells to TSTA was achieved
by incubation of lymphoid cells on growing monolayers of tumor cells.
The lymphoid cells were harvested after five days, purified by filtration through nylon wool columns (8) and tested for responsiveness to
TSTA by one or more of the methods mentioned above.

RESULTS AND DISCUSSION

With results obtained using anti-hamster T cell serum and thymectomized, lethally-irradiated, bone marrow-reconstituted (TIR) hosts,
we demonstrated that rejection of syngeneic SV40 tumors in inbred hamsters depended upon the presence of specifically sensitized T lymphocytes (3,8). More recently, we reported that specific cellular immunity to SV40 tumors could be induced in vivo by inoculation of syngeneic hosts with macrophages pulsed with soluble SV40 TSTA (10,11). SV40
tumor-specific immunity could not be induced with silica-treated macrophages nor when TIR hosts served as recipients of TSTA-pulsed macrophages. These findings demonstrated that macrophages were required
for induction of tumor-specific immunity, and strongly suggested that
macrophage-T cell cooperation occurred in the generation of such immunity. Activated macrophages were unable to prevent growth of SV40

Table 1.   Effects of Gamma Irradiation upon Hamster Spleen Cell Re-
           sponses to Mitogens and Alloantigens

Irradiation dose (rads)	Percent reduction of stimulation ratio				
	Con A[1]	PHA	PWM	LPS	MLR
0	--	--	--	--	--
500	-30	67	52	65	55
1000	-25	78	67	76	70
1500	N.T.	N.T.	N.T.	N.T.	97
2000	9	95	87	83	99
3000	94	98	96	96	100
4000	96	98	97	92	N.T.
5000	98	96	98	97	100

[1]Con A = Concanavalin A; PHA = phytohemagglutinin;
PWM = pokeweed mitogen; LPS = lipopolysaccharide;
MLR = mixed lymphocyte reaction.

tumors in normal syngeneic recipients, while specifically sensitized
T lymphocytes did so readily. These results confirmed our previous
finding that specifically sensitized T cells were required for rejection of SV40 tumors in syngeneic hosts (3,8).

In recent experiments to characterize the cellular responses of
hamsters to mitogens and alloantigens, we found marked differences in
responses, based upon the material used for stimulation and the dose
of irradiation to which the responding cells were exposed. These data,
shown for a typical experiment in Table 1, demonstrated clearly that
the blastogenic response to Con A, which we have shown previously to
be a T-cell mitogen in the hamster (8), was relatively more radioresistant than the responses to PHA, pokeweed mitogen or lipopolysaccharide. At 1000 rads, the stimulation ratio for Con A was actually
above control levels, while stimulation ratios for the other mitogens
were reduced by 70% to 80%, and at 2000 rads the stimulation ratio for
Con A was reduced from control levels by less than 10%, while stimulation ratios for the other mitogens were depressed by 85% to 95%. At
the same time, the cellular immune response to alloantigens (a T cell
response) in mixed lymphocyte culture was reduced by 70% and 99%, respectively. Those T cells that responded primarily to Con A thus differed in radiosensitivity from those responding to PHA, pokeweed mitogen or alloantigens, strongly suggesting involvement of different T
cell subsets in these cellular responses.

It has been reported that mouse lymphocytes subjected to 700 rads
of x-irradiation did not undergo blastogenesis (but were capable of
protein synthesis) when exposed to PHA (12), prompting some investigators to suggest that similarly treated sensitized lymphocytes could

Table 2. Effect of Gamma Irradiation upon Tumor Rejection by Sensi-
          tized Hamster Peripheral Blood Lymphocytes

MHA hamsters sensitized to:	Tumor cell challenge	Tumor incidence after irradiation at:		
		None	1000 rads	3000 rads
SV40 TSTA	MHST	0/8	1/8	8/8
	MHDB	8/8	7/8	8/8
MHDB TSTA	MHDB	1/8	---	---
	MHST	8/8	---	---

not kill syngeneic SV40 tumor cells (13). The data in Table 2, however, demonstrate convincingly that specifically sensitized hamster
peripheral blood lymphocytes given 1000 rads gamma irradiation had the
same ability as their unirradiated counterparts to prevent the growth
of SV40 tumors in normal syngeneic recipients. At 3000 rads, the point
at which the Con A response was suppressed by 94%, the specifically
sensitized T cells no longer prevented SV40 tumor growth. These
findings indicate that cytotoxic effector T cells are contained within
a T cell subset that is relatively radioresistant and primarily responsive to Con A.

     Further evidence of differences in hamster lymphoid cell popula-
tions involved in SV40 tumor rejection came from our findings that
whole peripheral blood lymphocyte and peritoneal exudate cell populations from specifically sensitized hamsters prevented the growth of
syngeneic SV40 tumors in vivo, whereas spleen and lymph node cells from

Table 3. Effect of Nylon Wool Column Filtration upon SV40-Specific
          Tumor Rejection by Sensitized Lymphoid Cells from Different
          Sources

Treatment of sensitized lymphoid cells	Tumor cell challenge	Tumor incidence with:			
		PBL[1]	PEC	Spleen	LN
None	MHST	0/8	0/8	7/8	8/8
	MHDB	8/8	7/8	8/8	8/8
Nylon column elution	MHST	0/8	0/8	2/8	3/8
	MHDB	8/8	7/8	7/8	8/8

[1]PBL = peripheral blood lymphocytes; PEC = peritoneal exudate cells;
LN = lymph node.

Table 4. Separation of SV40-Specific Cytotoxic Cells from Suppressor Cells by Nylon Wool Column Filtration

Lymphocytes sensitized to:	Whole spleen	Effluent spleen	Column-adherent spleen	PBL[1]	Tumor cell challenge	Tumor incidence
SV40 TSTA						
A	+				MHST	8/8
	+				MHDB	8/8
B		+			MHST	1/8
		+			MHDB	8/8
C			+		MHST	8/8
			+		MHDB	7/8
D				+	MHST	0/8
				+	MHDB	8/8
E		+	+		MHST	8/8
		+	+		MHDB	7/8
F			+	+	MHST	7/8
			+	+	MHDB	8/8
MHDB TSTA						
G		+			MHDB	1/8
		+			MHST	8/8
H		+	+[2]		MHDB	1/8
		+	+[2]		MHST	8/8

[1]PBL = peripheral blood lymphocytes.
[2]Cells from SV40TSTA-sensitized hamsters.

Table 5. Effect of Irradiation or Anti-T Cell Serum Treatment upon SV40-Specific Suppressor Cell Activity

Cells[1]	Whole spleen	Whole spleen (1000 R)	Non-adherent spleen	Adherent spleen	Adherent spleen (1000 R)	Adherent spleen (anti-T+C')	Tumor cell challenge	Tumor incidence
A	+						MHST	8/8
	+						MHDB	8/8
B		+					MHST	1/8
		+					MHDB	8/8
C			+				MHST	0/8
			+				MHDB	7/8
D				+			MHST	8/8
				+			MHDB	8/8
E					+		MHST	8/8
					+		MHDB	8/8
F				+		+	MHST	8/8
				+		+	MHDB	7/9
G			+		+		MHST	7/8
			+		+		MHDB	8/8
H			+			+	MHST	1/8
			+			+	MHDB	7/8
I			+				MHST	0/8
			+				MHDB	8/8

[1] Lymphocytes sensitized to SV40 TSTA

Table 6. Specific Rejection of Syngeneic SV40 Tumors by Hosts Sensitized with Syngeneic, Allogeneic or Xenogeneic SV40 Tumor Cells

Host	Sensitized in vivo with:	Tumor incidence after challenge with syngeneic tumor cells	
		MHST	MHDB
MHA/ssLAK	MHST	0/8	8/8
hamsters			
	MHDB	8/8	1/8
	CBSV	0/8	8/8
	CBDB	8/8	7/8
	VLM-S	0/8	7/8
	BMC	8/8	8/8
	None	8/8	8/8
		CBSV	CBDB
CB/ssLAK	CBSV	0/8	7/8
hamsters	CBDB	8/8	1/8
	MHST	0/8	8/8
	VLM-S	1/8	7/8
	None	8/8	8/8
		VLM-S	BMC
BALB/c mice	VLM-S	0/8	8/8
	BMC	8/8	1/8
	MHST	0/8	8/8
	CBSV	0/8	7/8
	None	8/8	7/8

these donors were inactive, unless filtered through nylon wool columns (Table 3). In order to determine whether the lack of anti-SV40 tumor reactivity in whole spleen and lymph node populations might be due to suppressor cells, nylon wool column-adherent spleen cells were admixed with reactive effluent spleen cells or with peripheral blood lymphocytes from hamsters specifically sensitized to SV40 TSTA. The data in Table 4 demonstrate that nylon wool column-adherent spleen cells abrogated the tumor cell growth inhibitory capacity of the immune lymphoid cells. Treatment of the column-adherent cells with anti-T cell serum and complement or with 1000 rads gamma irradiation eliminated the suppressor activity, thus indicating that the specific suppressor cells in this tumor system are radiosensitive T lymphocytes (Table 5).

Table 7. Specific Cellular Immune Response to Soluble SV40 TSTA in
          vitro by Peritoneal Exudate Cells from Hosts Sensitized in
          vivo with Syngeneic, Allogeneic or Xenogeneic SV40 Tumor
          Cells

Host	Sensitized with	Percent migration inhibition by soluble SV40 TSTA derived from:
		MHST
MHA/ssLAK	MHST	43
hamsters		
	MHDB	7
	CBSV	40
	CBDB	10
	VLM–S	39
	BMC	6
	None	9
		CBSV
CB/ssLAK	CBSV	45
hamsters		
	CBDB	11
	MHST	42
	VLM–S	35
	None	8
		VLM–S
BALB/c mice	VLM–S	52
	BMC	5
	MHST	46
	CBSV	43
	None	12

A recent report indicated that outbred hamsters generated cellular immunity to SV40 TSTA when the antigen was presented on SV40 tumor
cells of hamster but not mouse origin (14). In contrast, it was reported earlier (15) that immunization of outbred hamsters with human
SV40-transformed cells protected the sensitized animals against challenge with homologous SV40 tumor cells. Our results indicate that hamsters sensitized in vivo with SV40 tumor cells of syngeneic, allogeneic or xenogeneic origin specifically rejected direct challenge with
syngeneic SV40 tumor cells (Table 6). Similarly, peritoneal exudate
cells from such sensitized hosts responded specifically in vitro to
soluble SV40 TSTA of syngeneic origin, as determined by macrophage migration inhibition (Table 7). Finally, utilizing a newly developed

Table 8. Specific Rejection of Syngeneic SV40 Tumors in vivo by
          Lymphoid Cells Sensitized to SV40 TSTA in vitro

Lymphoid cell donors	Lymphoid cells sensitized on monolayers of:	Tumor cell challenge	Tumor incidence
MHA/ssLAK hamsters	MHST	MHST	2/8
		MHDB	8/8
	MHDB	MHST	8/8
		MHDB	3/8
	MKS	MHST	2/8
		MHDB	7/8
	BMC	MHST	8/8
		MHDB	8/8
BALB/c mice	MKS	VLM-S	0/8
		BMC	7/8
	MHST	VLM-S	0/8
		BMC	8/8
	MHDB	VLM-S	8/8
		BMC	7/8

method of in vitro sensitization to SV40 TSTA, we found that lymphoid
cells from MHA/ssLAK hamsters sensitized to SV40 TSTA on growing monolayers of syngeneic, allogeneic or xenogeneic SV40 tumor cells (Table
8) specifically prevented the growth of SV40 tumors in normal syngeneic recipients. This was also true when mouse lymphoid cells were
sensitized in vitro to SV40 TSTA (Table 8).

From the results of the experiments described above, we conclude
that:

1.   The rejection or growth of SV40 tumors in syngeneic hosts
results, in large part, from the interactions among cytotoxic T lymphocytes, suppressor T lymphocytes and macrophages. Both cytotoxic
and suppressor T cells demonstrate specificity for SV40 TSTA.
2.   Cytotoxic T cells can be distinguished from suppressor,
mixed lymphocyte reaction-responsive and perhaps other hamster T cell
subsets by their relative radioresistance, primary responsiveness to
Con A and non-adherence to nylon wool. In addition, cytotoxic T cells
were found in all peripheral lymphoid cell populations tested.
3.   Suppressor T cells, which specifically inhibit the anti-
tumor reactivity of cytotoxic T cells, are radiosensitive, nylon wool-
adherent, and were found in the spleens and lymph nodes but not in the
peripheral blood lymphocytes or peritoneal exudate cells of specific-

ally sensitized hamsters. Like cytotoxic T cells, suppressor T cells are sensitive to treatment with anti-T cell serum and complement.

4.   Despite the lack of antisera to lymphocyte cell surface differentiation antigens, subpopulations of hamster lymphocytes specifically reactive to SV40 TSTA can be defined and isolated on the basis of physical and functional properties and their roles in tumor immunity can be analyzed.

5.   The cellular immune response to SV40 TSTA, both in hamsters and in mice, appears not to be restricted by the major histocompatibility complex, whether in vitro or in vivo. These findings raise serious questions regarding the relevance of major histocompatibility complex-restricted killing of SV40 tumor cells in vitro to actual rejection of SV40 tumors by syngeneic hosts in vivo.

SUMMARY

Lymphoid cell cooperation and cellular immune recognition of SV40 tumor-specific transplantation antigen (TSTA) in syngeneic systems and across allogeneic and xenogeneic histocompatibility barriers were investigated. Previous work in our laboratory demonstrated that macrophages are required for the generation of T lymphocytes specifically sensitized to SV40 TSTA, and that rejection of syngeneic SV40 tumors is dependent upon the latter cells. Using in vivo and in vitro sensitization to SV40 TSTA, we now report that MHA hamster T lymphocytes cytotoxic (Tc) to syngeneic SV40 tumors were found in a fraction of lymphoid cells resistant to x-irradiation and selectively responsive to mitogens but unresponsive to allogeneic histocompatibility antigens. This finding, to the best of our knowledge, is thus far unique to hamsters. Tumor-specific reactivity of the Tc was inhibited by a second T cell subpopulation which was sensitive to x-irradiation, and which we have functionally defined as suppressor T cells (Ts). Ts cells adhered to nylon wool columns, were sensitive to treatment with anti-T cell serum and inhibited the SV40 tumor-specific reactivity of Tc cells. Ts cells were found in the spleens and lymph nodes of SV40 TSTA-immune hamsters but not in their peritoneal exudate cells or peripheral blood lymphocytes. Finally, MHA hamster lymphoid cells sensitized in vitro or in vivo with syngeneic, allogeneic (CB) or xenogeneic (BALB/c) SV40 tumor cells mediated specific rejection of syngeneic SV40 tumors in vivo and responded to soluble SV40 TSTA in vitro, thus demonstrating no histocompatibility restriction of the cellular immune response to SV40 TSTA. The results of these studies indicate that, in spite of the lack of antisera directed against lymphocyte cell surface differentiation antigens in the hamster, subpopulations of hamster lymphocytes specifically reactive to syngeneic SV40 tumor cells can be defined and physically isolated on the basis of functional properties, and their interactions in generating tumor-specific immunity can be studied both in vitro and in vivo.

REFERENCES

1. Stobo, J.D. Transplant Rev 11 (1972) 60.
2. Callard, R.E.; Basten, A. Eur J Immunol 8 (1978) 247.
3. Blasecki, J.W. J Immunol 119 (1977) 1621.
4. Blasecki, J.W.; Tevethia, S.S. Int J Cancer 16 (1975) 275.
5. Blasecki, J.W.; Tevethia, S.S. J Immunol 114 (1975) 244.
6. Blasecki, J.W.; Tevethia, S.S. J Immunol 110 (1973) 590.
7. Blasecki, J.W. et al. Immunol Commun 6 (1977) 567.
8. Blasecki, J.W.; Houston, K.J. Immunol 35 (1978) 1.
9. Houston, K.J.; Blasecki, J.W. J Natl Cancer Inst 63 (1979) 665.
10. Blasecki, J.W. In: Mechanisms of Immunity to Virus-Induced Tumors,
    ed. Blasecki. Marcel Dekker, Inc., New York, (1980) in press.
11. Blasecki, J.W. et al. In: Advances in Comparative Leukemia Re-
    search 1979, ed. Yohn, Lapin, Blakeslee. Elsevier North-Holland,
    Inc., New York, (1980) 309.
12. Salvin, S.B.; Nishio, J. J Exp Med 135 (1972) 985.
13. Tevethia, S.S. et al. In: Immunobiology of the Macrophage, ed.
    Nelson. Academic Press, New York (1976) 509.
14. Law, L.W. et al. Int J Cancer 22 (1978) 315.
15. Girardi, A.J. Proc Natl Acad Sci USA 54 (1965) 445.

NATURAL CYTOTOXICITY BY HAMSTER LYMPHOID CELLS FOR VIRUS-INFECTED AND TRANSFORMED CELLS

Robert N. Lausch, Nancy Patton, and Donna Walker

Department of Microbiology and Immunology,
College of Medicine, University of South Alabama,
Mobile, AL   36688

INTRODUCTION

Cell-mediated immunity is a significant aspect of the host re-sponse to herpes simplex virus (HSV) infection. Several investigators have shown that adoptive transfer of immune T lymphocytes will protect mice against virus challenge (1,2,3). More recently, in vitro studies have shown that draining lymph node (4,5) or spleen cells (6) from virus-sensitized hosts were specifically cytotoxic for HSV-infected cells. Substantial levels of lysis usually were not seen, however, unless the effector cells, identified as T lymphocytes (6,7) first had experienced some form of experimental manipulation such as incubation in vitro for a number of days.

Further studies have led to the recognition of a second popula-tion of lymphocytes with cytotoxic activity. These cells can be demon-strated readily in non-sensitized hosts (8,9) and therefore have been referred to as natural killer (NK) cells. They have a propensity for damaging or lysing a variety of target cells in vitro, notably tumor cells and cells harboring intracellular pathogens (10). In contrast to immune T-cell-mediated killing, NK attack appears to be non-specific and is not histocompatibility-restricted. It is important to assess what role NK cells may play in host resistance to virus infection. While studying the mechanism of resistance of HSV in the Syrian ham-ster, therefore, we examined NK activity. We found that cells from selected lymphoid tissues are highly cytotoxic for HSV-infected synge-neic target cells. This finding may explain why attempts to demon-strate HSV oncogenicity in vivo have been unproductive (11,12).

MATERIALS AND METHODS

The in vitro transformation of LSH hamster embryo fibroblasts (HEF) by SV40-adenovirus 7 hybrid virus (13), HSV-type 1 (14) and HSV-type 2 (15) have been described. All three cell lines were oncogenic in syngeneic hosts. The cells were grown in Dulbecco's medium supplemented with 5% to 10% fetal or newborn calf serum, 100 µg of streptomycin/ml, 100 IU of penicillin/ml, 300 µg of L-glutamine/ml, and 0.075% sodium bicarbonate. HSV type 1 strain 14-012 and vaccinia virus were grown and titrated in Vero cells. The inbred hamster strains LSH and MHA, and the random bred strain LVG, were obtained from Charles River, Newfield, N.J. The UT1 hamster strain was provided by Dr. J. Wayne Streilein, University of Texas Health Science Center at Dallas, Dallas, Texas.

Effector cells used in the ^{51}Cr-release assay were prepared aseptically. Cells were teased from the spleen, thymus, and cervical lymph nodes, washed repeatedly, resuspended in RPMI 1640 with 5% heated fetal calf serum, and adjusted to the desired concentration. To obtain peripheral blood lymphocytes (PBL), heparinized blood was layered on Ficoll-Hypaque (Pharmacia Chemicals, Piscataway, N.J.) and centrifuged at room temperature for 20 minutes at 1500 rpm. The white blood cell band was drawn off, washed, resuspended in medium, and adjusted to the desired concentration.

Some of the ^{51}Cr-release tests were done in 10 x 75 mm plastic tubes as described (16). Other tests were carried out in 3040 Falcon microtest II plates (Becton-Dickinson, Oxnard, Calif.). The desired target cells (1 x 10^6) were labeled with 100-200 µCi of ^{51}Cr (New England Nuclear, Boston, Mass.), then washed three times, and 1-2 x 10^3 cells in RPMI 1640 medium were placed in wells (0.2 ml per well). After overnight incubation the medium was discarded and cells were infected with 0.2 ml virus (5-10 PFU per cell). Following incubation of three to seven hours, the medium was discarded and 0.2 ml effector cells were added. Cultures then were incubated for various lengths of time depending on the experiment. At the completion of the incubation period the plates were centrifuged at 1200 rpm for 10 minutes, then 0.1 ml supernatant was drawn off and counted in a gamma counter. To determine maximum release, cells were lysed with 2.5% sodium dodecyl sulfate. The percent specific lysis was calculated as described (17). Results were evaluated statistically using Student's t test.

In some experiments virus-infected target cells were pretreated for one hour with 0.1 ml antiserum prepared in hamsters or rabbits by repeated immunization with HSV type 1 strain 14-012 or Patton, respectively. Then 0.1 ml effector cells were added and the test was completed as described above. In the antibody-mediated lysis tests, the complement source was Hartley guinea pig serum.

Table 1.   Cytotoxicity of Peripheral Blood Cells from Unsensitized
           Hamsters for HSV-1-Infected and Uninfected Syngeneic Tumor
           Cell Lines[1]

Test No.	Target cells	Transforming virus	Infected with HSV-1	E:T ratio	% specific lysis	p<
1	PARA-7	SV40	yes	100:1	53	0.001
			no	100:1	23	0.001
			yes	25:1	24	0.001
			no	25:1	9	0.001
2	14-012-8-1	HSV-1	yes	100:1	52	0.001
			no	100:1	25	0.001
			yes	25:1	38	0.001
			no	25:1	11	0.01
3	333-2-29,T-1	HSV-2	yes	100:1	31	0.001
			no	100:1	18	0.001
			yes	25:1	9	0.025
			no	25:1	8	0.005

[1]PBL donors were female LSH 12-15 weeks old.

RESULTS

In our initial studies, the lytic activity of PBL from normal LSH
hamsters for syngeneic target cells was examined using a 16-hour ^{51}Cr-
release assay.   Table 1 shows the results of tests using HEF transformed by SV40, HSV-1 or HSV-2 as target cells.   A modest susceptibility to lysis was usual but not invariable (Table 4).   On the other

Table 2.   Time Course of Specific ^{51}Cr Release from HSV-1-Infected
           and Uninfected Para-7 Cells Incubated with Normal PBL

Incubation period	E:T ratio	Target cells	
		HSV-1-PARA-7	PARA-7
4 hours	100:1	15[1] (0.001)[2]	9 (0.001)
	25:1	10 (0.025)	0
20 hours	100:1	39 (0.001)	27 (0.005)
	25:1	16 (0.025)	10 (0.005)

[1]% specific ^{51}Cr release.

[2]Values in parentheses are P value as determined by Student's t test.

Table 3. Natural Cytotoxic Cell Lysis by PBL from Various Strains of
Hamsters for HSV-1-Infected Para-7 Cells[1]

Lymphoid cells	E:T ratio	Hamster strain			
		LSH	MHA	LVG	UT1
PBL	200:1	41***[2]	60***	36***	44***
	50:1	34***	55***	26***	26***
	13:1	26***	27***	10*	14***
Thymus	200:1	7*	7	7	ND

[1]Male hamsters 15-17 weeks old were lymphoid cell donors.

[2]*P < 0.025; ***P < 0.001.

hand, substantial and consistent lysis was obtained if the tumor cells
first were infected with HSV. In the tests shown, cells were infected
3 to 16 hours before being used as target cells. Spontaneous ^{51}Cr-re-
lease from the infected cells (33% to 37%) was virtually identical to
the uninfected preparations (33% to 36%). Virus infection thus did
not produce an increase in leakage of label, i.e., the increased lysis
was real and not due to experimental artifact.

We examined the kinetics of the killing. Labeled fibroblasts were
incubated with normal PBL for four hours or overnight at the effector
to target cell ratios indicated (Table 2). Significant lysis was found
during short-term incubation in some tests. Substantially more lysis
was obtained, however, if the reaction was continued overnight. For
our further studies, the incubation period was limited to 16 hours because in this time frame the spontaneous release usually could be held
to $\leq$ 40%.

It was of interest to determine whether hamsters in general possessed blood cells naturally cytotoxic for HSV-infected cells. Table
3 shows a comparison of the lytic activity of four different strains.
It is evident that MHA, UT1, and LVG PBL were readily cytotoxic at
levels roughly comparable to that seen with LSH. In contrast, thymus
cells showed minimal activity.

Vaccinia virus, like HSV, replicates in hamster cells. We tested
whether cells infected with this virus and exhibiting cytopathology
were more sensitive to PBL attack than uninfected PARA-7 cells. Representative results are shown in Table 4. It was found that PBL that
readily lysed HSV-infected cells produced little or no lysis of vaccinia-infected targets. Virus infection per se thus does not increase
PARA-7 cell susceptibility to NK attack. Table 4 also shows that cervical lymph node cells, even at high effector to target cell ratios,
produced little or no lysis of HSV-infected cells. NK cells therefore
are not distributed uniformly among hamster peripheral lymphoid tissues.

Table 4. Selective Cytotoxicity of Peripheral Blood Cells from Un-
          sensitized Hamsters for Virus-Infected Syngeneic Target
          Cells

Test	Effector cells	E:T ratio	Target cells		
			HSV-1-PARA-7	Vaccinia-PARA-7	PARA-7
1	LN[1]	400:1	1	-5	-3
		200:1	6		-3
	PBL	200:1	28**[2]	2	2**
2	LN	400:1	7**	-5	ND
		200:1	5**	-7	
	PBL	200:1	56**	7	ND
		50:1	33**	5*	

[1]LN, lymph node.

[2]*P < 0.02; **P < 0.005.

Table 5. Natural Cytotoxicity of Hamster Peripheral Blood Lymphocy-
          tes: Effect of Anti-HSV Serum Pretreatment of Target Cells[1]

Test	Target cells exposed to:			% specific lysis	P <
	PBL	Anti-HSV	Complement		
1[2]	0	+	+	35	0.001
	0	+	+ heated	-3	NS
	+	0	0	41	0.001
	+	+	0	35	0.001
2[3]	0	+	+	65	0.001
	0	+	+ heated	-3	NS
	+	0	0	45	0.001
	+	+	0	34	0.005

[1]Target cells were HSV-1-infected PARA-7 cells.

[2]E:T ratio was 60:1; hamster antiserum (1:10); guinea pig complement (1:16).

[3]E:T ratio was 100:1; rabbit antiserum (1:10); guinea pig complement (1:16).

The foregoing results have shown that HSV-infected cells are susceptible to normal PBL attack. Could virus-specific antigens on the
cell surface be triggering an enhanced cytotoxic response? This question was probed by testing whether pretreatment of the target cells
with antibody to HSV would block cytotoxicity. The results of two
such tests are shown in Table 5. Test 1 shows that hamster antiserum
was able to lyse HSV-infected target cells in the presence of guinea
pig serum, establishing that the serum had antibody capable of binding
to the target cells. We found that antiserum-pretreated target cells
were lysed readily by PBL. The slight reduction (6%) in comparison to
the control was not statistically significant (p < 0.1). Similar results were obtained when the experiment was performed with HSV antiserum prepared in the rabbit (test 2). Pretreatment of HSV-infected
target cells with antiserum did not consistently block PBL cytotoxicity at a statistically significant level, nor did it enhance lysis.

DISCUSSION

In our experiments, PBL from untreated hamsters were able to
effect modest lysis of virus-transformed syngeneic target cells. A
sharp increase in lysis was obtained if the tumor target cells were
pre-infected with HSV. Several observations indicate that enhanced
lysis was not mediated by HSV-sensitized cytotoxic T cells. Firstly,
the killing was mediated by PBL from four different strains of hamster, none of which had knowingly been exposed to the virus. Hamsters
do not appear to be naturally sensitized to HSV, as only a small fraction had serum neutralizing antibody (4). Secondly, high levels of
cytotoxicity were seen consistently in tests with PBL conducted over
a more than six-month period. In contrast, hamsters deliberately immunized with HSV had only a transient cytotoxic response, detectable
principally in draining lymph node cells at a high ($\geq$ 200:1) effector:
target cell ratio (4; personal observations). Finally, preliminary
studies have indicated that the elevated lysis is not histocompatibility-restricted, not confined only to HSV-infected cells, and not
abrogated by guinea pig anti-hamster T cell serum (manuscript in preparation).

The enhanced lysis also is unlikely to be due to antibody-dependent cellular cytotoxicity (18,19). In our hands, sera from normal
donors have not mediated lysis in the presence of normal spleen or
lymph node cells (to be published). Moreover, pretreatment of infected target cells with sera hyperimmune to HSV did not enhance
killing by PBL (Table 5).

A detailed characterization of the effector cell(s) producing
lysis of HSV-infected and uninfected target cells needs to be made.
At present it seems likely that the killing is brought about by
NK cells in the blood. It has been shown (17) that hamsters do have
cells in the spleen and bone marrow (PBL not tested) spontaneously

cytotoxic for virus-transformed syngeneic lymphoma cells. Other investigators (20) also have described spleen cell lysis of syngeneic and allogeneic hamster target cells and noted that the activity increased after Pichinde virus infection. In our studies, killing was seen with effector cells from spleen and bone marrow (personal observations) as well as blood, but little activity was seen with lymph node or thymus cells. This distribution of NK activity is analogous to that reported for mouse and man (21).

It is not clear why infection of target cells with HSV results in increased lysis. Numerous studies have shown that HSV infection is accompanied by surface membrane changes such as appearance of virus-specific antigens and Fc receptors. One of these modifications or perhaps unmasking of cryptic host cell antigens may facilitate NK attack, or increase target cell sensitivity to lysis. Alternatively, it is possible that NK cells were activated during the incubation period by interferon induced in HSV-infected cells, as shown (22,23) in a human system. This explanation is attractive for two reasons. It accounts for the increased lysis with time of incubation; and, in those studies as in ours, enhanced lysis of vaccinia-infected cells was not seen. They found that, unlike HSV-infected cells, vaccinia-infected cells did not induce interferon. Studies to test whether hamster interferon plays a role in our model are in progress.

In summary, it is now clear that hamsters, like other species, possess effector cells spontaneously cytotoxic for virus-infected and transformed cells. It will be important to assess whether these cells exert a protective effect in vivo.

ACKNOWLEDGMENTS

The authors thank Dr. John Oakes for providing the rabbit anti-HSV serum, and for critically reviewing the manuscript. This work was supported by grant CA-23777 awarded by the National Cancer Institute.

REFERENCES

1.   Ennis, F.A. Infect Immun 7 (1973) 898.
2.   Oakes, J.E. Infect Immun 12 (1975) 166.
3.   Rager-Zisman, B.; Allison, A.C. J Immunol 116 (1976) 35.
4.   Hay, K.A.; Lausch, R.N. Int J Cancer 23 (1979) 337.
5.   Pfizenmaier, K. et al. Immunology 119 (1977) 939.
6.   Lawman, M.J.P. et al. Infect Immun 27 (1980) 133.
7.   Pfizenmaier, K. et al. Nature 265 (1977) 630.
8.   Herberman, R.B. et al. Int J Cancer 16 (1975) 216.
9.   Kiessling, R. et al. Eur J Immunol 5 (1975) 112.
10. Herberman, R.B.; Holden, H.T. Adv Cancer Res 27 (1978) 305.
11. Nahmias, A.J. et al. Proc Soc Exp Biol Med 134 (1970) 1065.

12. McCormick, K.J.; Trentin, J.J. Prog Exp Tumor Res 23 (1979) 13.
13. Lausch, R.H.; Rapp, F. Int J Cancer 7 (1971) 322.
14. Duff, R.; Rapp, F. J Virol 12 (1973) 209.
15. Rapp, F.; Duff, R. Cancer Res 33 (1973) 1527.
16. Laux, D.; Lausch, R.N. J Immunol 112 (1974) 1900.
17. Datta, S.K. et al. Int J Cancer 23 (1979) 728.
18. Shore, S.L. et al. Nature 251 (1974) 350.
19. Rager-Zisman, B.; Bloom, B.R. Nature 251 (1974) 542.
20. Gee, S.R. et al. J Immunol 123 (1979) 2618.
21. Herberman, R.B. et al. Immunol Rev 44 (1979) 43.
22. Santoli, D. et al. J Immunol 121 (1978) 526.
23. Santoli, D. et al. J Immunol 121 (1978) 532.

THE HAMSTER MAJOR HISTOCOMPATIBILITY COMPLEX AND ALTERNATE
MECHANISMS OF CELL-MEDIATED ANTI-VIRAL CYTOTOXIC ACTIVITY
IN THE SYRIAN HAMSTER

Mitchell J. Nelles and J. Wayne Streilein

Rosenstiel Basic Science Medical Research Center,
Brandeis University, Waltham, MA 02254 and the
Department of Cell Biology, University of Texas
Health Science Center at Dallas, Dallas, TX 75235

INTRODUCTION

Previous studies using the Syrian hamster (1,2,3) have partially
defined and characterized the major histocompatibility complex (MHC)
in this species. Although various cellular alloimmune reactivities
have been described in hamsters, it is not known whether any of these
responses result from allogeneic disparities encoded by class I MHC
loci analogous to the murine H-2K and H-2D.

We describe vaccinia virus-induced, cell-mediated cytotoxic activity in acutely infected hamsters. We hoped to ascertain the extent
of functional class I MHC molecule polymorphism in hamsters by the
ability of such molecules to promote and restrict T cell-mediated
cytotoxic activity. Contrary to mice and rats undergoing acute viral
infection (4,5), Syrian hamsters do not generate measurable spleen
cell cytotoxic T cell activity. It appears that the hamsters utilize
alternate mechanisms of cell-mediated, anti-viral cytotoxic activity,
not governed by the MHC. The significance of this observation is discussed in relation to hamster immunogenetics and viral immunity.

MATERIALS AND METHODS

Syrian hamster strains MHA, CB, UT, TX, and MIT were used. The
origin, stage of inbreeding, and alloreactive potential of these
strains have been described (6). Virus-induced cytotoxic activity was
assayed in a 16-hour ^{51}Cr release assay employing spleen cells effector and adherent target cells. The histological characterization and
strain of origin of the various target cells utilized have been de-

scribed (6). A specific goat anti-hamster T cell antiserum (GαHT)(7) was used to deplete spleen cell suspensions of functional T cell activity. Adult thymectomized hamsters were irradiated lethally and reconstituted with anti-T cell antiserum-treated bone marrow (8). Heat-aggregated human gamma globulin (HGG), an IgG fraction of a rabbit anti-hamster immunoglobulin antiserum (RαHIg) and pepsin-digested RαHIg (F(ab')$_2$-RαHIg) were used directly in the ^{51}Cr release assay.

RESULTS AND DISCUSSION

Acute virus infection in mice and rats elicits the production of cytotoxic T cells specific for the immunizing virus and genetically restricted in their cytolytic activity (4,5). Hamsters undergoing acute infection with vaccinia virus generate virus-induced cytotoxic activity whose virus-specificity and kinetics are similar to those in the mouse and rat (6).

Such cytotoxic activity, when described initially, was consistent with the belief that class I molecules in hamsters promoted virus-induced, T cell-mediated cytotoxic activity. We therefore wanted to determine whether such cytotoxic activity in hamsters was genetically restricted, as definitive evidence for the T cell nature of such cytotoxic activity. In this case, the inability of virus-induced cytotoxic effector cells of one strain to kill virus-infected target cells of a second strain would be taken as evidence for class I molecule polymorphism in this species.

Various alloreactive hamster strains were acutely infected with vaccinia virus and their spleen cells were assayed for cytotoxic activity against virus-infected target cells in reciprocal fashion (Table 1). Virus-induced cytotoxic activity was not restricted genetically among any of the combinations tested. This was rather surprising, because many of these combinations elicit strong, mutual mixed lymphocyte reactivity, graft-versus-host reactivity and skin graft rejection (1,2,3). In fact, alloantibody has been generated recently in some of the strain combinations employed (9).

Two different hypotheses may be advanced to explain the apparent lack of genetically restricted cytotoxic activity in hamsters. First, it is possible that all hamster strains studied share one or more class I encoded molecules. It is unlikely that such limited, or even non-existent, polymorphism reflects sampling error of animals derived from the wild, as these same strains are strongly alloreactive to each other. In any event, the first hypothesis predicts that virus-induced cytotoxic activity in hamsters is mediated in a classical manner by cytotoxic T cells.

The second, and alternate, hypothesis is that unlike mice and rats, hamsters do not utilize MHC-encoded class I molecules in response

Table 1. Studies on the Genetic Restriction of Vaccinia Virus-Induced
          Cell-Mediated Cytotoxic Activity in Hamsters

Effector[1] strain	% Specific ^{51}Cr release from target cells[2]							
	MHA		CB		UT		MIT	TX
	U	I	U	I	U	I	I	I
MHA	9	44	10	45	13	47	43	37
CB	15	70	16	68	31	61	58	54
UT	10	47	nd[3]	53	nd	45	42	40
MIT	9	44	1	34	11	46	37	30
TX	3	29	nd	30	nd	34	15	19

[1]Hamsters were inoculated intraperitoneally with approximately 1 x
10^7 PFU of vaccinia virus. Six days later, spleen cells were assayed
for cytotoxic activity in vitro in a 16-hour ^{51}Cr release assay at
an E:T ratio of 40.

[2]The following target cells were utilized: MHST (MHA), MC-4,(CB) MC-3
(UT), MIT fibroblast (MIT), and TX fibroblast (TX). Target cells
either were infected with vaccinia virus or were used without virus
infection. U = uninfected, I = infected.

[3]Not done.

to acute viral infection. This hypothesis also requires that cytotoxic
activity would be non-T cell in nature, as the MHC would play no part
in the promotion or restriction of cytotoxic activity.

    To decide between these two hypotheses, spleen cell suspensions
obtained from hamsters acutely infected with vaccinia virus were
treated in vitro with a specific anti-hamster T cell antiserum (GαHT)
in the presence of complement. Viable cells remaining after such
treatment were then assayed for cytotoxic activity in vitro in the
^{51}Cr release assay (Table 2). Immune spleen cell suspensions obtained
from virus-infected hamsters depleted of T cells exert unimpaired cytotoxic activity against syngeneic, virus-infected target cells (0%
to 9% decrease in activity compared to cells treated with normal serum
and complement). This same antiserum, however, inhibits 77% to 83%
of murine virus-induced cytotoxic activity, which is mediated predominantly by T cells (4). Thus, in contrast to the mouse and rat, in
the Syrian hamster vaccinia virus-induced cytotoxic activity is not
mediated by cytotoxic T cells.

    Although vaccinia virus-induced cytotoxic activity in hamsters
is not mediated directly by T cells, there is evidence for the participation of T cells in certain aspects of the immune response of acutely
infected hamsters. For instance, hamsters injected locally with live
vaccinia virus generate primary footpad swelling identical to that in
mice and rats (4,5,6,10). More importantly, such virus-induced footpad swelling is not seen in hamsters devoid of functional T cell ac-

Table 2. Differential Effects of an Anti-T Cell Antiserum on Hamster
and Mouse Vaccinia Virus-Induced Cytotoxic Activity

Effector[1]	Treatment	E:T Ratio	% Specific [51]Cr Release	% Decrease[2]
Hamster	NGS	13	55	--
		4	28	--
	GαHT	13	50	9
		4	45	0
Mouse	NGS	40	47	--
		13	30	--
	GαHT	40	11	77
		13	5	83

[1]MHA-strain hamsters and C3H-strain mice were inoculated intraperitoneally with vaccinia virus as in Table 1. Spleen cells were assayed
for cytotoxic activity six days later on syngeneic virus-infected
target cells in a 16-hour (hamster) and 4-hour (mouse) ^{51}Cr release
assay. Spleen cells were treated with either normal goat serum (NGS)
or a specific goat anti-hamster T cell antiserum (GαHT) in the presence of complement prior to incubation with target cells.

[2]As compared to NGS treatment.

tivity (8). Hamsters thus apparently are capable of utilizing certain
T cell subsets in the immune response to acute vaccinia virus infection.

The requirements for T cells in vivo for the generation of virus-
induced cytotoxic activity are presented in Table 3. In this case,
normal and thymectomized hamsters were acutely infected with vaccinia
virus. Six days later, spleen cell cytotoxic activity was assayed in
vitro as earlier, in the ^{51}Cr release assay. Thymectomized hamsters
generated significantly lower levels of cytotoxic activity (41% to 80%
decrease) than did virus-infected hamsters possessing an intact thymus.
T cells thus are required in vivo for the generation of a significant
portion of vaccinia virus-induced cytotoxic activity, although T cells
do not mediate such activity directly.

Even though hamster T cells do not mediate vaccinia virus-induced
cytotoxic activity directly, one still must account for the observed
virus specificity and kinetics of such responses in this species.
Since T cells are required in vivo for the generation of a significant
proportion of cytotoxic activity (41% to 80%), this might be related
to a requirement for helper T cells involved in production of antibody
to T cell dependent antigens (i.e. virus). In this case, cytotoxic
activity following acute infection with vaccinia virus could result
from antibody-dependent cell-mediated cytotoxicity (ADCC). Both the

Table 3.   Effects of Adult Thymectomy on Virus-Induced Cytotoxic
           Activity in Hamsters

| Experiment | Effector[1] | E:T Ratio | % Specific ^{51}Cr Release | | |
			Infected	Uninfected	% Decrease[2]
1	MHA Immune	13	59	7	--
		4	35	0	--
	TX Immune	13	35	3	41
		4	20	0	43
2	MHA Immune	13	42	4	--
		4	14	2	--
	TX Immune	13	24	1	42
		4	5	0	80

[1]MHA-strain hamsters with intact thymuses (MHA immune) and MHA-strain
hamsters lacking thymuses (TX Immune) were acutely infected with
virus as in Tables 1 and 2.   Cytotoxic activity was determined six
days later in a 16-hour ^{51}Cr release assay.

[2]As compared to MHA Immune spleen cell cycotoxic activity.

kinetics and specificity of virus-induced cytotoxic activity are consistent with such a mechanism.   In addition, ADCC could explain the
apparent lack of genetic restriction seen in hamsters.

Table 4 presents the results of an experiment to determine directly whether virus-induced cytotoxic activity in hamsters is ADCC in
nature.   Hamsters were acutely infected with vaccinia virus as before.
Six days later, spleen cells from these animals were assayed for cytotoxic activity in vitro against virus-infected target cells.   In addition to effector and target cells, some of the assay wells also contained various reagents capable of inhibiting ADCC (11,12).

Heat-aggregated human gamma globulin (HGG), at a final concentration of 6.7 mg/ml, inhibited cytotoxic activity by 54%.   Inhibition by
HGG presumably results from the blocking of K cell (effector cell in
ADCC) Fc receptors.   Since K cells exert their specific cytolytic potential by virtue of their Fc receptors' binding specific antibody,
such effector cells are rendered unable to interact with virus-infected target cells sensitized with anti-vaccinia antibody.

Also shown in Table 4 are results using anti-immunoglobulin reagents as inhibitors in the ^{51}Cr release assay.   In the case of an IgG
fraction of a rabbit anti-hamster immunoglobulin antiserum (RαHIg),
cytotoxic activity was inhibited by 58% at a concentration of 1.7
mg/ml.   The table also shows that such inhibition results from the ca-

Table 4.   Inhibition of Vaccinia Virus-Induced Cytotoxic Activity In
           Vitro

Effector[1]	Reagent[2]	% Specific [51]Cr Release	% Inhibition[3]
Normal	--	2	--
Immune	--	33	--
	HGG 6.7 mg/ml	15	54
	RαHIg 1.7 mg/ml	14	58
	F(ab')$_2$-RαHIG 1.7 mg/ml	19	42

[1]As in Tables 1-3, E:T ratio of 40.

[2]HGG, heat-aggregated human gamma globulin; RαHIg, IgG fraction of a
rabbit anti-hamster immunoglobulin antiserum; F(ab')$_2$-RαHIG, pepsin
digested RαHIg.

[3]As compared to immune spleen cells incubated with virus-infected
target cells in the absence of inhibitors.

pacity of the RαHIg reagent to interact with putative anti-vaccinia
antibodies, rather than functioning as an aggregated gamma globulin.
In this case, pepsin digests of RαHIg (F(ab')$_2$-RαHIg), which lack an
Fc piece, inhibit 42% of virus-induced cytotoxic activity at a concentration of 1.7 mg/ml. Thus, a significant portion of vaccinia virus-
induced cytotoxic activity in hamsters is inhibitable either with reagents that block Fc receptors or with reagents that bind hamster immunoglobulin. We conclude that virus-induced cytotoxic activity in
hamsters is at least part ADCC in nature.

Although hamsters acutely infected with vaccinia virus generate
ADCC, other mechanisms of cell-mediated cytotoxic activity also appear
to be operant. For example, thymectomized hamsters acutely infected
with vaccinia virus still generate levels of cytotoxic activity above
that seen in uninfected normal and uninfected thymectomized hamsters
(8).

Natural killer (NK) activity has been described recently in hamsters in two different systems. In one study (13), normal hamsters
were shown to possess cytotoxic activity against the SA7 hamster lymphoma. Another study (14) described NK activity in hamsters infected
with Pichinde virus. The presence of non-T cell-mediated cytotoxic
activity in vaccinia infected hamsters also has been documented (15),
although activity in this system appears to be macrophage mediated.

Table 5. NK Activity in Hamsters Following Acute Infection with
          Vaccinia Virus

| | | % Specific ^{51}CR Release | | |
| | | MHST | | SA7[2] |
Effector[1]	E:T	Infected	Uninfected	Uninfected
Normal	40	16	4	40
	13	11	4	nd[3]
	4	4	1	nd
Immune	40	85	16	59
	13	60	7	45
	4	21	3	13

[1]As in Tables 1-4.

[2]NK sensitive hamster target cell.

[3]Not done.

The experiment described in Table 5 was undertaken to ascertain
whether acute vaccinia virus infection in Syrian hamsters elicits detectable NK activity. Spleen cells from normal and acutely infected
(immune) hamsters were assayed for cytotoxic activity against uninfected and infected syngeneic target cells (MHST). Spleen effector
cells also were assayed for cytotoxic activity against uninfected SA7
target cells sensitive to the cytotoxic activity of hamster NK cells
(13). Although spleen cells from normal (uninfected) hamsters possess
considerable NK activity against SA7 target cells (40% specific ^{51}Cr
release at an E:T ratio of 40), this activity increases somewhat following infection with vaccinia virus (59% specific ^{51}Cr release at an
E:T ratio of 40). Thus, in addition to eliciting ADCC, acute infection with vaccinia virus apparently boosts NK activity in hamsters.

Although it now is understood why vaccinia virus-induced cytotoxic activity in hamsters is not genetically restricted (because K cells
derive their specificity solely from anti-vaccinia antibody), it is
not clear why hamsters do not, or cannot, generate detectable cytotoxic T cell-mediated activity following acute infection with vaccinia
virus. Assuming that the results presented for vaccinia virus in this
study are prototypic for hamsters infected with viruses in general,
perhaps a more fundamental defect lies at the heart of hamster viral
immunity. This defect may be related in some way to certain unique
attributes of the Syrian hamster MHC.

The following hypothesis is one of many that can be advanced to
explain the inability of hamsters to utilize cytotoxic T cells in response to acute vaccinia virus infection. Although Syrian hamsters

possess homologues of class I MHC encoded molecules (16), no evidence has been obtained documenting even limited polymorphism for such molecules in the hamster. This contrasts with studies in the mouse that clearly show extensive polymorphism for such MHC encoded molecules (17).

It has been suggested (18,19) that class I molecule polymorphism and the size of the T cell receptor repertoire (as manifested by diverse cytotoxic activity) are linked functionally and might have co-evolved. In other words, the ability of a species to generate cytotoxic T cell activity toward a multitude of viruses is dependent upon the maintenance of a polymorphic system of class I molecules. This hypothesis is more attractive because the cell-mediated response in mice after virus infection is mediated by T cells whose activities are promoted and restricted by such polymorphic class I MHC molecules (20).

Perhaps virus-induced T cell-mediated cytotoxic activity cannot be generated in hamsters undergoing acute infection with virus because the apparent lack of class I polymorphism in this species has left hamsters unable to develop a sufficient T cell receptor repertoire. As a result, hamsters might have been forced to employ alternate systems of cell-mediated anti-viral immunity that are neither governed by the MHC nor mediated by cytotoxic T cells.

Whatever the reason for the lack of a cytotoxic T cell response in hamsters undergoing acute infection with vaccinia virus, the alternate systems of cell-mediated anti-viral immunity appear to be quite effective, for hamsters are remarkably free of enzootic viruses (21, 22).

ACKNOWLEDGMENTS

The authors wish to thank Ms. Glenda Shroeder and Mr. Kevin Stasney for expert technical assistance, Dr. David Hart for the generous gifts of RαHIg and F(ab')$_2$-RαHIg, and Dr. William Duncan for collaboration in the production and testing of adult thymectomized hamsters. This work was supported in part by USPHS grants CA 09082 and RR 01133.

REFERENCES

1.   Duncan, W.R.; Streilein, J.W. J Immunol 118 (1977) 832.
2.   Duncan, W.R.; Streilein, J.W. Transplantation 25 (1978) 12.
3.   Duncan, W.R.; Streilein, J.W. Transplantation 24 (1978) 17.
4.   Doherty, P.C.; Zinkernagel, R.M. Transplant Rev 19 (1974) 89.
5.   Zinkernagel, R.M. et al. J Immunol 119 (1977) 1242.
6.   Nelles, M.J.; Streilein, J.W. Immunogenetics 10 (1980) 185.
7.   Nelles, M.J.; Streilein, J.W. Immunogenetics (1980) in press.

8.   Nelles, M.J. et al. J Immunol (1981) in press.
9.   Streilein, J.W.; Duncan, W.R. Immunogenetics 9 (1979) 563.
10. Tosolini, F.A.; Mims, C.A. J Infect Dis 123 (1971) 134.
11. Ziegler, H.K.; Henney, C.S. J Immunol 119 (1977) 1010.
12. Pearson, G.R. Curr Top Microbiol Immunol 80 (1978) 65.
13. Datta, S.K. et al. Int J Cancer 23 (1979) 728.
14. Gee, S.R. et al. J Immunol 123 (1979) 2618.
15. Chapes, S.K.; Tompkins, W.A.F. J Immunol 123 (1979) 303.
16. Phillips, J.T. et al. Immunogenetics 7 (1978) 445.
17. Klein, J. Biology of the Mouse Histocompatibility-2 Complex.
     Springer-Verlag (1975).
18. Blanden, R.V.; Ada, G.L. Scand J Immunol 7 (1978) 181.
19. Zinkernagel, R.M. Annu Rev Microbiol 33 (1979) 201.
20. Doherty, P.C. et al. Transplant Rev 29 (1976) 89.
21. Parker, J.C. et al. Bacteriol Proc 163 (1967).
22. Van Hoosier, G.L. et al. Lab Anim Care 20 (1970) 232.

NATURAL KILLER (NK) CELLS IN HAMSTERS AND THEIR MODULATION IN

TUMORIGENESIS

John J. Trentin and Surjit K. Datta

Division of Experimental Biology, Baylor College of Medicine
Houston, TX   77030

INTRODUCTION

Natural killer (NK) cells have been reported in several species
including mice, rats, hamsters, guinea pigs, miniature swine, chickens
and humans (1-14). These normal unsensitized lymphocytes exhibit cytolytic activity against a variety of targets including tumors and virus-
infected cells (15-18). NK cells that have been studied extensively
in mice and humans are small, non-adherent, non-phagocytic lymphocytes
that originate in the bone marrow (14,19-22). NK cells lack conventional levels of T- and B-cell surface markers. Human NK cells have
readily detectable Fc receptors on their surface, whereas mouse NK
cells may express only low concentrations of Fc receptor, which are
difficult to demonstrate (23). Recently it has been shown that NK
cells of both mice and humans may have a low level of T-cell markers
such as theta antigen and E rosette receptors, respectively (24,25).
NK-cell activity is age-related (1,2) and genetically controlled (26,
27).

Recently the phenomenon of genetic resistance (GR) to bone marrow transplantation (BMT) was compared with spleen NK cell-mediated
lysis of YAC-1 (28-30). There appears to be identity between the effector mechanisms of GR and NK-cell lysis of YAC-1 cells. Although
the biological significance of natural cytotoxicity is not fully
clear, it would appear to be a newly discovered, but perhaps more
primitive, effector mechanism of cell-mediated cancer immunity, different from the classical T, B and macrophage effector mechanisms.
We have previously reported natural cytotoxicity in hamsters (5) and
a relationship between GR to BMT and NK-cell lysis in mice (28,30).
In this paper we describe further studies to characterize NK cell activity in hamsters and its regulation during tumorigenesis, and dis-
cuss the role of GR to BMT as an NK cell-mediated lymphoma-leukemia
defense mechanism.

MATERIALS AND METHODS

(C57 X A)F_1 hybrid mice were bred in our specific pathogen free (SPF) inbred mouse colony. The mice were usually female and were about 3 months old unless otherwise specified.

Inbred LSH and random-bred Syrian golden hamsters were bred in our SPF hamster colony. Most of the experiments were done on 3- to 4-month-old animals of both sexes unless otherwise stated.

The cell line YAC-1, established from a Moloney virus-induced lymphoma of strain A mice, was provided by Dr. R. Kiessling of the Karolinska Institute, Stockholm, Sweden. It was maintained in RPMI 1640 medium supplemented with 10% fetal calf serum (FCS) and 50 µg erythromycin, 100 µg streptomycin and 25mM Hepes buffer per ml. The cell line K562, established from a patient with chronic myelogenous leukemia, was procured from Dr. K. C. McCormick of the Stehlin Cancer Foundation, Houston. It was maintained in RPMI 1640 medium containing 20% FCS, 50 µg erythromycin, 100 µg streptomycin and 25mM Hepes buffer per ml. The simian adenovirus$_7$ (SA_7) tumor and tissue culture cell line SA_7Tc have been described before (5).

Adherent cells were removed from spleen cell preparations by incubating 5×10^7 cells in 15 ml of medium in a tissue culture flask (75 cm^2 growth area). After incubating for 60 minutes, the nonadherent cells were decanted, washed once in medium and adjusted to the desired concentration.

For ammonium chloride treatment, 5×10^7 spleen cells were centrifuged and the pellet was resuspended in 5 ml of 0.174M Tris-NH_4Cl solution (pH 7.2) for 10 minutes at room temperature. Cells were washed once in the medium and adjusted to the desired concentration.

For culture, 5×10^7 spleen cells were incubated in 15 ml of medium in tissue culture flasks (75 cm^2 growth area) at $37^{\circ}C$ for about 20 hours. Suspensions were centrifuged and adjusted to the desired concentration.

Lymphocytes with receptors for the Fc portion of IgG were depleted by absorption on EA monolayers as described (8,31).

For trypsin treatment, 5×10^7 spleen cells suspended in PBS were centrifuged and the pellet was resuspended in 5 ml of 0.25% trypsin in PBS and incubated at $37^{\circ}C$ for 30 minutes. The cell suspension was washed once in the medium and adjusted to the desired concentration.

Radiation, cyclophosphamide, silica and carrageenan treatments have been described before (5,30).

The NK-cell assay employing ^{51}Cr release by labelled YAC-1 target cells and mouse spleen cells, and by labelled SA$_7$ target cells and hamster spleen cells, has been described before (5,30). The ^{51}Cr release assay employing xenogeneic K562 target cells and hamster spleen cells was done as for mouse YAC-1 target cells except for minor modifications. The incubation period was 16 to 18 hours instead of four hours for YAC-1 cells.

Genetic resistance to bone marrow transplantation was done by spleen colony assay as described earlier (32,33).

RESULTS AND DISCUSSION

Genetic Resistance to Marrow Transplantation and Natural Killer Cell Activity in Mice

The several shared features of the phenomena of GR to BMT in vivo and of spleen NK cell-mediated lysis of YAC-1 lymphoma cells in vitro are presented in Table 1. Like GR to BMT, spleen NK cell activity was found to appear abruptly at about 3 weeks of age and to be radio-resistant to 1100 R whole-body irradiation. But whole-body irradiation to 2200, 4400 and 6600 R increasingly inhibited both spleen NK-cell activity and GR to BMT. Treatment of mice with cytoxan and the macrophage inhibitors silica and carrageenan abrogated or inhibited both GR to BMT and NK cell activity, silica being least effective in both systems. Similar observations have been made in another study (29). These many unique characteristics common to both GR to BMT in vivo and NK-cell lysis of YAC-1 in vitro suggest that the effector mechanism may be the same in both systems. NK-cell activity seems to represent an in vitro correlate of GR to BMT.

The possible role of GR to BMT as a natural lymphoma-leukemia defense mechanism also was analyzed. The C57 strain of mice and its hybrids express strong GR to BMT and are resistant to spontaneous leukemia. Fractionated whole-body irradiation (4 x 225 R per week) breaks GR to BMT and GR to spontaneous leukemia. Resistance to growth of AKR lymphoma was tested in "responder" (C57 X AKR) and "non-responder" (C3H X AKR) hybrid mice, according to the scheme depicted in Fig. 1. Lethally irradiated (C57 X AKR)F$_1$ mice show genetic (hybrid) resistance to C57, but not to AKR, parental marrow. Lethally radiated (C3H X AKR)F$_1$ hybrids do not have GR to BMT from either of their parental strains. Intravenously transplanted AKR lymphoma cells produced lymphomatous spleen colonies and mortality in irradiated (C3H X AKR)F$_1$ hybrids but not in irradiated (C57 X AKR)F$_1$ hybrids. Thus "responder" (C57 X AKR)F$_1$ hybrids can recognize and reject AKR lymphoma cells, but not normal AKR bone marrow cells. A normal biological role of lymphoma-leukemia surveillance was postulated for genetic resistance

Table 1.   Comparison of Genetic Resistance to C57 Bone Marrow Transplantation in vivo, with Spleen NK Cell-Mediated Lysis of YAC-1 Lymphoma Cells in vitro in (C57 X A)F$_1$ Mice

Mice and treatment	In vivo		In vitro	
	Genetic resistance	Percent abrogation of genetic resistance[1]	YAC-1 lysis[5]	Percent inhibition of YAC-1 lysis[2]
12-18 days old	Absent[3]		Absent	
22-30 days old	Present[3]		Present	
Young adult	Present[3]		Present	
Young adult + 1100 R treated	Not abrogated[3]	0	Not inhibited	0
Young adult + 2200 R treated	Abrogated[3]	19	Inhibited	66
Young adult + 4400 R treated	Abrogated[3]	92	Inhibited	76
Young adult + 6600 R treated	Abrogated[3]	100	Inhibited	100
Young adult + cytoxan treated	Abrogated[4]	59	Inhibited	76.3
Young adult + carrageenan treated	Abrogated[4]	77	Inhibited	73.2
Young adult + silica treated	Abrogated[4]	24	Inhibited	26

[1]Calculated on the basis of microscopic spleen colony number of experimental and control mice.

$$\left(\frac{\text{C57 colonies in treated CA F}_1 \text{ mice}}{\text{C57 colonies in C57 mice}} \times 100 \right)$$

[2]Calculated on the basis of percent lysis of YAC-1 target cells.

$$\left(\frac{\text{\% lysis of normal} - \text{\% lysis of treated mice}}{\text{\% lysis of normal untreated mice}} \right) \times 100$$

[3]Prior experiment.
[4]Concurrent experiment.
[5]Effector to target ratio was 100:1.
From Biomedicine 31 (1979) 62.

to marrow transplantation, directed at antigens which, like TL, are expressed on normal hemopoietic cells of some strains, but only on leukemic cells of other strains (34,35).

Natural Killer Cell Activity in Hamsters

We previously reported NK cell activity in hamsters against SA$_7$ lymphoma target cells (5). It was found that NK cell activity was much higher in random-bred (38.2% lysis) than in inbred (14.9% lysis) hamsters. There was much day to day variation in the range of percent lysis between experiments. NK-cell activity could be inhibited by unlabelled SA$_7$ target cells in a dose-dependent fashion. NK cell activity was high in spleen and bone marrow, intermediate in mesenteric lymph nodes, peritoneal exudate cells, and peripheral blood, with little or none in thymus. NK cell responses were detected as early as in the first week (four to seven days) after birth and as late as 1½ to 2 years of age. NK cell activity was low in young animals and increased progressively with age (up to 1 or 1½ years), but in some 2-year-old random-bred hamsters, it had apparently returned to a level found in adult 3- to 4-month-old hamsters.

Many similarities in the pattern of NK cell responses have been reported in many species, including hamsters (1-10). The age and tissue distribution of NK reactivity in hamsters, however, differs from that of mice and rats. In mice, NK-cell activity appears abruptly at 3 weeks of age, peaks at 6 to 8 weeks and declines thereafter (15). In hamsters, activity was detected in 4-day-old infants and 2-year-old hamsters. There appear to be progressive increases with age to 1½ years, but in some 2-year-old hamsters tested, NK activity was at the same level as in 3- to 4-month-old hamsters. The mouse NC (Natural Cytotoxic) cells that are active against chemically induced sarcoma

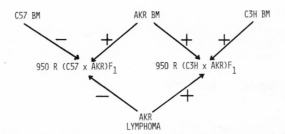

Fig. 1:   Schema of take (+) or rejection (-) of intravenously transfused inbred parental bone marrow (BM) or lymphoma cells in lethally irradiated (950 R ^{137}Cs, total body) (C57 X AKR)F$_1$ responder mice and (C3H X AKR)F$_1$ nonresponder mice.

Table 2. Characteristics of Hamster NK Cells[1]

Characteristics	% Lysis[2]	
	Untreated	Treated
Effective after removal of adherent cells	18.8	38
Resistant to trypsin in vitro	10.5	10.9
Resistant to NH_4Cl in vitro	10.5	9.9
Lost at $37^{\circ}C$ in vitro	21.8	3.1
Positive for Fc receptors		
Exposed to E monolayer	51.4	62.6
Exposed to EA monolayer	51.4	11.5
Resistant to 600 R in vivo	9.1	13.9
Resistant to 1100 R in vivo	14.2	14.9
Susceptible to cytoxan in vivo	21.7	1.4
Susceptible to carrageenan in vivo	21.7	16.5

[1]Pooled spleen cells from 2- to 3-month-old inbred LSH hamsters were used.

[2]Effector to target cell ratio was 100:1.

target cells (36) appear at birth and persist in old age. High NK activity also has been reported in older rats (4). Similarly, human NK reactivity has been detected over a wide age range, including umbilical cord blood (37,38), and in young and adult donors (11,13). No significant relationship between the level of NK activity and the age of donor appears to exist in humans (11-13). The prevalence of NK-cell activity in hamsters over a wide age range, including old age, may have significance in terms of the low incidence of spontaneous tumors in this species (39). The tissue distribution of hamster NK cells differs from that of mice and rats, being as high in bone marrow as in spleen. In the mouse and rat, bone marrow has low reactivity, even though spleen NK-cell reactivity has been shown to be marrow-dependent or -derived (21,22). But, as in hamsters, NK reactivity of the mouse was high in bone marrow and in spleen. Low NK activity has been found recently in hamster bone marrow (7). There is also a conflicting report of the presence of significant levels of NK-cell activity among thymocytes in rats (4). Some of the different results regarding the organ distribution of NK cells may be due to basic differences among species, or to the heterogeneity of NK cells associated with the use of different target cells in different studies.

Characteristics of Hamster NK Cells

Various characteristics of hamster NK cells are summarized in Table 2. NK-cell lysis was mediated by non-adherent cells. NK activity was resistant to trypsin and NH_4Cl treatment but was lost after incubation at $37^{\circ}C$ for 20 hours. Depletion of Fc receptor-bearing

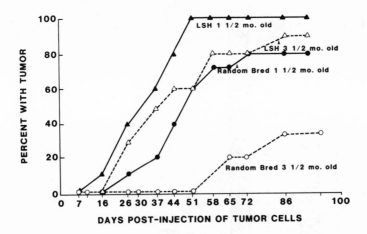

Fig. 2: Tumor growth in inbred LSH or random-bred hamsters. Ten ham-
        sters of either inbred LSH or random-bred origin, 1½ and 3½
        months old, were injected SC with 2 x 10^5 cultured SA7 tumor
        cells in 0.5 ml. Animals were observed weekly for the appear-
        ance of transplanted tumor.

lymphocytes on EA monolayers markedly reduced NK-cell lysis, suggesting
that hamster NK cells possess Fc receptors. Exposure of hamsters to
600 R or 1100 R whole-body irradiation did not diminish NK-cell lysis.
Treatment of hamsters intraperitoneally (IP) with 500 mg of cyclophos-
phamide/kg or 5 mg of carrageenan abrogated NK-cell activity, cytoxan
being more effective than carrageenan. Thus, hamster NK cells share
the major characteristics of mouse NK cells. They are nonadherent, resistant to NH_4Cl and trypsin treatment, are lost by preincubation at
$37^{\circ}C$ for 20 hours, and possess Fc receptors (19,20,23). Lack of surface immunoglobulin on hamster as well as mouse NK cells has been reported (6,7). It is not known whether hamster NK cells express low
levels of thymic antigen surface marker as is reported in the mouse
(24). NK-cell activity in hamsters is radioresistant to 1100 R whole-
body irradiation and susceptible to cytoxan and the macrophage inhibitor carrageenan, as in the mouse (28-30). There is evidence that interferon stimulates NK activity (40,41). Macrophages may be involved
in NK activity by virtue of their ability to produce interferon (15).

Correlation Between the Level of NK-Cell Activity and Resistance to
Tumor Development

    We have shown previously that random-bred hamsters have higher
NK-cell activity than inbred LSH hamsters, and that NK activity increases progressively with age in either strain of hamsters (5). To

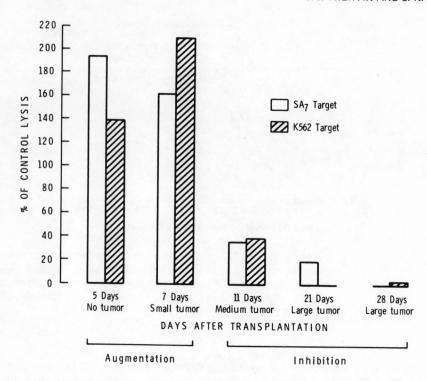

Fig. 3:   NK-cell activity in random-bred hamsters following SC inocu-
          lation of 10^7 cultured SA$_7$ tumor cells. E:T ratio was 100:1.

investigate the possible correlation between the level of NK-cell activity and relative resistance to tumor development, 10 inbred LSH
or random-bred hamsters, either 1½ or 3½ months old, were inoculated
subcutaneously (SC) with 2 x 10^5 SA$_7$ tumor cultured cells in 0.5 ml
medium and observed weekly for the appearance of tumors. Results are
presented in Fig. 2.   Random-bred hamsters 3½ and 1½ months old were
more resistant to tumor development than inbred hamsters of similar
ages. Further, 3½-month-old hamsters of both inbred and random-bred
origin had fewer tumors than 1½-month-old hamsters of the same strain.
This suggests that resistance to transplanted tumor development may be
associated with the level of NK-cell activity, but the possible role
of T cells and macrophages is not excluded. Studies in mice have also
shown that animals with higher levels of NK activity are more resistant to tumor development than animals with low NK activity (15,27,42,
43). Levels of NK activity among strains of mice have been found to
correlate inversely with their susceptibility to fatal infection with
herpes simplex virus type 1 (44,45).

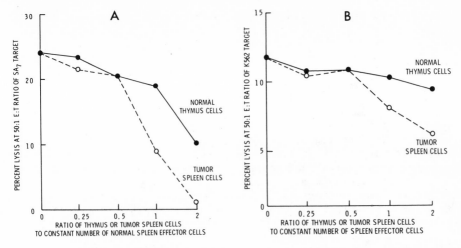

Fig. 4: NK-cell activity of mixtures of spleen cells from normal and
         SA$_7$ tumor-bearer hamsters at a constant E:T ratio of 50:1.
         To a constant number of normal spleen cells were added vary-
         ing numbers of either spleen cells from tumor-bearers or thy-
         mocytes from normal hamsters, so that their ratios to normal
         spleen cells were 0.25:1, 0.5:1, 1:1 and 2:1. A. NK-cell
         activity against SA$_7$ target. B. NK-cell activity against
         K562 target.

Effect of Tumor Growth on NK-Cell Activity

Adult random-bred hamsters were given a transplant of 10^7 SA$_7$
tumor cultured cells SC and their spleen cell-mediated cytotoxic activity was measured at various days post-transplant, along with normal
age-matched controls. In addition to the SA$_7$ target, against which
specific T-cell immunity may also have been induced, cell-mediated cytotoxicity was also tested against an unrelated (human) target, K562,
to assess NK-cell activity more directly, rather than a combination
of NK and immune T-cell cytotoxic activity. Five and seven days post-
transplant of SA$_7$ cells, when there was little or no visible tumor, NK-
cell activity was greatly augmented. But on or later than day eleven
post-transplant, when the tumor was medium or large in size, cell-
mediated cytotoxicity was greatly suppressed (Fig. 3). The suppression
of NK-cell activity in tumor-bearing hamsters prompted us to investigate whether the suppression is due to suppressor cells. A cell mixture protocol was used to test the ability of spleen cells from tumor
bearers to suppress NK cell-mediated lysis by normal spleen cells. The
E;T ratio of normal spleen cells was kept constant at 50:1, and to
this were added graded numbers of spleen cells from tumor bearers so
that ratios of spleen cells from tumor-bearer to normal spleen cells
were 0.25:1, 0.5:1, 1:1 and 2:1. As a control for cell crowding

effects, normal thymus cells (having no NK-cell activity) were added
to a constant number of spleen cells at similar ratios. NK-cell activity of these mixtures was tested against SA_7 and the xenogeneic
target K562. Results are presented in Fig. 4 A and B. Addition of
spleen cells from tumor-bearing hamsters at ratios of 1:1 and 2:1 reduced NK-cell lysis of SA_7 and K562 target cells beyond the inhibiting
effect of normal thymus cells. In our preliminary study we found
that serum from large SA_7 tumor-bearers suppressed NK-cell activity
of normal spleen cells against SA_7 target cells. These results suggest that during tumorigenesis, NK-cell responses may be regulated by
suppressor or inhibitor cells, as well as by serum factors. Both suppressor cells and serum factors are known to regulate tumor-immune T-
cell responses in many tumor systems (46,47). Suppression of NK-cell
responses in tumor-bearers may have implications for tumor progression
if NK cells play a role in surveillance against tumors.

ACKNOWLEDGMENT

This work was supported by USPHS grants CA 12093, CA 03367, and
K6 CA 14219 from the National Cancer Institute.

REFERENCES

1.   Herberman, R.B. et al. Int J Cancer 16 (1975) 216.
2.   Kiessling, R. et al. Eur J Immunol 5 (1975) 112.
3.   Nunn, M.E. et al. J Natl Cancer Inst 56 (1976) 393.
4.   Shellam, G.R.; Hogg, N. Int J Cancer 19 (1977) 225.
5.   Datta, S.K. et al. Int J Cancer 23 (1979) 728.
6.   Gee, S.R. et al. J Immunol 123 (1979) 2618.
7.   Tompkins, W.A.F. et al. J Immunol (1980) in press.
8.   Altman, A.; Rapp, H.J. J Immunol 121 (1978) 2244.
9.   Koren, H.S. et al. Proc Natl Acad Sci USA 75 (1978) 5127.
10. Sharma, J.M.; Coulson, B.D. J Natl Cancer Inst 66 (1979) 527.
11. Oldham, R.K. et al. J Natl Cancer Inst 55 (1975) 1305.
12. Takasugi, M. et al. Cancer Res 33 (1973) 2898.
13. Rosenberg, E.B. et al. J Natl Cancer Inst 52 (1974) 345.
14. West, W.H. et al. J Immunol 118 (1977) 355.
15. Herberman, R.B.; Holden, H.T. Adv Cancer Res 27 (1978) 305.
16. Kiessling, R.; Haller, O. In: Contemporary Topics in Immuno-
     biology 8, ed. Hanna. Plenum Press, New York (1978) 305.
17. Welsh, R.M.; Zinkernagel, R.M. Nature 268 (1977) 646.
18. Santoli, D.G. et al. J Immunol 121 (1978) 526.
19. Herberman, R.B. et al. Int J Cancer 16 (1975) 230.
20. Kiessling, R. et al. Eur J Immunol 5 (1975) 117.
21. Haller, O. et al. J Exp Med 145 (1977) 1411.
22. Haller, O.; Wigzell, H. J Immunol 118 (1977) 503.
23. Herberman, R.B. et al. J Immunol 119 (1977) 322.
24. Herberman, R.B. et al. Int J Cancer 19 (1977) 555.

25. Kay, H.D. et al. J Immunol 118 (1977) 2058.
26. Kiessling, R. et al. Int J Cancer 15 (1975) 933.
27. Petranyi, G. et al. Immunogenetics 3 (1976) 15.
28. Trentin, J.J. et al. In: Experimental Hematology Today, ed.
     Baum and Ledney. Springer-Verlag, New York (1977) 179.
29. Kiessling, R. et al. Eur J Immunol 7 (1977) 655.
30. Datta, S.K. et al. Biomedicine 31 (1979) 62.
31. Kedar, E. et al. J Immunol 112 (1974) 1231.
32. McCulloch, E.A.; Till, J.E. J Cell Comp Physiol 61 (1963) 301.
33. Rauchwerger, J.M. et al. Biomedicine 18 (1973) 109.
34. Gallagher, M.T. et al. Biomedicine 25 (1976) 1.
35. Gallagher, M.T. et al. In: Proceedings of the Conference on
     Immuno-aspects of the Spleen, ed. Battisto and Streilein.
     North-Holland Publishing Company, Amsterdam (1976).
36. Stutman, O. et al. J Immunol 121 (1978) 1819.
37. Campbell, A.C. et al. Clin Exp Immunol 18 (1974) 469.
38. Jondal, M.; Pross, M. Int J Cancer 15 (1975) 596.
39. Van Hoosier, G.L. et al. In: Defining the Laboratory Animals.
     National Academy of Sciences, Washington, D.C. (1971) 450.
40. Oehler, J.R. et al. Int J Cancer 21 (1978) 210.
41. Gidlund, M. et al. Nature 273 (1978) 759.
42. Kiessling, R. et al. Int J Cancer 17 (1976) 1.
43. Haller, O. et al. Nature 270 (1977) 609.
44. Lopez, C. Fed Proc 37 (1978) 1560.
45. Rager-Zierman, B.; Allison, A. Fed Proc 38 (1979) 1466.
46. Hellström, K.E.; Hellström, I. Adv Cancer Res 12 (1969) 167.
47. Broder, S. et al. J Natl Cancer Inst 61 (1978) 5.

PREVENTION OF PRIMARY SIMIAN ADENOVIRUS TYPE 7 (SA7) TUMORS IN HAMSTERS BY ADOPTIVE TRANSFER OF LYMPHOID CELLS: ROLE OF DIFFERENT CELL TYPES

Surjit K. Datta, John J. Trentin and Kenneth J. McCormick

Division of Experimental Biology, Baylor College of Medicine
Houston, TX   77030

INTRODUCTION

Malignant neoplasms in general acquire neo-antigens, usually called tumor-specific transplantation antigen (TSTA). Chemically induced tumors usually exhibit antigens unique to each tumor, whereas tumors induced by a virus share a common antigen specific for that virus regardless of the histological type of tumor or host species in which the tumor was induced (1-3). These TSTA invoke an immune response, mainly of cell-mediated type. The immune control or progressive growth of the tumor depends upon many factors including strength of the cellular immune response (degree of sensitization of lymphoid cells), "sneaking through" or appearance of serum blocking factor (1, 3-5), and suppressor cells (6-8). It has generally been accepted that thymus-dependent lymphocytes (T) are primarily responsible for rejection of tumors (9-15). There is considerable evidence that macrophages also contribute an important effector mechanism against tumors (16). Recently, natural killer (NK) cells are also thought to be involved in tumor surveillance (17-19). Most of the studies of effector mechanisms of tumor immunity have been carried out in vitro, using various cytotoxicity assays. To assess the role of in vivo cell-mediated immune responses in tumor immunity, two main approaches usually have been used. One consisted of studying the influence of immuno-suppression (x-irradiation, thymectomy, anti-lymphocyte serum) on the development of tumors (20-24). The alternate approach is to augment cellular immune responses either through non-specific stimulation such as Bacillus Calmette-Guerin (BCG), Corynebacterium parvum (CP), poly I:C, etc. (25-28), or through adoptive transfer of specifically sensitized lymphoid cells (29-31).

We studied the role of immunological factors in resistance to primary tumor development by simian adenovirus type 7 (SA7) in ham-

165

sters. Newborn hamsters are highly susceptible, whereas adult hamsters are resistant, to primary oncogenesis by SA$_7$ virus (32). To understand the role of cell-mediated immune responses in age-related resistance to SA$_7$ virus oncogenesis, a system of adoptive transfer of lymphoid cells from adult to newborn hamsters was employed. Adoptively treated newborn hamsters should be analogous to immunologically competent adults, but in addition should have a sufficient number of target cells for induction of neoplasia by SA$_7$ virus. This report describes the effect of adoptive transfer of normal or sensitized lymphoid cells on the development of primary tumor by SA$_7$ virus in susceptible hamsters.

MATERIALS AND METHODS

Inbred LSH hamsters were obtained from the closed SPF hamster colony of the Division of Experimental Biology. Adult hamsters (1½ to 4 months old) of both sexes served as donors, and neonatal hamsters as recipients.

The simian adenovirus$_7$ (SA$_7$) was propagated in BSC-1 cells and assayed in Vero cells. Titer of the virus was 10^8 plaque-forming units per milliliter (PFU/ml).

An SA$_7$ tumor was originally induced in an inbred LSH hamster by inoculation of 10^7 PFU of SA$_7$ virus subcutaneously (SC) into 3- to 4-day-old hamsters. The tumor was serially transplanted into syngeneic weanling hamsters. A tissue culture cell line (SA$_7$Tc) was derived from the transplanted tumor and maintained by serial passage in Eagle's MEM containing 10% fetal calf serum and antibiotics. Chicken embryo lethal orphan (CELO) virus-induced liver tumor (CILT) was derived from a hepatocellular carcinoma induced in an inbred LSH hamster following SC inoculation of CELO virus into newborn hamsters.

Peritoneal exudate cells (PEC) were induced either by inoculation of 3 to 4 ml of thioglycollate medium (Difco) or a 10% solution of proteose peptone (Difco). PEC were collected at day 1, 2 and 3 after stimulation by washing the peritoneal cavity with 5 to 10 ml of Hank's balanced salt solution (HBSS) or phosphate buffered saline solution (PBS). The peritoneal washings were filtered through four to six layers of gauze, spun and resuspended. The cell suspension was passed through a 200-mesh stainless steel screen fitted in a Swinney filter holder, and adjusted to the desired concentration. Spleen or thymus fragments were pressed through 50-mesh screen into the medium and the cell suspension was passed through a 200-mesh screen fitted in a Swinney filter holder. The suspended cells were washed once by spinning down and adjusted to the desired concentration.

Litters of newborn hamsters, 3 to 5 days old, were divided into groups in such a way that litters born on different days were spread

as equally as possible throughout all the groups. Usually 20 infants
were selected per group, but actual numbers varied depending upon availability. Groups of newborn hamsters were injected intraperitoneally
(IP) with 0.1 ml of PBS or cell suspensions such as PEC, spleen or
thymus cells, etc., and a day later were challenged with SA$_7$ virus or
tumor cells. At about 3 weeks of age, animals of each group were
weaned, separated into sexes and observed for the development of tumors.
Statistical analysis was done by means of Fisher's exact probability
(one-tailed) test to determine whether the tumor incidence was significantly lowered in experimental groups, as compared to control groups.

RESULTS

Effect of Transfer of Normal PEC, Spleen Cells and Thymocytes on the Development of Primary Tumors

     Groups of newborn hamsters were inoculated IP with PBS, 1 or 5 x
10^7 one-day PEC, 5 x 10^7 spleen cells, and a mixture of 2.5 x 10^7
spleen and 2.5 x 10^7 one-day PEC. A day after the transfer of cells,
animals were challenged SC with 10^7 PFU of SA$_7$ virus and observed for
the development of tumors. Results are shown in Fig. 1. At eight weeks
post-injection of SA$_7$ virus, onset of tumor development was delayed in
all groups of animals that received different types of cells as compared to PBS controls. Only 5 x 10^7 PEC (P = < 0.02) or a mixture of
2.5 x 10^7 spleen cells and 2.5 x 10^7 PEC (P = < 0.02) significantly delayed or inhibited the development of tumors up to 32 weeks after injection of virus. Morphological analysis of one-day PEC after Giemsa

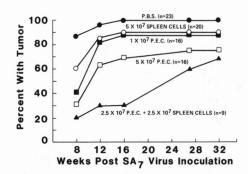

Fig. 1: Effect of adoptive transfer IP of one-day PEC, spleen cells
         and PEC plus spleen cells from normal adult hamsters into 3-
         to 5-day-old hamsters, on the development of primary SA$_7$
         tumors following SC inoculation of 10^7 PFU of SA$_7$ virus a
         day later.

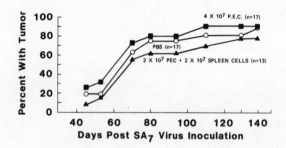

Fig. 2: Effect of adoptive transfer IP of two–day PEC, or PEC plus
        spleen cells from normal adult hamsters into 3– to 5–day–old
        hamsters, on the development of primary SA$_7$ tumors following
        SC inoculation of 5 x 10^6 PFU of SA$_7$ virus a day later.

staining showed that the exudate contained about 65% to 70% neutrophils
and 30% to 35% mononuclear cells.

In other experiments, with a similar type of protocol, the effect
of PEC collected either two or three days after stimulation (containing
80% to 90% mononuclear cells) was tested on primary tumor development.
After adoptive transfer of two– or three–day PEC or spleen cells, hamsters were challenged with 5 x 10^6 PFU of SA$_7$ virus. Both two– and
three–day PEC failed to inhibit the development of primary SA$_7$ tumors
(Fig. 2,3).

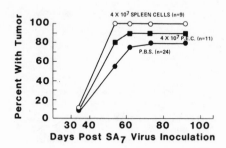

Fig. 3: Effect of adoptive transfer IP of three–day PEC, or spleen
         cells from normal adult hamsters, into 3– to 5–day–old ham-
         sters, on the development of primary SA$_7$ tumors following SC
         inoculation of 5 x 10^6 PFU of SA$_7$ virus a day later.

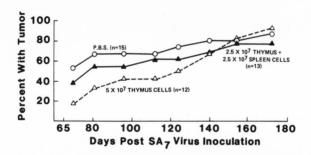

Fig. 4:   Effect of adoptive transfer IP of thymocytes, or thymocytes
          plus spleen cells from normal adult hamsters, into 3- to 5-
          day-old hamsters, on the development of primary SA$_7$ tumors
          following SC inoculation of 5 x 10^6 PFU of SA$_7$ virus a day
          later.

     The adoptive transfer of 5 x 10^7 thymocytes or a mixture of 2.5
x 10^7 thymocytes and 2.5 x 10^7 spleen cells did not inhibit the development of primary SA$_7$ tumors (Fig. 4).

Effect of Transfer of Normal One-day PEC or Spleen Cells on the Development of Transplanted Tumors

     Groups of 6- to 7-day-old newborn hamsters were given IP adoptive
transfer of 5 x 10^7 one-day PEC or spleen cells and a day later were
challenged with 500 SA$_7$ tumor tissue culture cells. The results are
shown in Fig. 5. Though it appears that both PEC and spleen cells
exert some inhibitory effect on the development of transplanted tumor,
the difference was not statistically significant.

Effect of Transfer of Sensitized Spleen Cells on the Development of
Primary Tumors

     Adult hamsters were sensitized with either SA$_7$ virus or SA$_7$ trans-
planted or primary tumors, and their spleen cells were used in transfer
experiments. For virus immunization, hamsters were injected IP three
times biweekly with 10^8 PFU of SA$_7$ virus. As controls, 10^8 sheep red
blood cells (SRBC) or tissue culture fluid (TCF) collected from uninfected BSC-1 monolayers, treated in a similar way as for the preparation of virus, were used. One week after the last immunization, spleen
cells from immunized hamsters were adoptively transferred to neonates
that were challenged a day later with 5 x 10^6 PFU of SA$_7$ virus. Three
x 10^7 spleen cells sensitized with SA$_7$ virus significantly inhibited
primary SA$_7$ tumor development (P = < 0.05) compared to normal spleen

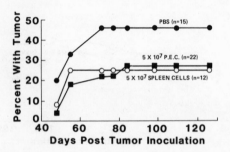

Fig. 5:   Effect of adoptive transfer IP of one-day PEC, or spleen
          cells from normal adult hamsters, into 6- to 7-day-old ham-
          sters, on the development of transplanted SA$_7$ tumors following
          SC inoculation of 500 SA$_7$ tissue culture cells a day later.

cells, whereas 3 x 10^7 SRBC-sensitized or 5 x 10^7 TCF-sensitized spleen
cells had no effect. (Fig. 6, A and B)

      Sensitization of spleen cells against transplanted SA$_7$ tumor was
achieved by giving a transplant of SA$_7$ tumor to adult hamsters, and
spleen cells from hamsters developing a small tumor were tested for
the prevention of primary tumor development.   Specificity of the experiment was controlled by studying the protective effect of spleen
cells from hamsters bearing a small unrelated transplanted tumor, CILT.
Four x 10^7 spleen cells sensitized by SA$_7$ tumor significantly inhibited
the development of primary SA$_7$ tumor (P = < 0.01) compared to PBS controls, whereas 4 x 10^7 spleen cells sensitized to the unrelated CILT
tumor did not have any effect (Fig. 7, A and B).

      To study the effect of spleen cells sensitized by primary SA$_7$
tumor, 3- to 5-day-old newborn hamsters were given 10^7 PFU of SA$_7$
virus.   About seven weeks later, spleen cells and one-day PEC from
hamsters having developed small primary tumors were studied for their
inhibitory effect on SA$_7$ primary tumor development.   5 x 10^7 and 2.5
x 10^7 spleen cells were highly effective in preventing tumor development (P = < 0.001), and 5 x 10^7 PEC had a slight retarding effect on
tumor incidence (Fig. 8).

      Spleen cells from adult hamsters immunized by transplanted SA$_7$
tumor were exposed to 950 R.   Both irradiated and non-irradiated spleen
cells were used in adoptive transfer studies.   Five x 10^7 non-irradiated spleen cells significantly inhibited tumor development (P = <
0.05).   Irradiated spleen cells gave a slight but nonsignificant inhibiting effect (Fig. 9).

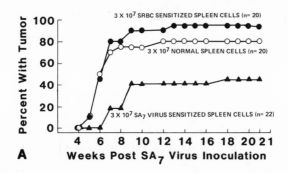

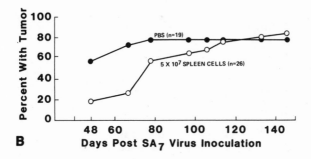

Fig. 6: Effect of adoptive transfer IP of normal, or SA₇ virus-sensi-
         tized, or SRBC-sensitized spleen cells (A), and tissue cul-
         ture fluid-sensitized spleen cells (B) from adult hamsters,
         into 3- to 5-day-old hamsters, on the development of primary
         SA₇ tumors following SC inoculation of 5×10^6 PFU of SA₇
         virus a day later.

DISCUSSION

     We investigated the role of immunological factors in resistance
to primary SA₇ tumors by adoptive transfer of various immunocompetent
cells to newborn hamsters. Infant hamsters offer advantages over
adults, being extremely sensitive to malignant tumor induction by
viruses and lacking mechanisms that control expression and outgrowth
of transformed cells. Newborn hamsters were given an adoptive transfer of spleen, thymus and PEC (collected one, two, and three days
after stimulation), and a day later were challenged with SA₇ virus
or tumor cells. Spleen cells, thymocytes and two- to three-day PEC
from normal adult hamsters did not inhibit tumor development, whereas
one-day PEC retarded or inhibited primary tumor development. The
cellular composition of one-day PEC consisted of 65% to 70% neutrophils in contrast to 80% to 90% lymphoid cells in two- to three-day
PEC. The observation that normal lymphoid cells from immunocompetent

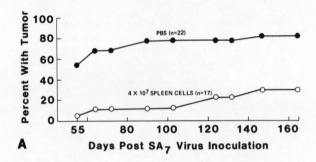

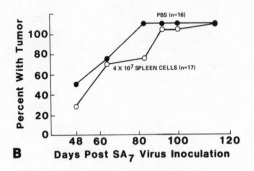

Fig. 7:   Effect of adoptive transfer IP of SA₇ tumor-sensitized spleen
          cells (A), or CELO tumor-sensitized spleen cells (B), from
          adult hamsters bearing transplanted tumors, into 3- to 5-day-
          old hamsters, on the development of primary SA₇ tumors
          following SC inoculation of 5 x 10⁶ PFU of SA₇ virus a day
          later.

hamsters failed to protect susceptible infant hamsters against tumor
development is in contrast to reports in mice and rats, in which
normal lymphoid cells lowered the incidence of polyoma tumors in
intact mice and rats inoculated at birth, or in thymectomized mice
inoculated during the first week of life (29,31,33).   The failure to
confer protection by transfer of normal immunocompetent cells could
be due either to failure of sensitization of effector cells or to inhibition of effector function by suppressor cells.   Retardation of
tumor development by one-day PEC containing about 70% neutrophils
could be due to some effect on the oncogenic potential of virus or
to cytotoxic effect on neoplastic cells in the host.   One-day PEC
were cytotoxic to SA₇ target cells in an in vitro NK cell assay (data
not shown).   It has been reported that mouse PEC rich in neutrophils
(90%) after stimulation with polyvinylpyrrolidinone (PVP) were cytotoxic to mouse tumor target cells in vitro (34).

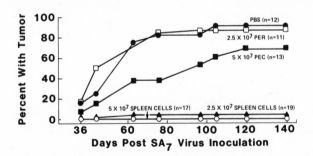

Fig. 8: Effect of adoptive transfer IP of SA7 primary tumor sensitized spleen cells, or PEC from adult hamsters bearing primary SA7 tumor, into 3- to 5-day-old hamsters, on the development of primary SA7 tumors following SC inoculation of
5 x 10⁶ PFU of SA7 virus a day later.

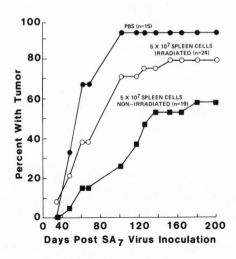

Fig. 9: Effect of adoptive transfer IP of irradiated or non-irradiated SA7 tumor-sensitized spleen cells from adult hamsters
bearing transplanted tumors, into 3- to 5-day-old hamsters,
on the development of primary SA7 tumors, following SC inoculation of 5 x 10⁶ PFU of SA7 virus a day later.

Contrary to non-effect of normal lymphoid cells, spleen cells from hamsters sensitized either with SA_7 virus or tumor conferred a marked protection against primary SA_7 oncogenesis. The conferred resistance was specific, as spleen cells sensitized to unrelated cells (SRBC) or tumor (CILT) showed no effect on tumor development. This is in accordance with the results obtained in the rat-polyoma tumor system in which adoptive transfer of specifically sensitized lymphoid cells to newborns reduced the incidence of primary polyoma tumors, even if the cells were transferred three weeks after inoculation of newborns with polyoma virus (31). Similar observation was made in immunodepressed mice inoculated with polyoma or Moloney sarcoma virus and afterwards immunologically restored with specifically sensitized lymphoid cells (29).

Our results indicate that protection conferred by spleen cells sensitized by SA_7 tumor could be largely abolished by irradiation of spleen cells with 950 R. Both classical T and B cells are radiosensitive, whereas macrophages and NK cells are radioresistant. It is not possible to point out the types of cells that mediate protection against SA_7 oncogenesis from our study. Reports from other studies that used different tumors in mice, rats, and hamsters, however, indicate mainly the involvement of T cells in tumor rejection responses (9,15). In analogy, it could be speculated from our results that the major component of protection against SA_7 oncogenesis has been contributed by radiosensitive cells, probably T cells, but a minor part of protection might have come from radioresistant cells, such as macrophages and NK cells, as radiation of spleen cells did not completely abolish the conferred resistance.

Susceptibility of newborn hamsters to primary oncogenesis could be due to failure of sensitization, or inhibition of effector function of sensitized cells, or both, as well as to rapid development of neoplastic clones.

ACKNOWLEDGMENTS

This work was supported by USPHS grants CA 12093, CA 03367, and K6 CA 14219 from the National Cancer Institute.

REFERENCES

1.   Klein, G. Annu Rev Microbiol 20 (1966) 223.
2.   Law, L.W. Cancer Res 26 (1966) 551.
3.   Law, L.W. Cancer Res 29 (1969) 1.
4.   Hellström, K.E.; Hellström, I. Adv Cancer Res 12 (1969) 167.
5.   Prehn, R.T. Science 176 (1972) 170.
6.   Gorczynski, R.M. J Immunol 112 (1974) 1826.
7.   Kirchner, H. et al. J Exp Med 139 (1974) 1473.

8. Broder, S. et al. J Natl Cancer Inst 61 (1978) 5.
9. Cerottini, J.C.; Bruner, K.T. Adv Immunol 18 (1974) 67.
10. Herberman, R.B. et al. J Natl Cancer Inst 51 (1973) 1509.
11. LeClerc, J.C. et al. Int J Cancer 11 (1973) 426.
12. Gorczynski, R.M. J Immunol 112 (1974) 533.
13. Berenson, J.R. et al. J Immunol 115 (1975) 234.
14. Glaser, M. et al. J Immunol 116 (1976) 1507.
15. Blasecki, J.W. J Immunol 119 (1977) 1621.
16. Levy, M.H.; Wheelock, E.F. Adv Cancer Res 20 (1974) 131.
17. Kiessling, R.; Haller, O. In: Contemporary Topics in Immuno-
    biology, 8, ed. Hanna. Plenum Press, New York (1978) 171.
18. Herberman, R.B.; Holden, H.T. Adv Cancer Res 27 (1978) 305.
19. Datta, S.K. et al. Int J Cancer 23 (1979) 728.
20. Law, L.W.; Dawe, C.J. Proc Soc Exp Biol Med 105 (1960) 414.
21. Vandeputte, M. et al. Life Sci 2 (1963) 475.
22. Agnew, H.D. Proc Soc Exp Biol Med 125 (1967) 132.
23. Vandeputte, M. Transplant Proc 1 (1969) 100.
24. Allison, A.C.; Law, L.W. Proc Soc Exp Biol Med 127 (1968) 207.
25. Mathé, G. et al. Br J Cancer 23 (1969) 814.
26. Larson, C.L. et al. Proc Soc Exp Biol Med 140 (1972) 700.
27. Woodruff, M.F.A. Transplant Proc 7 (1975) 229.
28. Vandeputte, M. et al. Eur J Cancer 6 (1970) 323.
29. Law, L.W. et al. Proc Natl Acad Sci USA 57 (1967) 1068.
30. Fefer, A. Int J Cancer 5 (1970) 327.
31. Vandeputte, M.; Datta, S.K. Eur J Cancer 8 (1972) 1.
32. Hatch, G.G. et al. Fed Proc 29 (1970) 371.
33. Hirsch, M.S. et al. J Immunol 108 (1972) 649.
34. Burton, R.C. et al. Br J Cancer 37 (1978) 806.

A RELATIONSHIP BETWEEN SV40-TRANSFORMED CELL SUSCEPTIBILITY TO

MACROPHAGE KILLING AND TUMOR INDUCTION IN RODENTS

James L. Cook, John B. Hibbs, Jr., and Andrew M. Lewis, Jr.

Veterans Administration Hospital and University of Utah
Medical Center, Salt Lake City, UT 84113 and
National Institute of Allergy and Infectious Diseases,
National Institutes of Health, Bethesda, MD 20014

INTRODUCTION

Simian virus 40 (SV40) is a papovavirus that induces tumors in
golden Syrian hamsters and transforms cells from many species in tissue
culture (1). The ability of SV40-transformed hamster cells, but not
cells from other species transformed by SV40, to induce tumors in the
host (2) implies that in transformation of hamster cells, SV40 may induce a species-specific change that renders the neoplastic cells resistant to rejection by the host. Previous studies by the authors suggested that LSH hamster cells transformed by adenovirus 2 (Ad2, a
human virus not oncogenic in newborn hamsters) (3,4) are susceptible
to rejection by a thymus-dependent, cell-mediated host response(5,6,7).
The resistance of SV40-transformed LSH cells to rejection by syngeneic
animals and the recent observation that SV40-transformed LSH cells
induce tumors in histoincompatible CB hamsters almost as efficiently
as in syngeneic animals (8) support the hypothesis that SV40 alters
the efficiency with which the hamster cells it transforms are recognized or destroyed by the host.

To evaluate the reasons for the apparent resistance of SV40-
transformed hamster cells to host cell-mediated defenses, we have
studied the effects of "activated" macrophages from animals with chronic intracellular infections on SV40- and Ad2-transformed rodent cells.
The target cells evaluated showed three different transformed cell
phenotypes when inoculated into immunocompetent animals--nononcogenic,
oncogenic in the host of origin but not in the histoincompatible host,
and oncogenic in both the host of origin and the histoincompatible
host--and permitted study of relative susceptibilities of these dif-

177

ferent target cell types to killing by activated macrophages. Activated macrophages are one of the effector cell components of cellular
immune reactions shown to inhibit the growth of, or to lyse, neoplastic cells in vitro. The tumoricidal effect of these activated macrophages is mediated by a nonphagocytic mechanism that requires intimate
contact with target cells (9; Fig. 1). In this report we present evidence that resistance to the cytolytic effect of tumoricidal, activated macrophages is one of the mechanisms by which SV40-transformed
hamster cells may evade destruction by the host.

MATERIALS AND METHODS

     A detailed description of materials and methods for the experi-
ments presented here has been published (10,11). Briefly, peritoneal
exudate cells (PEC) were harvested from female ICR or C3H/HeN mice or
from random bred (RGH) or inbred LSH Syrian hamsters with chronic, in-

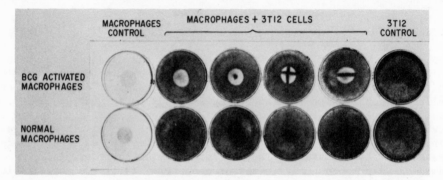

Fig. 1:   Photo of cells in Petri dishes, demonstrating importance of
           contact in macrophage mediated cytotoxicity. Peritoneal
           cells from BCG-infected or normal BALB/c mice (6 x 10^5) in
           0.1 ml of Dulbecco's modified Eagle's medium with 10% fetal
           bovine serum were added to center of 35mm plastic Petri
           dishes for one hour at 37°C in 95% air-5% CO$_2$ to allow for
           macrophage adherence. Nonadherent cells were washed from
           each dish, leaving a central monolayer of macrophages re-
           stricted to the size of the 0.1 ml drop in which they were
           added. Periphery of dishes remained free of macrophages.
           A rubber policeman was used to remove macrophages from the
           centrally located monolayer, creating several varieties of
           macrophage-free areas. Target cells (1 x 10^5 BALB/3T12) were
           added in 2 ml of medium and attached evenly to bottom of
           Petri dishes, then stained with Giemsa after 60 hours of
           culture. Multilayers of 3T12 target cells stain darkly.

traperitoneal (IP) infections with <u>Bacillus</u> <u>Calmette-Guerin</u> (BCG) or
<u>Toxoplasma</u> <u>gondii</u> three days after intraperitoneal inoculation of 10%
proteose peptone. Macrophage monolayers (4×10^6 PEC per 16-mm well)
washed free of non-adherent cells were cultured under conditions previously shown to be optimal for the destruction of SV40-transformed
mouse cells (12). In vitro macrophage-mediated tumor cell killing was
quantitated by measuring ^{3}H-TdR release from prelabeled, virus-transformed target cells (6×10^4 cells per 16-mm well) following 48 hours
of cocultivation with activated mouse or hamster macrophages. The results of cytotoxicity experiments also were evaluated visually after
fixing and staining the remaining cells at the end of each experiment.

The properties of the virus-transformed target cell lines evaluated in these experiments are described in Table 1. The TCMK-1 line
was derived from SV40-transformed mouse kidney cells (13). The THK-1$_t$
line originated from a subcutaneous random bred hamster tumor induced
by the THK-1 line (14) of SV40-transformed hamster kidney cells.
Ad2HTL3-1 is a tissue culture line from the 36th in vivo LSH weanling
passage of a subcutaneous tumor originally induced in LSH newborn hamsters by the Ad2HE3 line of Ad2-transformed LSH hamster embryo cells
(5). The other cell lines listed in Table 1 were derived by in vitro
transformation of embryo cells from the listed species and strains
using the viruses designated in the names of the cell lines (e.g.,
SV40RE1 = SV40-transformed Sprague-Dawley rat embryo cell line number
1).

RESULTS AND DISCUSSION

Nine SV40- or Ad2-transformed cell lines from different rodent
species were used in these studies (Table 1). All of these lines contained virus-specific, nonvirion T antigens (Table 1, columns 3 and 4).
No tumors developed following subcutaneous inoculation of 10^8 viable
TCMK-1, SV40RE1, SV40RE2, or Ad2HE7 cells into adult animals of the
species and strain of origin (Table 1, column 5). The Ad2HTL3-1 cell
line, which had been adapted to induce tumors in adult, syngeneic LSH
hamsters by serial in vivo passage, did not induce tumors when inoculated subcutaneously (10^7 cells/animal) into histoincompatible CB hamsters (Table 1, column 6). Conversely, all of the SV40-transformed
LSH hamster cell lines tested (SV40HE1, SV40HE2 and SV40HE3) induced
subcutaneous tumors in both syngeneic LSH and histoincompatible CB
hamsters with approximately equal efficiency (Table 1, columns 5 and
6; the differences between the $TPD_{50}LSH$ and $TPD_{50}CB$ were not significant, $p = 0.15$). The SV40-transformed random bred hamster cell line,
THK-1$_t$, also induced tumors efficiently in CB hamsters.

To study the effects of activated macrophages on these transformed
cell lines, several series of experiments were performed. In the
first three experimental series, activated mouse macrophages were used
as effector cells. In experiments in which nononcogenic SV40-trans-

Table 1. Virus-Specific Antigen Content and Tumor-Inducing Capacity of Virus-Transformed Rodent Cells

Cell line	Species/strain of origin	Presence of virus-specific T antigen by FA[1]		No. cells $(\log_{10})$/TPD$_{50}$[2] in:	
		SV40	Ad2	Host of origin	Histoincompatible host (strain)
TCMK-1	Mouse/C3H/Mai	95	0	>8.5[3]	
SV40RE1	Rat/Sprague-Dawley	95	0	>8.5	
SV40RE2	Rat/Sprague-Dawley	95	0	>8.5	
SV40HE1	Hamster/LSH	95	0	4.2	5.0 (CB)
SV40HE2	Hamster/LSH	95	0	3.6	5.5 (CB)
SV40HE3	Hamster/LSH	95	0	3.5	3.5 (CB)
THK-1	Hamster/NIH	95	0	<2.5	<2.5 (CB)
Ad2HE[†]	Hamster/LSH	0	95/95	>8.5	
Ad2HTL3-1	Hamster/LSH	0	45/45	4.1	>7.5 (CB)

[1]FA (indirect fluorescent antibody) reactions expressed as the percent positive cells. For Ad2 T antigen, numerator = percent cells with cytoplasmic bodies, denominator = percent cells with positive nuclei. 0 = < 0.01%.

[2]No. cells $(\log_{10})$/TPD$_{50}$ = number of tissue culture cells required to produce subcutaneous tumors in 50% of surviving animals. For tumor challenge procedure, see reference 5.

[3]TPD$_{50}$ > 8.5 = no tumors developed during a three-month observation period following subcutaneous challenge with 10^8 tissue culture cells.

(unpublished data)

formed mouse target cells, TCMK-1, were destroyed after 48 hours of
cocultivation with activated mouse macrophages, many SV40HE1 cells,
exposed to the same macrophage populations, remained (Fig. 2; Table 2,
experimental series 1). Over 90% of the SV40HE1 target cells were
viable by trypan blue exclusion at the end of the cocultivation period,
and when macrophage-exposed SV40HE1 cells were reseeded as suspensions
of single cells in fresh medium, macroscopic target cell colonies were
visible within three to seven days. Cocultivation of SV40HE1 cells
with activated mouse macrophages thus had resulted in transient cytostasis but relatively inefficient cytolysis of the target cell population.

To evaluate the possibility that the apparent resistance of this
SV40-transformed hamster cell line to activated mouse macrophage-mediated cytolysis was a result of the inability of activated macrophages
to destroy xenogeneic SV40-transformed cells (a conclusion which previous reports [15] suggest is unlikely), the effects of activated
mouse macrophages on SV40-transformed mouse (TCMK-1), hamster (SV40HE1),
and nononcogenic rat (SV40RE1 and SV40RE2) cells were compared (Table
2, experimental series 2. Only SV40RE1 is shown. Specific release
with SV40RE2 = 93.6 $\pm$ 3.5%.) These experiments showed that, while
activated mouse macrophages killed SV40-transformed, xenogeneic rat
cells as well as TCMK-1 cells, the effectors were relatively ineffective in destroying SV40HE1 cells, in spite of the marked cytostasis
caused by these effectors (Fig. 2). Thus it appeared that the inability of activated mouse macrophages to lyse SV40HE1 cells was not
due merely to the derivation of the target cells from a different species.

The finding that the SV40HE1 cell line was relatively resistant
to activated macrophage-induced cytolysis implied that this phenotype
may be a general property of SV40-transformed hamster cells. To test
this hypothesis, three other SV40-transformed hamster cell lines were
evaluated for susceptibility to activated mouse macrophage-induced destruction (Table 2, experimental series 3). Two of these lines,
SV40HE2 and SV40HE3, arose under agar from different clones of transformed cells in the same transformation experiment from which the
SV40HE1 line was derived. All four of the SV40-transformed hamster
lines in these experiments were significantly less susceptible to the
tumoricidal effect of activated mouse macrophages than was the TCMK-1
line (p < 0.001), suggesting that the resistant phenotype is not a
unique property of SV40HE1 or of transformed LSH cells (THK-1$_t$ was derived from random bred hamsters). While all of the SV40-transformed
hamster lines tolerated exposure to activated mouse macrophages much
better than did TCMK-1 cells, there was significant variability in
the degree of lysis in the different hamster lines. This finding suggests that the SV40HE1, SV40HE2 and SV40HE3 lines are the products of
different transformation events, and that there may be phenotypic variability in different cells transformed by the same viral inoculum.

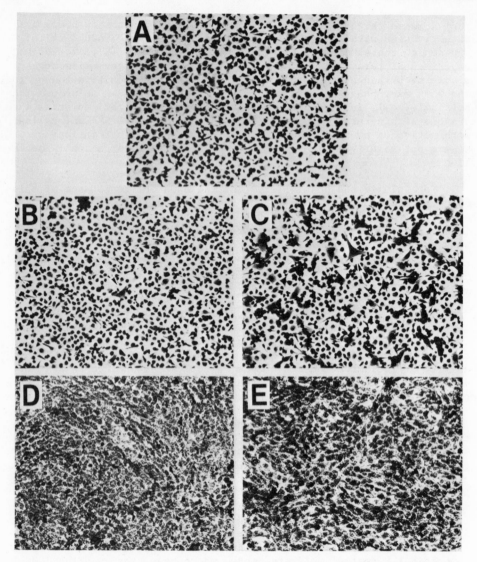

Fig. 2:   Results of cocultivation of BCG-activated C3H/HeN macro-
           phages with target cells for 48 hours. a. Macrophage mono-
           layer cultured without target cells. x 80. b. TCMK-1 cells
           incubated with macrophage population shown in a. Residual
           target cell, center (arrow). x 80. c. SV40HE1 cells incu-
           bated with macrophage population shown in a. Numerous target
           cells throughout field (arrow). x 10. d. TCMK-1 cells incu-
           bated alone. x 80. e. SV40HE1 cells incubated alone. x 80.
           (Reduced 14% for reproduction.)

Table 2. Specific Release of ^{3}H-thymidine from SV40-Transformed Mouse, Rat, and Hamster Cells Cocultured with Activated[1] Mouse Macrophages

Expt.[3] series no.	Percent specific ^{3}H-thymidine release[2]					
	TCMK-1	SV40RE1	SV40HE1	SV40HE2	SV40HE3	THK-1$_t$
1 (6)	85.2 ± 3.4		11.9 ± 1.5			
2 (4)	95.4 ± 2.3	89.2 ± 5.7	11.6 ± 1.7			
3 (5)	93.7 ± 3.2[4]		16.8 ± 2.1	47.7 ± 2.1	28.6 ± 3.4	27.8 ± 3.4

[1]Macrophage monolayers were prepared from peritoneal cells from inbred C3H/HeN or random bred ICR female mice 17-22 days after I.P. infection with 10^7 Pasteur strain BCG or 8-20 weeks after IP infection with the C56 strain of Toxoplasma gondii.

[2]Percent spontaneous release (mean ± SEM) of the target cells in these experiments was as follows: TCMK-1: 13.8 ± 1.2; SV40RE1: 23.7 ± 2.2; SV40HE1: 13.8 ± 1.0; SV40HE2: 15.2 ± 1.3; SV40HE3: 11.7 ± 2.5; THK-1$_t$: 14.1 ± 1.4

[3]Number in parentheses = number of experiments in the series.

[4]Significance of the differences in the percent specific release for these cell lines was as follows: TCMK-1 vs. each hamster line: p < 0.001; SV40HE1 vs. SV40HE2: p < 0.001; SV40HE1 vs. SV40HE3 or THK-1$_t$: p < 0.05; SV40HE2 vs. SV40HE3 or THK-1$_t$: p < 0.01.

(unpublished data)

Although activated mouse macrophages effectively lysed xenogeneic, SV40-transformed rat cells (Table 2), it was still possible that the inefficient destruction of SV40-transformed hamster cell lines was due to the species difference between the effector and target cells and not an inherent resistance of the target cells. Therefore, the previously described experiments were repeated using activated macrophages from BCG-infected random bred (RGH) and inbred (LSH) golden Syrian hamsters (Table 3). Several observations derive from these data. First, macrophages from uninfected hamsters injected with peptone had little cytolytic effect when cocultivated with TCMK-1 or SV40HE1 cells, while peptone-elicited macrophages from BCG-infected hamsters effectively lysed TCMK-1 but not SV40HE1 cells (Table 3, experimental series 1). Second, the general pattern of target cell susceptibility to activated macrophage-induced cytolysis using hamster macrophages was similar to that seen in the experiments in which activated mouse macrophages were used; SV40-transformed mouse and rat cells were susceptible, while SV40-transformed hamster cells were relatively resistant (Table 3, experimental series 2-4). In contrast to the experiments in which activated mouse macrophages were used as effector cells (Table 2), however, there was no significant difference in the percent specific release from SV40HE1 and SV40HE2 target cells cocultured with activated hamster macrophages. The reasons for this difference are unknown. Third, two different lines of LSH hamster embryo cells transformed by Ad2 (Ad2HE7 and Ad2HTL3-1) were as susceptible to activated hamster macrophage-induced lysis as SV40-transformed mouse or rat cells (Table 3, experimental series 3 and 5). Ad2HE7 does not induce tumors in syngeneic newborn hamsters (5). Ad2HTL3-1 induces tumors in adult syngeneic hamsters; however, unlike SV40HE1 and SV40-HE2, this line will not induce tumors in histoincompatible adult CB hamsters (Table 1). Fourth, activated macrophages which are syngeneic to the SV40-transformed hamster cell lines (SV40HE1 and SV40HE2 are of LSH origin), when compared to macrophages from random bred hamsters, did not cause increased lysis of these targets (Table 3, experimental series 6).

These data support the conclusion that SV40-transformed hamster, but not mouse or rat, cells are resistant to the tumoricidal effects of activated macrophages irrespective of histocompatibility differences between effector and target cells. The susceptibility of the two Ad2-transformed LSH cell lines to lysis suggests further that the resistant phenotype is SV40-specific and that resistance to macrophage-mediated destruction does not correlate with tumor-inducing capacity in the syngeneic adult host.

The recent observation that SV40-transformed, inbred LSH hamster cells were able to induce tumors in histoincompatible CB hamsters almost as efficiently as in syngeneic animals (8) suggested that SV40 either may alter the immunologic recognition of the hamster cells it transforms or may modify the cells in such a way that they can with-

Table 3. Specific Release of ^{3}H-thymidine from SV40-Transformed Mouse, Hamster, and Rat Cells and Ad-2 Transformed Hamster Cells Cocultured with Activated Hamster Macrophages

Expt. series no.[2]	PEC source	Percent specific ^{3}H-thymidine release[1]							
		TCMK-1	SV3T3	SV40HE1	SV40HE2	SV40RE1	SV40RE2	Ad2HE7	Ad2HTL3-1
1 (3)	Peptone-RGH	12.8±2.5[3]		3.5±1.8					
	BCG-RGH	91.1±3.5		13.9±3.5[4]					
2 (5)	BCG-RGH	98.5±0.9	98.0±0.5	25.1±2.1[4]					
3 (4)	BCG-RGH	97.9±2.0		25.2±2.1[4]		97.6±0.9	90.9±1.0		
4 (6)	BCG-RGH	94.5±2.9		14.2±3.1[4]	14.3±2.6[4]				
5 (6)	BCG-RGH			16.2±3.2[4]				95.8±4.2	96.2±2.1
6 (2)	BCG-RGH	91.3±8.7		16.5±9.4[4]	12.5±5.6[4]				
	BCG-LSH	98.0±1.4		11.6±4.6[4]	13.7±2.9[4]				

[1]Percent spontaneous release (mean ± SEM) of the target cells in these experiments was as follows: TCMK-1: 20.8±1.1; SV3T3: 19.5±2.4; SV40HE1: 11.0±0.8; SV40HE2: 13.9±1.9; SV40RE1: 27.6±3.4; SV40RE2: 29.0±4.0; Ad2HE7: 12.8±1.7; Ad2HTL3-1: 18.5±2.1

[2]Number in parentheses = number of experiments in the series.

[3]Mean ± SEM percent specific release.

[4]Mean percent specific release of the SV40-transformed hamster lines is significantly lower than that from the other lines tested (p < 0.001).

(unpublished data)

stand an attack by the cell-mediated host defenses. The data presented here, which show that SV40-transformed hamster cells are relatively resistant to in vitro cytolysis by the activated macrophage, suggest that the latter postulated SV40 mechanism may operate in vivo. While Ad2HE7 will not induce tumors in immunoincompetent newborn syngeneic LSH hamsters (5), Ad2HTL3-1 is oncogenic for weanling LSH animals but not weanling histoincompatible CB hamsters (Table 1); both of these cell lines are sensitive to activated macrophage-induced cytolysis (Table 3). These data suggest that resistance to cytolysis may correlate with an SV40-transformed LSH hamster cell line's ability to induce tumors in CB hamsters and that this macrophage cytolysis assay offers an in vitro model which may be useful in defining reasons for the survival and proliferation of SV40-transformed hamster cells in what one would predict to be a hostile environment--the histoincompatible host.

As previous in vivo studies suggest that macrophages play an important role in the host response to SV40-transformed mouse cells (16, 17), the resistance of SV40-transformed hamster cells, but not mouse or rat cells, to activated macrophage-induced cytolysis also may offer one explanation for the species-specific oncogenicity of this DNA virus. The SV40-transformed mouse, rat, and hamster cells used in these studies all contain serologically detectable, virus-specific T antigens; the function of these proteins, however, is still being defined. If SV40 T antigens are responsible for the resistant phenotype of transformed hamster cells, there may be a functional difference in the T antigens expressed in cells from different species that has not been detected serologically.

Others have postulated different mechanisms by which SV40-transformed cells might evade the host immune response, such as insufficient amounts of virus-specific transplantation antigen in the developing focus of tumor cells to sensitize the host; blocking antibody protecting the antigenic sites of transformed cells from recognition by host effector cells (18); and development of suppressor cells which reduce the intensity of the host cellular immune response to transformed cells (19,20). None of these mechanisms is incompatible with the existence of an inherent resistance of SV40-transformed hamster cells to the mechanisms by which activated macrophages cause tumor cell lysis. If, in addition to antigenic changes which might result during the transformation process, neoplastic cells acquire a heritable resistance to destruction by activated macrophages and possibly other types of effector cells such as cytotoxic lymphocytes and natural killer cells, then rejection of the incipient malignancy would be more difficult. An understanding of the mechanisms by which tumor cells resist host defenses such as activated macrophage-induced cytolysis could prove useful in defining alterations in the tumor cell microenvironment which might enhance the effect of the host response and result in tumor destruction.

ACKNOWLEDGMENTS

This work was supported by the Veterans Administration, Washington, D.C., by American Cancer Society Grant CH-139, and by NIH training grant 5-T-32-AI07011.

REFERENCES

1. Butel, J.S. et al. Adv Cancer Res 15 (1972) 1.
2. Eddy, B.E. Prog Exp Tumor Res 4 (1964) 1.
3. Trentin, J.J. et al. Science 137 (1962) 835.
4. Huebner, R.J. In: Perspectives in Virology, ed. Pollard, Vol.5. Academic Press, New York (1967) 147.
5. Cook, J.L.; Lewis, A.M., Jr. Cancer Res 39 (1979) 1455.
6. Cook, J.L. et al. Cancer Res 39 (1979) 3335.
7. Cook, J.L. et al. Cancer Res 39 (1979) 4949.
8. Lewis, A.M., Jr.; Cook, J.L. Proc Natl Acad Sci 77 (1980) 2286.
9. Hibbs, J.B., Jr. Nature [New Biol] 235 (1972) 48.
10. Hibbs, J.B., Jr. et al. Science 197 (1977) 279.
11. Cook, J.L. et al. Proc Natl Acad Sci (in press).
12. Hibbs, J.B., Jr. Science 180 (1973) 868.
13. Black, P.H.; Rowe, W.P. Proc Soc Exp Biol Med 114 (1963) 721.
14. Black, P.H.; Rowe, W.P. Proc Natl Acad Sci USA 50 (1963) 606.
15. Fidler, I.J. et al. Cell Immunol 38 (1978) 131.
16. Tevethia, S.S. et al. In: Immunobiology of the Macrophage, ed. Nelson. Academic Press, New York (1976) 509.
17. Howell, S.B. et al. Int J Cancer 14 (1974) 662.
18. Tevethia, S.S. In: Viral Oncology, ed. Klein. Raven Press, New York (1980) 581.
19. Glaser, M. J Exp Med 149 (1979) 774.
20. Chen, H. et al. Eur J Immunol 9 (1979) 80.

SECTION IV

PULMONARY IMMUNOLOGY

Chairpersons:

Joan Stein-Streilein

Timothy Sullivan

IMMUNE RESPONSES RELATED TO THE HAMSTER LUNG

Joan Stein-Streilein, Mary F. Lipscomb, and David A. Hart

Departments of Microbiology and Pathology
University of Texas Health Science Center at Dallas
Dallas, TX   75235

INTRODUCTION

The respiratory tract is exposed continuously to immunogenic and infectious agents. The host controls these potentially harmful agents by nonspecific and immune defense mechanisms. It is known that nonspecific mechanisms involve filtration, mucocilliary movement and active phagocytosis and that these nonspecific defenses may be amplified and directed by specific immune responses (1). The lower respiratory tract generally is protected by the defense mechanisms of the upper respiratory tract. This protection, however, is not always complete, and it now appears that the lower respiratory tract (lung) may have unique mechanisms for protection (2).

Although many studies dissect the fundamentals of immune responses in systemic lymphoid tissues (3), much less information is available concerning immune interactions in the lung. It is known that both local and systemic immunity may defend the lung (4), but how these two systems interact is not as well understood.

The purpose of the present studies was to develop an experimental model in hamsters to investigate the immune response following presentation of antigen to the lower respiratory tract, and to evaluate the interdependence of the local and systemic response to the antigen. The hamster is a particularly useful model for studying immune responses related to the lung for three important reasons: 1. it is relatively easy to inoculate substances into its trachea; 2. the hamster carries a low endogenous bacterial and viral load (5); and 3. the relative quantity of lung lymphoid tissue resembles that in the human lung.

The development of immunity to the particulate antigens, sheep erythrocytes (SRBC), and to influenza virus (PR/8/34 strain HONI), was investigated in the hilar lymph nodes and other lymphoid tissue in several inbred strains of hamsters. While the hilar lymph nodes are not the lung per se, evidence suggests that the response in the draining nodes may reflect the immune status of the lung (6).

Three aspects of our investigations in pulmonary immunology are included in this report. First, we describe the development of the hamster model with a particulate antigen, SRBC; second, we analyze splenic involvement in a local pulmonary response to SRBC; and third, we demonstrate that the hamster is an excellent model for influenza infections, and describe preliminary results from our immunological studies showing both cellular and humoral immune responses to influenza virus inoculated intratracheally.

MATERIALS AND METHODS

Female MHA, LSH and LHC hamsters (Charles River, N.Y.) weighing between 80 and 100 g were used throughout the study.

Adult hamsters were splenectomized under ether anesthesia through an incision in the shaved left lateral flank. The splenic pedicle was tied off, the spleen removed and the wound sutured. Sham-operated hamsters underwent a similar procedure except the pedicle was not tied and the spleen was not removed. Animals were allowed to rest 14 to 30 days before they were used in experiments.

Sheep erythrocytes (SRBC) were obtained from Colorado Serum Co. (sheep no. 446) or from a sheep (no. 80) maintained by the University of Texas Health Science Center at Dallas Animal Resources Center. Sheep blood was stored in sterile Alsever's solution. Before use, the SRBC were washed three times in basic saline solution (BSS). Dilutions of antigen were made assuming that 1 ml of packed SRBC contained 10^{10} cells. Preliminary experiments using antigen concentrations of 10^7, 10^8 and 10^9 indicated that 10^9 SRBC was optimal for inducing an AFC response in the hilar lymph nodes and spleen if inoculated intratracheally. Optimal concentration for inducing only a local response was 10^8 SRBC.

Influenza virus (PR/8/34 HON1) was purchased from American Type Culture Collection (Rockville, Md.) and was grown in embryonated chicken eggs by standard procedures (7). Virus was stored at -70°C after quick freezing in liquid nitrogen. Hemagglutination titers using chicken erythrocytes were performed before and after freezing (7).

Intratracheal inoculation was accomplished by inoculating 0.1 ml of antigen into a catheter placed inside a cannula that had been inserted into the trachea of hamsters anesthetized with chloral hydrate.

The optimal anesthetic dose of chloral hydrate (.036% solution) was
0.1 ml per 10 g body weight. Intravenous inoculation was accomplished
by injection of the antigen through a 30-gauge needle placed in the
saphenous vein. Intraperitoneal inoculation was through a 23-gauge
needle inserted into the peritoneal cavity through the abdominal wall.
Hamsters were anesthetized with ether for these inoculations.

Groups of 15 to 20 animals were immunized on day 0. Panels of
one to four animals were killed on specified days. Lymphoid tissue
harvested included peripheral lymph nodes (inguinal, bracheal, axil-
lary, cervical and cheek pouch; cervical and cheek pouch nodes were
not included in some of the experiments using PR/8/34 as antigen),
mesenteric lymph nodes, hilar lymph hodes, Peyer's patches and spleen.
Single cell suspensions were prepared as described (8). For experiments using SRBC, cell counts were done with a Coulter Counter and
viabilities were determined with a Cytograf A6300. When virus was used
as the antigen, cell counts were done by phase microscopy and viabilities were determined by means of trypan blue exclusion.

Target erythrocytes were prepared as described (9), using 2- to
4-week-old pooled SRBC (Colorado Serum Co.). In brief, SRBC were washed
three times in Veronal buffered saline, pH 7.2 (VBS) and pelleted at
500 x g. The packed cell volume of SRBC was treated with 1 volume of
5×10^{-4}M KIO_4 in VBS and 10 volumes of influenza virus in alloantoic
fluid. The quantity of virus was not less than 4×10^3 hemagglutination units (HAU) per 0.1 ml packed SRBC. The mixture was allowed to
stand for 10 minutes at room temperature. Cells were washed with VBS
and resuspended in a final volume 1:15, SRBC:BSS.

Direct antibody-forming cells (AFC) were quantitated by a slide
modification of the Jerne Plaque assay (10). Indirect AFC to SRBC
were developed by a second incubation of these slides with rabbit anti-
hamster immunoglobulin (Cappel Laboratory, Downingtown, Pa.) and complement (guinea pig serum, Pel-Freeze Biologicals, Rodgers, Ark.).
Direct AFC to virus-coated SRBC were quantitated as indicated above.
Indirect AFC, however, were developed by adding the facilitating antibody (1:3000 dilution) directly to a duplicate set of slides, in which
the complement was omitted. Slides were incubated for two hours before
incubation in a 1:20 dilution of complement:BSS. Indirect AFC were
determined by subtracting the quantity of direct AFC recorded on the
first set of slides, which contained complement without facilitating
antibody. Nonspecific plaques were developed by use of horse erythrocytes. As a control for the virus experiments, preliminary experiments indicated an absence of plaques developing to allantoic fluid-
coated erythrocytes.

To measure cellular immune responses, cells were counted and resuspended at 10^6/ml RPMI 1640 containing 25mM HEPES buffer and supplemented with 300 µg glutamine/ml, 200 units penicillin/ml, 100 µg strep-
tomycin/ml, 500 µg gentamycin/ml and either zero or 10% heat inacti-

vated fetal calf serum (FCS: Microbiological Associates, Inc.,Bethesda, Md.). Aliquots (0.2 ml) were added to round-bottom microtiter wells and 10 µl of 0.4 mg/ml or 0.2 mg Con A (Sigma, St. Louis, Mo.)/ml, 10 µl virus (25 HAU), or 10 µl allantoic fluid were added to each well. Cultures were incubated 72 hours at $37^{\circ}C$ in 5% CO_2. Eighteen hours before harvest, 0.5 µCi of tritiated thymidine was added to each culture. The cultures were collected on an automated cell harvester and counted in a scintillation counter. Cultures were done in triplicate and data expressed as a stimulation index (counts per minute in the experimental animal/counts per minute in the control). Preliminary experiments with nonimmune cells or cells from hamsters inoculated with allantoic fluid verified that a stimulation index of ≥ 3.0 in the presence of virus indicated specific reactivity for all lymphoid tissues.

Hamster tissue was fixed in 10% buffered formalin, paraffin embedded, sectioned and stained with hematoxylin and eosin by standard techniques. Lung tissue was not inflated prior to fixation.

RESULTS

Description of the Hamster Lung Model

MHA hamsters were inoculated intratracheally or intravenously (IT or IV) with 10^9 SRBC as described (11). Lymphoid tissue was removed from individual hamsters at various times after inoculation. The lymph nodes draining the lung were observed for hypertrophy. The hilar and mediastinal lymph nodes were grossly enlarged by days 4 and 7 after IT immunization; no comparable hypertrophy was noted after IV inoculation. The number of lymphocytes recovered from the pool of hilar lymph nodes (HLN) removed from each animal correlated with the visible enlargement (Table 1). Although lymph node enlargement per se does not prove that an immune response has occurred, the preferential enlargement of nodes draining the site of SRBC inoculation indicates that a response has been elicited.

Another parameter used to measure an immune response was quantitation of the number of AFC in the various lymphoid tissues. Initial experiments were performed to identify the target lymphoid tissues and to correlate them with the route of antigen inoculation. Of all the lymphoid tissues tested, peripheral, mesenteric, and hilar lymph nodes, Peyer's patches, and spleen, specific AFC were detected only in HLN and spleen when 10^9 SRBC were inoculated either IT or IV.

An optimal concentration of 10^9 SRBC was deposited in the lower lung by intratracheal inoculation. Specific AFC were assayed in the HLN and spleen of individual hamsters. Local inoculation of SRBC consistently induced an AFC response in the HLN by day 4 (Figure 1). At later times, an increase in this response correlated with the concomitant development of an AFC response in the spleen. The hamsters re-

Table 1.   Effect of IT Inoculation on Draining Lymph Node Hypertrophy

Route of inoculation	[SRBC]	Cells ± SEM x 10^6/HLN[1] Day of harvest				
		4	7	14	21	28
IT	10^9	17±2	16±3	8±1	6±2	6±2
IV	10^9	5±2	4±2	2±2	2±0.2	4±0.2

[1]HLN = Hilar lymph nodes.

sponded in either of two ways: Group I responded with both a local (hilar) and systemic (spleen) response. Group II had a detectable AFC response only in the HLN. An increase in the quantity of direct AFC by day 7 was seen only in group I. This observation is consistent with the hypothesis that the spleen may serve as a repository of IgM AFC for the animal.

Indirect AFC were developed by incubation of the slides previously developed for IgM AFC with rabbit anti-hamster immunoglobulin and complement. There was no evidence of a splenic influence on the quantity of indirect AFC that developed in the HLN. The indirect specific AFC response in the HLN after IT inoculation of SRBC was similar for animals with and without a splenic AFC response (Fig. 1).

For comparison, another panel of animals was inoculated with 10^9 SRBC directly into the femoral vein. Specific AFC were quantitated for HLN and spleen at various times post-inoculation. Systemic immunization effectively induced direct AFC in the spleen (Fig. 2). Direct AFC also were seen regularly in the HLN after IV inoculation of SRBC, but the number rarely rose above 1% of the total specific AFC response of the animal. There was no hilar lymph node hypertrophy nor any augmentation of the quantity of AFC in the HLN on any day tested if the antigen was inoculated IV. These observations suggest that there is a threshold antigen level necessary for sustaining the local immune response which must accompany the systemic immunization in order to augment the HLN direct AFC response.

The kinetics of the indirect AFC response elicited after IV inoculation of SRBC were similar to those after local immunization (Fig. 1, 2). The numbers of indirect AFC found in the HLN were the same after both routes of immunization but the IV route was more efficient in producing indirect specific AFC in the spleen than the IT route.

These studies demonstrated that local and systemic routes of inoculation can elicit both a local pulmonary and a systemic immune response to particulate antigens. These responses, however, were both qualitatively and quantitatively different. Furthermore, the spleen

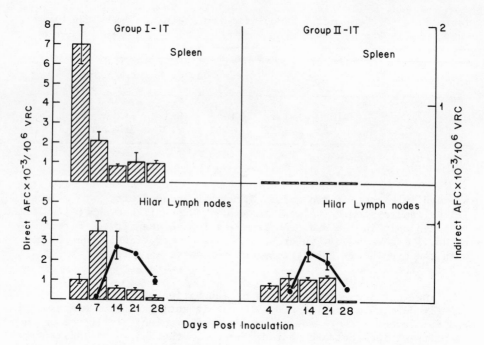

Fig. 1:   AFC response to intratracheal inoculation: MHA female ham-
           sters were inoculated intratracheally with 10^9 SRBC on day
           0. At various times post-inoculation hilar lymph nodes and
           spleen were assayed for direct AFC, slashed bars, left hand
           ordinate, and indirect AFC, dotted line, right hand ordinate.
           VRC = viable recovered cells.

appeared to play a pivotal role in quantitative enhancement of the
local response. Our next studies were designed to address the issue
of splenic involvement in the local response.

Splenic Influence on Development of AFC in Hilar Lymph Nodes

We studied local immune response after splenectomy or deliberate
concomitant splenic immunization.

Panels of animals were splenectomized or sham splenectomized 30
days prior to IT inoculation of 10^9 SRBC. HLN and spleen cells were
assayed for direct AFC on days 4, 7, 14 and 21 post-inoculation. In
both experimental and control animals, AFC were present in HLN by day
4 (Fig. 3). The presence of the spleen in the sham-operated hamsters,
however, did not appear to affect the quantity of AFC observed in the

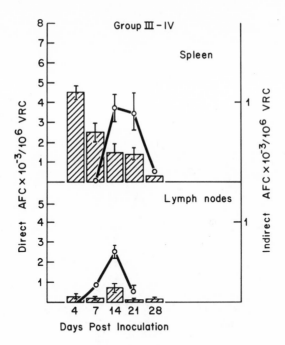

Fig. 2:   AFC response to intravenous inoculation. MHA female ham-
          sters were inoculated intravenously with 10^9 SRBC on day 0.
          At various times post-inoculation, hilar lymph nodes and
          spleen were assayed for direct AFC, slashed bars, left hand
          ordinate; and indirect AFC, dotted line, right hand ordinate.
          VRC = viable recovered cells.

HLN on day 7; nor did any of these hamsters show a splenic IgM AFC response. Experiments, therefore, were designed to ensure that a splenic
response was achieved regularly.

     To ensure the active participation of the spleen in a locally in-
duced immune response, normal hamsters were immunized both IT and IV
with 10^9 SRBC, and the kinetics of the appearance of direct AFC was
followed. The quantity of direct AFC in the HLN was significantly
greater in these animals than that seen the same day in the HLN of
animals that did not demonstrate a splenic response (Fig. 3).

     The non-IgM AFC response was evaluated in the same hamsters by
developing the indirect plaques with facilitating antibody. The non-
IgM response generally was unaffected by the presence or absence of
a spleen, nor was it affected by the presence or absence of an ongoing
IgM AFC response in the spleen. Splenectomized hamsters, however,
had an increased number of indirect AFC in their hilar lymph nodes
as compared to normal hamsters, suggesting that a negative influence

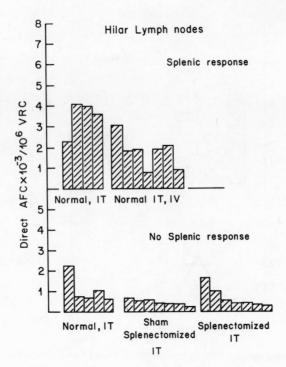

Fig. 3: AFC response in hilar lymph nodes, day 7 post IT inocula-
         tion: Normal, sham splenectomized or splenectomized MHA
         hamsters were inoculated IT with 10^9 SRBC. Another panel
         of normal hamsters received 10^9 SRBC, IT and IV. Hilar lymph
         nodes were assayed for direct AFC on day 7 post-inoculation.
         Each slashed bar represents the AFC response of an individ-
         ual animal.

has been removed (suppressor cells). These data suggest that local
and systemic immunization conspire to provide maximal protection of
the lower respiratory tract.

The Influenza Model

    We next studied the immune response to a natural infective
agent of the lung. We have found that influenza in hamsters is a
useful model for the human disease.

    All inbred hamsters (MHA, LSH, LHC) inoculated IT with 0.1 ml of
virus in allantoic fluid containing 256 HAU of virus became ill but
survived. Sick animals were listless and lost weight. Lungs observed
at 5, 7, and 14 days post-infection were heavy, firm, and hemorrhagic.

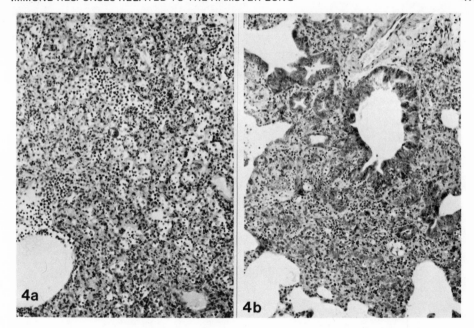

Fig. 4:   a.   MHA hamster lung, day 5 after intratracheal inoculation
               of influenza virus. Destruction of bronchiolar epithel-
               ium, marked interstitial edema and mononuclear infil-
               trates in alveolar septa, intra-alveolar spaces and peri-
               bronchiolar connective tissue. Magnification x 10.
          b.   MHA hamster lung, day 7 post-infection. Prominent
               squamous metaplasia of bronchiolar epithelium with con-
               tinuing prominent mononuclear infiltrates in alveolar
               spaces and interstitial tissue.

     Histologic study of MHA hamsters showed changes similar to those
described during influenza pneumonia in humans (13). At day 5, both
lungs showed widespread involvement with destruction of bronchiolar
epithelium, and interstitial and intra-alveolar mononuclear cell infiltrates with hemorrhage (Fig. 4a). By day 7 there was evidence of
bronchiolar epithelial regeneration with metaplastic changes in bronchioles and alveolar ducts (Fig. 4b). At day 14 there were still
widespread mononuclear infiltrates, and squamous metaplasia of terminal airways. Diffuse perivenular lymphocytic infiltrates were prominent by day 7 and were still present at day 14. Although bronchiolar
epithelium showed regenerative activity, the lack of resolution of
the alveolar infiltrates indicated either continuing viral infection
or sufficient damage to cause fibrosis of much of the lung.

Table 2. Development in Inbred Hamsters of Antibody-Forming Cells to Influenza (PR/8/34)[1]

Strain	No. animals	Tissue	Direct AFC/Organ ± SEM x 10^{-3}		
			Day 4	Day 7	Day 14
MHA	2	Hilar	127.0 ± 37.0	61.0 ± 22.0	2.8 ± 0.2
		Spleen		13.0 ± 10.0	0
LSH	2	Hilar		3.9 ± 0.1	(0.9)[2]
		Spleen		(0.6)[2]	5.4 ± 0.2
LHC	4	Hilar		73.0 ± 11.0	0.8 ± 0.2
		Spleen		35.0 ± 99.0	11.0 ± 6.0

Strain	No. animals	Tissue	Indirect AFC/Organ ± SEM x 10^{-3}	
			Day 7	Day 14
LSH	2	Hilar	(0.5)[2]	(1.6)[2]
		Spleen	0	(15.7)[2]
LHC	4	Hilar	110.0 ± 36.0	2.0 ± 1.6
		Spleen		23.0 ± 6.0

[1]Animals inoculated IT with 0.1 ml allantoic fluid containing 256 HAU influenza PR/8/34.

[2](Results from one animal.)

Table 3.   The Incidence of Specific Proliferative Responses to
           Influenza Virus in Inbred Hamsters

| Strain | Lymphoid Tissues Assayed at | | | | | |
| | 1 week[1] | | | 2 weeks[1] | | |
	Hilar LN	Spleen	Peripheral LN	Hilar LN	Spleen	Peripheral LN
MHA & LSH	5/5	1/6	2/6	2/2	3/3	1/3
LHC	2/6	6/6	1/6	–	–	–

[1]Number of animals with S.I. > 3.0 over the total number of animals
tested.   S.I. of non-immunized or allantoic fluid-immunized hamsters
in response to 25 HAU of virus < 3.0.

Three different inbred strains of hamsters (MHA, LSH, LHC) were
inoculated intratracheally with 256 HAU of live virus in 0.1 ml of
allantoic fluid.   Hamsters were killed on day 4, 7, or 14 post-inoculation.   Lymphoid tissues were harvested aseptically and assayed for
the development of AFC and virus-dependent antigen reactive T cells
(^{3}H-TdR incorporation).

All three strains responded to the virus deposited in their lungs
with development of direct and indirect AFC (Table 2).   By day 7 post
IT inoculation of 256 HAU of PR/8/34, the direct AFC response appeared
in both hilar lymph nodes and spleen, indicating the development of
a systemic as well as a local response to the virus.

Whether the AFC response appeared in the peripheral lymph nodes
(PLN) was dependent on the inclusion of cervical and cheek pouch nodes
in this lymph node pool.   These nodes, which drain the upper respiratory tract, were included initially and an AFC response was recorded
in the pooled PLN.   Because such a response might merely reflect drainage of the virus from the upper respiratory tract into the cervical
nodes rather than lymphoid traffic through the PLN, in subsequent experiments the PLN pool did not include the cervical or cheek pouch
nodes.   Under these circumstances an AFC response did not develop in
the PLN (data not shown).

All three inbred strains of hamsters responded to the virus deposited in their lungs by developing specifically sensitized T-lymphocytes as assayed by ^{3}H-TdR incorporation after 72 hours of culture
with or without the virus antigen.   Preliminary evidence suggests some

minor strain differences. Specific stimulation was always present in
HLN of MHA and LSH hamsters at both one and two weeks after IT inoculation (Table 3). Although responses were not detected in the spleen
of many animals at one week, a specific splenic response was present
in three of three animals at two weeks. In the LHC strain, in contrast, the HLN response was inconsistent at one week (two of six animals), but the spleen showed uniform response. Too few animals of this
strain have been tested to generalize about the response at two weeks.

These studies suggest that there are strain differences in the
generation of cells in the HLN and spleen which will respond to viral
antigens with a positive proliferative response at one week. These
differences may reflect the route or rate of spread of the virus in
the three strains; additional panels of animals must be tested, however, to determine whether these differences are consistent.

We conclude from these studies of intratracheal inoculation of
influenza virus in hamsters that the hamster provides a model to study
an influenza disease similar to human influenza in syndrome and severity. Preliminary studies involving T and B lymphocyte responses to
the virus suggest that there are both cellular and humoral components
to the immune response. Both the local and systemic immune systems
appear to interact in this response, since intratracheal inoculation
induces AFC and specifically sensitized T lymphocytes in the spleen as
well as the hilar lymph nodes.

DISCUSSION

This study has shown that the hamster is an excellent model for
studying immune responses related to the lung. We observed that the
local and systemic routes of inoculation can elicit both a pulmonary
and systemic response (10). This was found for both particulate antigens tested. With the possible exception of the cervical lymph nodes,
it appears that the AFC response was restricted primarily to the hilar
lymph nodes and the spleen. The observation that AFC in the hilar
lymph nodes do not circulate to the peripheral or mesenteric nodes,
together with morphologic evidence that cells that differentiate in
the hilar lymph nodes may preferentially home to the lung (6), suggests that these nodes may command a central role in a lymphoid traffic loop for the lung similar to the central role that mesenteric
lymph nodes play in the lymphocyte traffic of the gut (13).

The studies with sheep erythrocytes demonstrated a central role
for the spleen in the regulation of both the quantity and quality of
the AFC response induced in the HLN after local inoculation of antigen.
The results of these studies differ from those of most earlier studies
concerned with the role of the spleen in immune responsiveness in two
ways: 1. as far as we know, the IT route of inoculation was not used
in the previous studies and represents an unexplored physiological

route of antigen presentation; 2. in addition to studying the local immune response after surgical removal of the spleen, the present studies evaluated the local immune response in the presence of deliberate splenic immunization coincident with local immunization.

Classically, the physiological role of a particular organ or system has been evaluated in part by surgical removal of the structure in question and subsequent assessment of the animal without it. Such a procedure, however, fails to evaluate the possibility that one facet of the physiological role of an organ may involve activation in order to induce a regulatory function. In the present studies, the greatest AFC responses were recorded in animals that displayed a concomitant direct AFC response in their spleens (11). This suggests that a natural function of the spleen may be to influence a local response by seeding differentiated IgM AFC to distant lymphoid tissue where antigen may be trapped.

While the studies with influenza virus are preliminary, they do support the working hypothesis that the local and systemic immune systems conspire in immune responses related to the lung. Whereas 0.02 HAU of the PR/8/34 strain are lethal for mice (unpublished observations), hamsters tolerate 256 HAU. Although they get severe pneumonitis, they survive. Thus, the hamster model for influenza appears more akin to human influenza than the devastating disease that develops in mice in response to PR/8/34. In addition, hamsters with this disease show both a demonstrable AFC response and evidence for expanding clones of specific T lymphocytes in the hilar lymph nodes and spleen, as well as evidence for specific T cells throughout the lymphoid system. These data suggest that both local and systemic immune systems are induced during a local pulmonary infection with influenza. How these systems interact for maximal protection of the lung and the intact animal is the central issue of our continuing investigations using intratracheal inoculation of influenza virus in hamsters.

ACKNOWLEDGMENTS

The authors thank Jan Frazier, Nanette Broyles and John Rubinow for their invaluable technical assistance and Daisi Marcoulides for typing the manuscript. This work was supported in part by Public Health Grant AI-11851; HL-23870 from the National Institutes of Health.

REFERENCES

1.   Green, G.M.; Jakob, G.J. Annu Rev Respir Dis 115 (1977) 479.
2.   Kaltreider, H.B. Am Rev Respir Dis 113 (1976) 347.

3. Fudenberg, H.H. et al., ed. Review of Basic and Clinical Immu-
    nology. Lange Medical Publication, Los Altos, Calif. (1976).
4. Waldman, R.H.; Ganguly, R. J Infect Dis 130 (1974) 419.
5. Toolan, H. Fed Proc. 37 (1978) 2065.
6. Brownstein, D.G. et al. Am J Pathol 98 (1980) 499.
7. Lennett, E.H. et al., ed. Manual of Clinical Microbiology. Ameri-
    can Society for Microbiology, Washington (1974) 678.
8. Billingham, R.E.; Silvers, W.K. In: Transplantation of Tissues
    and Cells. Wistar Institute Press, Philadelphia (1966) 90.
9. Russell, S.M. et al. J Gen Virology 27 (1975) 1.
10. Jerne, N.K. et al. In: Cell Bound Antibodies, ed. Amos and
    Kaprowski. Wistar Institute Press, Philadelphia (1963) 109.
11. Stein-Streilein, J. et al. Infect Immun 24 (1979) 145.
12. Stein-Streilein, J. et al. Infect Immun 24 (1979) 139.
13. Spencer, H. Pathology of the Lung. W.B. Saunders Co. (1977) 203.
14. Waksman, B.H.; Ozer, H. Prog Allergy 21, ed. Kallos et al.
    Karger, Basel (1976) 1.

FUNCTIONAL HETEROGENEITY OF ALVEOLAR MACROPHAGES

Bruce S. Zwilling and Laura B. Campolito

Department of Microbiology, College of Biological
Sciences, and Comprehensive Cancer Center,
The Ohio State University, Columbus, OH 43210

INTRODUCTION

The alveolar macrophage is the first line of defense against in-
haled toxicants, infectious organisms and inert dusts. While much
attention has been paid to the mechanisms of activation of peritoneal
macrophages, little information is available concerning those of the
alveolar macrophage. Alveolar macrophages have been reported to
differ from peritoneal macrophages in many respects, including their
response to lymphokines (1,2). It has been reported that lower respiratory tract infections can activate alveolar macrophages (3), and
that intratracheal injection of <u>Mycobacterium</u> <u>bovis</u> (strain BCG) can
induce tumor cell destruction by macrophages isolated from the lung
(4). It is not clear, however, whether functionally distinct states
of macrophage activation, analogous to those identified for murine
peritoneal macrophages, can occur in the lung. We therefore have
sought to define functional characteristics of alveolar macrophages
after immunization of hamsters with BCG and to correlate these characteristics with the state of activation. Our results indicate that
macrophages derived from the lung of hamsters show alterations in
functional capacity which may indicate different states of activation.

MATERIALS AND METHODS

Outbred male Syrian golden hamsters (strain LVG/LAK), 8-10 weeks
old, were obtained from Charles River, Wilmington, Mass. They were
immunized intratracheally with 1×10^6 colony forming units (cfu)
<u>Mycobacterium</u> <u>bovis</u> (strain BCG) (TMC1029, Trudeau Institute, Saranac
Lake, N.Y.). Six weeks later and five days prior to use, the ham-

sters were rechallenged intratracheally with BCG. They were killed by an intraperitoneal injection of Brevatal-sodium and the lungs, with trachea, were removed. The lungs taken from immune-rechallenged, immune, or control animals were lavaged with 10 ml Hanks balanced salt solution (BSS) pH 5.5 as described (4). Macrophages were purified by adherence onto 35-mm tissue culture dishes (Corning). Monolayers were adjusted to contain 3 x 10^5 macrophages, more than 95% pure by morphologic criteria. Macrophages were cultured in McCoy's 5a medium containing 20% fetal calf serum (GIBCO), glutamine, penicillin, streptomycin and gentamycin.

The tumoricidal capacity of the lung macrophages was determined using the tritiated thymidine release method (4). The tumor cells, 25th to 80th passage cells derived from a benzo(α)pyrene-induced adenocarcinoma of the lung and designated LG1002, have been described (5). The effect of lipopolysaccharide (LPS) on the tumoricidal capacity of the macrophages was tested using LPS from Escherichia coli 0111:B4 (Westphal) (Difco, Detroit, Mich.).

The phagocytic capacity of the macrophages was determined using opsonized sheep red blood cells (SRBC) (1/1200, rabbit anti-SRBC IgM, Cappel, Downington, Pa.) labelled with ^{51}Cr (6). After incubation for 45 minutes at 37°C, the unphagocytized SRBC were lysed with Tris-NH$_4$Cl, the monolayers digested with 0.39N KOH, and the radioactivity retained by the monolayers assessed in a Packard Autogamma. Phagocytosis was expressed as the counts per minute in monolayers of macrophages. The bactericidal capacity was determined as described (7). Macrophages were allowed to phagocytize Listeria monocytogenes organisms for 30 minutes. The cultures were washed vigorously to remove unphagocytized organisms and incubated for another three hours without antibiotics. The number of intracellular Listeria organisms was determined for both time periods by lysing the macrophages and culturing the surviving organisms for 48 hours on trypticase soy agar plates. The data are expressed as the $\log_{10}$ number of surviving intracellular bacteria at 30 minutes and at $3\frac{1}{2}$ hours.

The response of alveolar macrophages to two complement-derived chemoattractants, used as zymosan activated hamster serum (ZAHS) and lymphocyte derived chemotactic factor (LDCF), was determined as described (8). The bottoms of blind well chemotactic chambers (Wallabs, Fairfax, Calif.) were filled with a 1:10 dilution of ZAHS (fresh serum incubated with 1 mg zymosan [Sigma]/ml for one hour), or with a 1:2 dilution of LDCF (culture fluid from BCG-immune lung cells at 1 x 10^6/ml incubated with 100 µg purified protein derivative [PPD, Connaught]/ml for 24 hours), or with medium as a control. The well was covered with a 5-µm Nucleopore filter (Wallabs, Lot 54AOC27) and the top of the chamber secured tightly. A 0.2-ml volume of the cell suspension was added to each chamber (3 x 10^5 macrophages) and incubated for three hours in air at 37°C. The filters were fixed in methanol and removed, and the cells were stained with Wright's stain.

The number of macrophages migrating through the filter in 20 oil immersion fields was counted.

RESULTS

    Alveolar macrophages from hamsters immune to BCG and rechallenged
intratracheally with BCG five days prior to assay destroyed 21.1%
of the tumor cells, while alveolar macrophages from other treatment
groups failed to exert any demonstrable tumoricidal activity (Fig. 1).
When 0.001 µg LPS was added to the culture medium, 34.7% of the tumor
cells were destroyed; 73.3% were destroyed in cultures containing 10
µg of LPS. The addition of LPS to cultures containing alveolar macro-

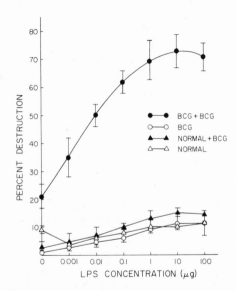

Fig. 1:   Lipopolysaccharide modulation of alveolar macrophage tumor
           cell destruction. Alveolar macrophages from hamsters immu-
           nized intratracheally with 1 x 10⁶ cfu BCG six weeks pre-
           viously and receiving an intratracheal rechallenge five
           days before assay (BCG + BCG); from immunized but not re-
           challenged hamsters (BCG); from hamsters injected five days
           previously (Normal + BCG); and from untreated animals (Nor-
           mal) were incubated with ³H-TdR-labeled tumor cells. After
           six days the radioactivity released into the supernatant
           fluid was determined and the cytotoxicity expressed as a
           percent of the total incorporated radioactivity. The radio-
           activity released by the tumor cells was less than 10% of
           the total.

Table 1. Effect of BCG Treatment on the Phagocytic Capacity of
          Alveolar Macrophages

Treatment	Phagocytosis of EA IgG[1]
BCG + BCG	3072 ± 134^2
BCG	2076 ± 8^3
Normal + BCG	1541 ± 152
Normal	1325 ± 236

Monolayers of alveolar macrophages obtained from BCG-treated or control hamsters were incubated for 45 minutes with opsonized sheep red
blood cells. The unphagocytized erythrocytes were lysed with Tris-
NH_4Cl, the monolayer digested and the intracellular radioactivity determined.

[1]Mean $\pm$ SD of triplicate counts of intracellular 51Cr SRBC.

[2]$p < .01$ vs normal and normal + BCG, BCG.

[3]$p < .05$ vs normal and normal + BCG.

phages from immune or normal hamsters or from normal hamsters that
had received BCG five days previously did not affect the tumoricidal
capacity of these macrophages.

    The phagocytic capacity of alveolar macrophages from BCG-immune
and immune-rechallenged hamsters was greater than that of alveolar
macrophages from control groups (Table 1). In contrast, only alveolar macrophages from immune-rechallenged hamsters destroyed significantly more intracellular Listeria organisms (Fig. 2). Only 2.5 x
10^5 viable organisms remained in these macrophages after three hours
of incubation, while as many as 1.3×10^6 viable organisms were recovered from alveolar macrophages from the other treatment groups.
The macrophages from immune-rechallenged animals reduced the number
of viable organisms by 2 logs, while the macrophages from the immune
hamsters or from control hamsters reduced the viable intracellular
organisms by only 0.5 log.

    The data in Fig. 3 show that significantly greater numbers of
alveolar macrophages from immune-rechallenged hamsters migrated
through a Nucleopore filter in response to ZAHS (2200 cells/20 oil
immersion fields) than did macrophages from the other treatment
groups. Results were similar when lymphocyte supernatants were used
as the chemotactic stimulant, Fig. 4; 1280 macrophages migrated in
20 fields compared to 200 to 400 cells in 20 fields from the other

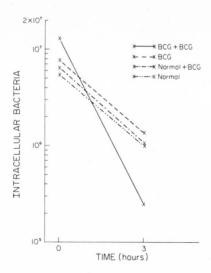

Fig. 2:   The effect of BCG treatment on the destruction of intra-
           cellular _Listeria_ _monocytogenes_ by hamster alveolar macro-
           phages. Hamsters were treated as described in Fig. 1.
           Alveolar macrophages were allowed to adhere for 30 minutes
           and _L_. _monocytogenes_ organisms were added. Cultures were
           incubated for 30 minutes more to allow for phagocytosis,
           and the unphagocytized organisms removed by vigorous wash-
           ing. Cultures were incubated for three hours more, the
           macrophages lysed and the surviving intracellular bacteria
           enumerated by plate count.

treatment groups. Macrophages from the lungs of BCG-immune hamsters
also showed significantly greater response to ZAHS (but not to LDCF)
than did macrophages from the control groups.

    To insure that the response was truly chemotactic and not due to
increased random migration of the BCG-activated cells, a gradient analysis was performed by varying the concentration of ZAHS above and below
the filter (Table 2). As the concentration of chemoattractant above
the filter was diluted to less than the concentration below the filter,
more cells migrated through the filter toward the area of increased
concentration.

DISCUSSION

    Functional heterogeneity between macrophage populations derived
from different anatomic locations is well documented (1). Alveolar
macrophages are reported to differ from peritoneal macrophages with

Table 2.   Response of Hamster Alveolar Macrophages to Chemotactic
           Gradient

Dilution of chemoattractant above filter	Dilution of chemoattractant below filter			
	1:10	1:40	1:160	Medium
1:10	398+98	276+134	301+71	205+113
1:40	659+163[1]	539+79	359+143	261+101
1:160	844+318[1]	560+180	300+95	241+172
Medium	1455+365[1]	1303+317[1]	702+166[1]	255+146

Dilutions of zymosan-activated hamster serum (ZAHS) were added to the
bottom of blind well chemotactic chambers. The macrophages were suspended in dilutions of ZAHS before addition of the cells to the upper
portion of the chambers. After incubation the cells migrating to the
lower portion of the filter were counted.

[1]Significant by Student's t test.

regard to energy metabolism, bactericidal capacity, and response to
chemotactic stimuli and to lymphokines. In the peritoneal cavity, differences in functional capacity have been reported between resident,
elicited and activated macrophages (9). A functional heterogeneity
within subpopulations of activated peritoneal macrophages also has
been reported (10,13). Much information has accumulated concerning
the relationship of peritoneal macrophage tumor cell destruction to
other parameters of peritoneal macrophage function (9). No information is available, however, that compares the functional capacities of
different activation states of alveolar macrophages with their tumoricidal capacity.

    The results of this investigation indicate that three functionally
distinct populations of macrophages isolated from the lung can be identified based on the prior exposure of the lung to BCG infection. One
population, recently arrived from the blood and obtained from the
lungs of BCG immune-rechallenged hamsters, was capable of destroying
tumor cells, was responsive to LPS activation, had increased phagocytic and bactericidal capacity and had a greatly enhanced capacity
to respond to two chemotactic stimuli. The second population, resident
alveolar macrophages obtained from BCG-immune hamsters, was not capable of destroying tumor cells and was not activated by LPS. The
latter cells differed from resident alveolar macrophages from untreated
or rechallenged control animals, which showed an increased phagocytic
capacity to SRBC and a somewhat greater chemotactic response to ZAHS.

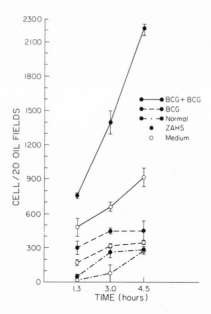

Fig. 3: The effect of BCG treatment on the chemotactic response of hamster alveolar macrophages to zymosan-activated hamster serum. Hamsters were treated as described in Fig. 1. A 1:10 dilution of ZAHS was placed below the filter in a blind well chemotactic chamber. Alveolar macrophages (0.3×10^6 in 0.2 ml) were placed above the filter and the cultures incubated at $37^{\circ}C$ in air for up to 4 1/2 hours. The cells were fixed with methanol and stained with Wright's stain, and the number of cells migrating to the underside of the filter was counted in 20 oil immersion fields.

Most studies assessing the effects of BCG treatments on alveolar macrophage function have used macrophages from animals immunized intravenously with killed BCG and rechallenged intratracheally (14). Our investigation, in contrast, used intratracheal instillation of viable BCG for both immunization and rechallenge. We felt that this was important because it has been reported by several laboratories that more effective protection of the lung was achieved when animals were immunized initially via the lung rather than by other routes (15,16).

Information regarding the LPS responsiveness of the hamster is confusing. One study (17) reported that LPS was mitogenic for hamster lymphocytes. Other investigators (18) were unable to obtain a mitogenic response with LPS and also could not produce polyclonal activa-

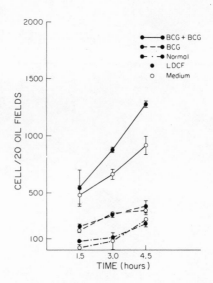

Fig. 4:   The effect of BCG treatment on the chemotactic response of
           hamster alveolar macrophages to lymphocyte-derived chemotac-
           tic factor. See Fig. 3 for description. Lymphocyte-derived
           chemotactic factor produced by PPD-stimulated lung lavage
           lymphocytes from tuberculin-sensitized hamsters.

tion. LPS did induce a good antibody response. Our observation that
high doses of LPS enhanced the tumoricidal capacity of alveolar macrophages obtained from immune-rechallenged hamsters is similar to other
observations (19) in LPS unresponsive C3H/HeJ mice. Somewhat surprising was the finding that a single injection of BCG did not induce
tumoricidal macrophages: Alveolar macrophages become responsive to
LPS only after the induction of an inflammatory exudate by rechallenge
with BCG. This suggests that the tumoricidal macrophage may have
arrived in the lung recently and that rechallenge with BCG resulted
in the partial activation of a macrophage population, rendering them
responsive to endotoxin activation. Investigation in our laboratory
using alveolar macrophages from BCG-immune or from normal hamsters
supports the latter hypothesis (Panke and Zwilling, submitted for publication).

    There has been some debate concerning the chemotactic responsive-
ness of alveolar macrophages to serum-derived chemotaxins. It has been
suggested that resident alveolar macrophages respond poorly to serum-
derived and lymphocyte-derived chemotactic factors (20). It would
appear from our studies that only inflammatory lung macrophages were
capable of responding to both serum-derived and lymphocyte-derived

stimuli. Resident macrophages from immune hamsters responded weakly to ZAHS but not to LDCF. This suggests that these alveolar macrophages may have undergone a partial activation. Our studies support findings (20) that resident populations from untreated animals are relatively unresponsive to serum-derived and lymphocyte-derived chemotactic factors.

Our investigation indicates that populations of lung macrophages can be identified that are analogous to the resident elicited and activated peritoneal macrophages identified in murine models. An experimental hamster model avoids the susceptibility to respiratory diseases shown by rabbits and provides greater numbers of cells than are obtainable from mice.

ACKNOWLEDGMENTS

The authors wish to thank Sharon Kerns for her assistance in preparing this manuscript. This work was supported by National Institutes of Health, Research Grant CA16342 and by Grant IM-208 from the American Cancer Society.

REFERENCES

1. Walker, W.S. In: Immunobiology of the Macrophage, ed. Nelson. Academic Press, New York (1976) 91.
2. Leu, R.W. et al. J Exp Med 136 (1972) 589.
3. Truitt, G.L.; Mackaness, G.B. Am Rev Respir Dis 104 (1971) 829.
4. Zwilling, B.S.; Campolito, L.B. J Immunol 119 (1977) 838.
5. Bakaletz, A.P.; Zwilling, B.S. Ohio J Sci 79 (1979) 126.
6. Schmidke, J.R.; Simmons, R.C. J Natl Cancer Inst 54 (1965) 1379.
7. Simon, H.; Sheagren, J.N. Infect Immun 6 (1972) 101.
8. Snyderman, R.; Pike, M. In: In Vitro Methods in Cell Mediated and Tumor Immunity, ed. Bloom and David. Academic Press, New York (1976) 651.
9. Meltzer, M.S.; Stevenson, M.M. Cell Immunol 35 (1978) 99.
10. Walker, W.S. J Reticuloendothel Soc 20 (1976) 57.
11. Weinberg, D.S. et al. Cell Immunol 38 (1978) 94.
12. Lee, K.C. et al. Cell Immunol 42 (1979) 28.
13. Miller, G.A. et al. J Reticuloendothel Soc 27 (1980) 167.
14. Moore, V.L.; Myrvik, Q.N. J Reticuloendothel Soc 21 (1977) 131.
15. Jargenson, P.F. et al. J Infect Dis 128 (1976) 730.
16. Waldman, R.H. et al. Cell Immunol 3 (1972) 294.
17. Hart, D.A. et al. Fed Proc 37 (1978) 2039.
18. Ahmed, A. et al. Fed Proc 37 (1978) 2045.
19. Ruco, L.P.; Meltzer, M.S. Cell Immunol 41 (1978) 35.
20. Daubin, J.F.; Daniele, R.P. Am Rev Respir Dis 117 (1978) 673.

ANTI-VIRAL CYTOTOXIC LYMPHOCYTE RESPONSE IN HAMSTERS

WITH PARAINFLUENZA VIRUS TYPE 3 INFECTION

Frederick W. Henderson

Department of Pediatrics
University of North Carolina School of Medicine
Chapel Hill, NC 27514

INTRODUCTION

The Syrian hamster is a useful model for experimental studies of immunity to agents causing acute respiratory disease because it is susceptible to several significant human pathogens, including influenza A viruses, parainfluenza virus 3 (P3), and Mycoplasma pneumoniae. The importance of cell-mediated immune mechanisms in respiratory virus infections remains an unresolved issue. A developing body of clinical experience suggests that cellular immune competence is required for resolution of respiratory syncytial virus, influenza A, and parainfluenza 3 infections in man. Prolonged infections with these agents have been identified in children with inborn and acquired disorders of cellular immunity (1). Recent studies of influenza A infection in mice suggest that a local cytotoxic T lymphocyte response may contribute to termination of intrapulmonary virus replication (2). Determination of the relative and quantitative significance of the cellular response, however, has proven difficult. Futhermore, since most studies of influenzal immunity employ "mouse-adapted" alveolar-tropic strains of virus, conclusions reached from these studies may not be directly applicable to other viral agents that infect the lung. We have examined the pulmonary cellular immune response of hamsters to P3 infection in order to develop a better understanding of immunity to viral infection of intrapulmonary airways (3).

MATERIALS AND METHODS

Male inbred MHA and CB and outbred golden Syrian hamsters were obtained from Charles River Breeding Laboratories (Wilmington, Mass.).

Primary kidney cell cultures were prepared using organs obtained from
3-week-old animals. Ten- to 12-week-old hamsters acutely infected
with test viruses were used as immune cell donors. Breeding colonies
of each strain were known to be infected with Sendai virus, and all
animals screened (approx. 30) had serum CF antibodies to Sendai virus.

Ether-anesthetized animals were infected by intranasal inocula-
tion of 10^4 to 10^6 tissue culture infectious dose$_{50}$ (TCID$_{50}$) of test
viruses in a volume of 0.2 ml. The viruses employed were human parainfluenza virus type 3 (NIH reference strain), influenza A/PR/8/34 (WHO
reference strain), and murine parainfluenza virus type 1--Sendai. The
influenza strain was partially adapted to hamsters by four serial lung
passages in adult animals; P3 and Sendai were not hamster-adapted.
Immune effector cells, to be assayed for cytolytic function, were obtained by endotracheal bronchoalveolar lavage using five 3-ml volumes
of Ca^{++}-Mg^{++} free PBS-2% HI-FCS. For a single experiment, lung wash
cells from two to six animals were pooled to give sufficient cell numbers for study.

Monolayers of second-passage syngeneic hamster kidney cells grown
in flat-bottom 96-well microtiter plates were used for target cells
in the cytotoxic assay. Target cells were infected with virus (multiplicity of infection, 10 to 1) six hours before overlaying effector
cells. Targets were labelled with ^{51}Cr by adding 2 μCi of Na^{51}Cr in
saline to each monolayer for two hours at $37^{\circ}C$. Cells were washed
four times to remove excess label, and immune cells were added immediately thereafter. An effector to target cell ratio of 10-20:1 and
an incubation time of 16 hours were used in most experiments. Cell-
free supernatants were counted in a gamma spectrometer, and results
expressed as percent chromium released calculated as follows:

$$\frac{\text{Experimental release - spontaneous release}}{\text{Total release - spontaneous release}} \times 100$$

Phagocytic cells were identified by incubating lung lavage cells
in a 0.1% suspension of latex particles for 45 minutes at $37^{\circ}C$. Fc
rosettes were prepared using sheep erythrocytes sensitized with hamster anti-SRBC serum according to established methods (4).

RESULTS AND DISCUSSION

The cytotoxic assay developed was modeled after successful systems
designed to detect virus-specific cytotoxic T cells in experimental
infection models, usually in mice (5). These studies had established
that maximum levels of cytotoxic T lymphocyte activity usually were
found approximately one week after acute infection. In initial experiments it was determined that bronchoalveolar lavage cells obtained
from MHA hamsters six days after infection with P3 mediated specific
cytolysis of P3-infected secondary MHA hamster kidney cells. Lung

lavage cells from infected animals did not lyse uninfected targets
and cells from uninfected animals failed to injure infected or control
monolayers.

The temporal course of the development and regression of the cytotoxic intrapulmonary immune response to P3 is shown in Fig. 1. Also
shown are lung virus titers on days 3 through 6 post-infection. Minimal levels of cytotoxic activity were detectable by day 4 after infection. Between 96 and 120 hours there was an influx of cytotoxic
effectors into the lumina of airways and alveoli, resulting in maximum levels of cytotoxicity between days 5 through 7 post-infection.
The cytotoxic response had waned to approximately one-half of peak
levels by day 10 and was no longer detectable on day 14. Peak lung
virus titers were found on days 3 and 4 post-infection. The mean concentration of virus had declined by approximately 90% on day 5 and infectious P3 was no longer recovered from a 10% lung suspension on day
6. The data demonstrate the close temporal correspondence between the
developing cellular response and the termination of virus replication.

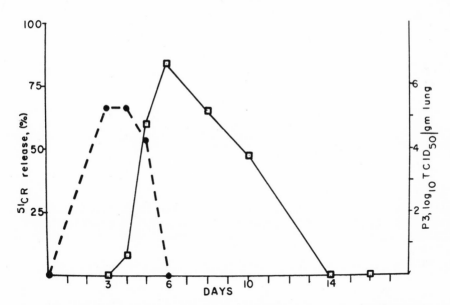

Fig. 1:   Correlation of broncho-alveolar cell cytotoxicity (%^{51}Cr
           release □---□) with parainfluenza 3 (P3 ●---●   ) virus
           titers in hamster lung suspension. Cytotoxicity data points
           represent the median of an average of five experiments;
           virus titers are geometric means of four animals at each
           sample time. (Reproduced with permission, Am Rev Resp Dis)

The specificity of the response was determined by comparing the cytolytic function of P3 and influenza A/PR/8/34 immune effector cells for target cells infected with P3, A/PR/8/34, and Sendai virus. Homologous cytotoxicity was consistently in the 65% to 95% release range. No ^{51}Cr release was seen when P3 immune cells were tested on influenza-infected cells or when influenza immune cells were assayed on P3 infected targets. Consistent partial lysis of Sendai-infected targets was mediated by P3 immune cells but not influenza effectors, which agrees with the known serologic relatedness of P3 and Sendai.

The relevance of histocompatibility antigens to expression of the cytolytic response was addressed by comparing the cytotoxicity of effector cells from P3-infected MHA, CB, and outbred Syrian hamsters when assayed on four different types of target cell monolayers (Table 1). No restriction òf cytotoxicity was found among the various hamster effector:target tissue combinations tested. Cytotoxicity was completely abrogated when immune cells were assayed on infected xenogeneic tissue. The susceptibility of the monkey and bovine kidney cells to P3 infection was determined by conventional hemadsorption tests, and their susceptibility to lysis was confirmed using antibody-complement mediated killing. The temporal aspects and the virus specificity of the response are compatible with a T cell response; the

Table 1.   Tissue Antigen-Related Specificity of Cytotoxic Response

Effector mechanism	[51]Cr release from target cells (%)[1]			
	MHA hamster	Outbred hamster	Rhesus monkey	Bovine (MDBK)
Immune cells[2]				
MHA hamster	82	81	0	0
CB hamster	69	--	--	--
Outbred hamster	82	78	0	0
Immune serum				
Human serum, fresh			55	36
Human serum, complement-inactivated			0	0

[1]Secondary kidney cells or cell line (MDBK) infected with parainfluenza virus type 3

[2]Bronchoalveolar lavage cells obtained six days after infection of hamster strains listed with parainfluenza virus type 3.

(Modified and reproduced with permission, Am Rev Resp Dis)

requirement for species identity between effectors and targets is even
stronger evidence that the assay measured a T cell effector function.
The lack of allogeneic restriction of cytotoxicity implies that MHA,
CB, and outbred Syrian hamsters share major histocompatibility antigens.

Preliminary work has been done to characterize further the changes
in the lung lavage cell population during infection and to identify
the cytotoxic effector cell. The total number of cells recovered by
lavage increased approximately three-fold from control to peak day 6
values. The greatest increase occurred between days 4 and 5, and most
of the increase was accounted for by lymphocytes. Cells were fractionated by removing the adherent cell population by incubation on a nylon
fiber column. The non-adherent effluent cells were non-phagocytic,
as assessed by latex particle ingestion, and no longer contained cells
with the capacity to form Fc rosettes. Enhanced killing was observed
when these cells were compared with unseparated lung lavage cells. An
attempt was made to demonstrate antibody-dependent cellular cytotoxicity, using non-immune lung lavage cells with hamster P3 immune sera,
both day 6 and day 14 samples. No target cell lysis was seen. The
distribution of cytotoxic cells was examined by comparing the cytolytic function of lung lavage cells with that of spleen cells. Levels
of cytotoxicity mediated by spleen cells were approximately one-fourth
the levels generated by lung lymphocytes.

These studies show that a lymphocyte-mediated virus-specific cytotoxic immune response is generated in the lungs of hamsters during
acute P3 infection. The evidence suggests strongly that T lymphocytes
mediate most of the observed effects. The lack of allogeneic restriction of cytotoxicity suggests that the hamster strains used share
major histocompatibility antigens.

REFERENCES

1.   Fishaut, M. et al. J Pediatr 96 (1980) 179.
2.   Yap, K.L.; Ada, G.L. Scand J Immunol 7 (1978) 389.
3.   Henderson, F.W. Am Rev Resp Dis 120 (1979) 41.
4.   Handbook of Experimental Immunology: Cellular Immunology, ed.
     Weir. Blackwell Scientific, Oxford (1978).
5.   Doherty, P.C. et al. Transplant Rev (1976) 89.

MECHANISMS OF INFLAMMATION IN LUNG TISSUE

Donald L. Kreutzer, Usha Desai, William H. J. Douglas, and
Mark Blazka

Department of Pathology, University of Connecticut
Health Center, Farmington, CT 06032 and
Department of Anatomy, Tufts Medical Center,
Boston, MA 02111

INTRODUCTION

Inflammation can be seen as a balance of pro-inflammatory and
anti-inflammatory reactions, with pro-inflammatory reactions involved
in the initiation and amplification of inflammation via mediators
(chemotactic and vasopermeability factors) and tissue injury (by loss
of cell function and death). Anti-inflammatory reactions, on the
other hand, will suppress inflammation by inactivation of these mediators (via chemotactic factor inactivator [CFI] and anaphylatoxin inactivator), thus reducing the delivery of destructive enzymes and
products of activated leukocytes (1). Although basic mechanisms of
inflammatory processes are beginning to be reasonably well understood
in the kidney, relatively little is known about inflammation in the
lung. Insult to the lung, whether immunologic, infectious or environmental, often will activate intrinsic systems such as the complement
system, which generates vasopermeability and chemotactic factors.
These factors will recruit leukocytes and serum factors into the lung
which will directly damage lung structure and function. In addition,
these recruited leukocytes have the potential capacity to amplify inflammatory reactions and tissue injury by various mechanisms: 1. release of lysosomal enzymes; 2. production of free radicals and other
factors that damage structural elements; 3. the activation or direct
cleavage of complement, complement components, or other lung consti-
tuents into active chemotactic factors; 4. activation of other inflammatory pathways such as coagulation; and 5. stimulation of resident
lung cells such as macrophages or type II cells to elaborate preformed (chemotactic factors) and precursor (C3 and C5) inflammatory
mediators which would increase the recruitment of leukocytes (PMN's

and monocytes) into the lung. At the same time, anti-inflammatory
modulators such as the CFI system (serum and cell-derived CFI's)
serve to regulate and limit the inflammatory reactions by inactivat-
ing the chemotactic factors, thus blocking the influx of leukocytes
into the lung (2). When pro-inflammatory and anti-inflammatory reactions are properly balanced, inflammation will occur with minimal
damage to healthy tissue. Uncontrolled, these inflammatory reactions
can destroy healthy tissue with resulting loss of normal lung architecture and function.

The purpose of these studies is to begin to gain basic insights
into the biochemical and biological mechanisms by which acute inflammatory reactions are initiated and modulated within the lung, and by
the lung. To achieve these ends, we have begun investigating the potential roles and sources of chemotactic factors and complement components within normal and injured lung tissue.

MATERIALS AND METHODS

Male Syrian golden hamsters, outbred Mesocricetus auratus,
weighing 95 to 150 g were obtained from Charles River Laboratories
(Wilmington, Mass.).

All chemotactic factors used were assayed by the modified Boyden
chamber technique and by the lysosomal enzyme release assay (3,4).
Glycogen-induced rabbit and hamster peritoneal PMN leukocytes were
used as indicator cells.

The chemotactic fragment of C5 (C5fr) was generated from zymosan-
treated human serum containing 1M epsilon-aminocaproic acid and isolated by gel filtration as described (5). The synthetic chemotactic
peptide N-formyl-methionyl-leucyl phenylalanine (F-Met-Leu-Phe) was
kindly provided by Dr. Elmer Becker (University of Connecticut Health
Center, Farmington, Conn.). A stock solution of F-Met-Leu-Phe (0.1M)
was made with dimethyl sulfoxide (DMSO) containing 2 mg bovine serum
albumin/ml in phosphate buffered saline (PBS) (6). All chemotactic
activity was expressed in units of ED_{50}, with one ED_{50} of chemotaxis
defined as the amount of chemotactic agent required for half maximal
chemotactic response in the Boyden chamber assay (7).

The fifth component of complement (C5) was isolated from human
serum as described (8). The fourth component of complement (C4) was
purified from human serum as described (9). Human serum albumin
(HSA) in purified crystalline form was obtained from Penta Biochemi-
cals (Kankakee, Ill.). Crystalline bovine serum albumin (BSA) was
purchased from Sigma Chemical Company (St. Louis, Mo.). Hamster serum
albumin (HaSA) was isolated from pooled normal hamster serum using
affi-gel blue (Biorad Laboratories, Rockville Centre, N.Y.); the
purity of this protein was determined by SDS polyacrylamide gel elec-

trophoresis (Biorad Laboratories, Rockville Centre, N.Y.). Serum al-
bumins were dissolved in phosphate buffered saline (pH 7.4) at concentrations of 2 and 20 mg protein/ml. Hamster serum albumin was
radiolabeled with carrier-free ^{125}I using the chloramine T method
(10).

Instillation of various test samples in anesthetized hamsters
was accomplished by the intraperitoneal injection of 5 to 7 mg keta-
mine hydrochloride (Ketaject, Bristol Laboratories, Syracuse, N.Y.).
Under direct laryngoscopic visualization, a 300-µl bolus of solution
containing the test reagent was instilled intratracheally through an
18-gauge polypropylene catheter. Just before instillation, the solutions and buffers were adjusted as necessary to physiologic pH
(7.4) and conductivity. Chemotactic preparations containing 600 to
1000 ED_{50} doses in buffered saline were instilled intracheally during
inspiration, with permeability changes and PMN influxes quantitated
by use of ^{125}I-hamster albumin and ^{111}In-hamster PMN's as we have described recently (11,12).

All preparations of chemotactic factors and control solutions,
which were used for intrapulmonary instillation, were assayed for endotoxin content by the Limulus lysate assay (13). The endotoxin content of all the samples used ranged between 3 and 10 ng endotoxin per
0.3 ml. Intratracheal instillation of 1 ng to 100 ng of bacterial
endotoxin from Escherichia coli 0111B4 (Difco Co., Detroit, Mich.)
into 25 hamsters failed to induce significant inflammatory changes
in the lung, as reflected by permeability changes or PMN influx.

In all radioactivity studies (^{111}In-PMN and ^{125}I-HaSA) involving
hamsters, the initial experimental data are calculated as the total
radioactivity in the individual lung divided by the radioactivity in
1 ml of blood from the corresponding hamster. The final data then
are expressed as the ratio of the experimental value (lung/blood) to
the control value (lung/blood). Thus, values greater than one indicate increased accumulation of radioactivity, and values less than
one indicate decreased accumulation of radioactivity in experimental
animals, relative to buffer-instilled controls. No significant difference in levels of radioactivity was seen between buffer-instilled
and noninstilled hamster lungs. Each data point represents at least
four to eight animals with standard error of the mean indicated.

Type II Pneumocyte Cultures

Human fetal lung (18 to 20 weeks of gestation) was obtained following elective abortion. Under sterile conditions, large airways
and pulmonary vessels were removed, leaving tissue consisting primarily of lung parenchyma. This tissue was gently minced into 1-3mm fragments and transferred to an Erlenmeyer flask. The mince was washed
three times with RPMI 1640 tissue culture medium, and then an enzyme

solution consisting of 0.1% collagenase (type I, Worthington Biochemical Co.), 0.1% trypsin (1:250 DIFCO) and 1% chicken serum
(Gibco Co.) in calcium-magnesium-free Hanks' saline was added. The
dissociation procedure consisted of a series of 15-minute incubation
at 37°C. Following each incubation, the cell suspension was harvested and filtered through a 41-μm nylon screen (Nitex HC3-41,
Tetko Inc.) into a 50-ml centrifuge tube on ice. An equal volume of
chilled culture medium supplemented with 10% selected fetal bovine
serum (FBS) and antibiotics (antibiotic-antimycotic mixture 100 x,
Gibco Co., 10 ml/liter medium) was added and the cells were stored
on ice. Upon completion of the dissociation procedure, the cell suspension was centrifuged at 220 x g for six minutes and the pellet resuspended in serum-supplemented medium. Cell viability was assayed
by erythrosin B dye exclusion. Cell viabilities of 70% to 80% were
achieved routinely. The cells were centrifuged a second time (220 x
g, 6 minutes) and the cell pellet was incubated for one hour at 37°C.

Following the incubation, the cells were resuspended in a volume
of serum-supplemented culture medium to yield 1.0 x 10^7 viable cells
per 50 μl. The suspension was inoculated (50-μl aliquots) onto the
surface of individual 2-cm^2 pieces of media-hydrated gelfoam collagen
sponge (Upjohn). Two cultures were placed in a 100-mm culture dish,
and the cultures were incubated at 37°C in a humidified atmosphere
of 5% CO_2 in air for one hour to allow the cells to attach to the sub-
strate. Twenty milliliters of serum-supplemented culture medium were
added and the cultures incubated for 48 hours. At this time they were
placed on a rocker platform set at three cycles per minute, for the
duration of the experiment. Culture medium was replaced every other
day, and the cultures were allowed to grow for one week in vitro.
After this seven-day period, the cultures were transferred to serum-
free RPMI 1640 culture medium containing ^{14}C-amino acids (5 μCi/ml).
On day 10 in vitro, the serum-free culture medium was harvested and
stored frozen at -55°C until analyzed.

Synthesis and elaboration of C3 and C5 by cultured type II pneumocytes was detected by double immunoprecipitation of concentrated
(500x) ^{14}C-labeled culture supernatants with specific anti-C3 and
anti-C5 antibody. Immunoprecipitation of ^{14}C-C3 or ^{14}C-C5 by the
specific antisera was detected by radioautography of the double immunoprecipitates (14).

RESULTS

Within five minutes after intratracheal instillation of 600 ED_{50}
units of C5fr, there was moderate perivascular edema and intravascu-
lar margination of PMN's within alveolar spaces. By 20 minutes these
features were more intense; at 60 minutes and at four hours there was
diffuse and confluent intra-alveolar accumulation of PMN's and persistent perivascular edema (Fig. 1). When 1000 ED_{50} C5fr was in-

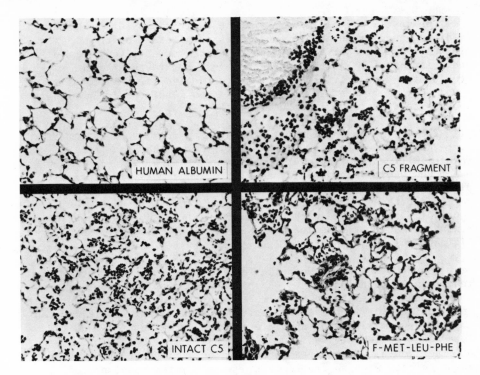

Fig. 1: Sections of lungs from hamsters injected intratracheally
         four hours earlier with 20 mg human serum albumin, 1000
         ED_{50} C5fr, 200 µg human C5, or 432 µg F-Met-Leu-Phe. The
         albumin-injected animals show histologic changes in the
         lung, whereas animals injected with C5fr, intact C5, or
         F-Met-Leu-Phe show diffuse intra-alveolar infiltrates of
         PMN's.

stilled, all of the changes described above were observed, but they
appeared with greater rapidity and greater intensity. The most
striking difference observed with the higher dose of C5fr was the extensive, confluent nature of the intra-alveolar PMN infiltrates and
the prominence of proteinaceous edema fluid in alveolar spaces. Phos-
photungstic acid-hematoxylin (PTAH) stain indicated the presence of
fibrin in this fluid.

    The reactions induced by the peptide F-Met-Leu-Phe were quanti-
tatively and qualitatively similar to those induced by C5fr. The
only difference was a lack of obvious margination of PMN's along ves-
sel walls adjacent to bronchioles (Fig. 1).

The instillation of 200 µg intact C5 into hamster lungs caused mild perivascular edema and occasional margination over the first 20 minutes. Between one and four hours there was an intense and diffuse accumulation of PMN's in alveolar spaces. Perivascular edema was also prominent. Very little evidence of intra-alveolar hemorrhage was found. Of all the proteins instilled into lung, the inflammatory responses to C5 were most marked (Fig. 1).

The intratracheal instillation of either: 2 or 10 mg human albumin; 200 µg human IgG; 200 µg human C4; or saline alone failed to invoke significant inflammatory reactions in lungs. Except for infrequent PMN's within alveolar spaces, the lungs were histologically indistinguishable from those of animals injected intratracheally with saline, or those of uninstilled hamsters. An additional group of four animals instilled with DMSO-Alb in saline (at the same final concentration as that used in the F-Met-Leu-Phe solutions) showed no significant pulmonary changes (Fig. 1).

Quantitation of chemotactic factor- and C5-induced inflammatory reactions was done using ^{125}I-hamster albumin as a permeability marker and ^{111}In-labeled hamster PMN's as an index of leukocyte influx into the lungs. In these radioactivity studies, the individual animals were normalized for absolute radioactivity infused, and accumulated lung radioactivity. The final data are expressed as a ratio of experimental values over control values. Thus, control values are equal to one, with an experimental value greater than one indicating increased accumulation of radioactivity in the lung. We first quantitated the C5-induced PMN influx into the hamster lungs using the ^{111}In-labeled cells. At four hours post-instillation, the C5 induced nearly a four-fold increase in lung-associated radioactivity, compared to control lungs. Similar increases in radioactivity were induced by the preformed C5 chemotactic factor and the synthetic chemotactic peptide F-Met-Leu-Phe (Table 1). Interestingly, only relatively minor permeability changes were induced in the lungs by the instilled C5, with usual values ranging between 1 and 2. These data not only demonstrate the technical and theoretical aspects of quantitating permeability changes and PMN influxes induced by chemotactic factors and C5, but also clearly dissect into independent events the permeability changes and the PMN influx that occur during inflammatory reactions in lung tissue.

One of our initial questions was whether these C5-induced inflammatory reactions were totally modulated by the instilled C5, or initiated by the C5 and then amplified or modulated in vivo by the hamster's own complement system. Initially, we depleted hamsters of 95% to 99% of their serum complement levels with cobra venom factor (CVF). This depletion of serum complement had no effect on C5-induced PMN accumulation as judged by histology or ^{111}In-PMN accumulation (15). CVF depletion of hamster complement had no effect on chemotactic factor- (and F-Met-Leu-Phe)-induced lung inflammation (15). One pos-

Table 1. Quantitation of Pulmonary Inflammatory Reactions in Hamster Lung

Material injected into lung[1]	Inflammatory reaction[2]	
	Permeability ^{125}I-hamster albumin	PMN influx (^{111}In-PMN)
	Ratio relative to uninstilled controls	
Control saline	1.0	1.0
C5fr (5000 ED_{50})	1.4 + .01	3.8 + .26
Intact C5 (300µg)	2.2 + .28	3.8 + .58
F-Met-Leu-Phe	2.0 + .47	2.5 + .40

[1]Materials were instilled intratracheally in volumes of 0.3 ml.

[2]Four hours after instillation into lung.

sible interpretation of these data is that the hamster serum complement is not important in the initiation or amplification of the chemotactic factor- or C5-induced reactions, and that these inflammatory reactions are initiated and modulated in the lung itself. These data suggest that the modulation and amplification of inflammatory reactions by the lungs may be achieved by the elaboration of pro-inflammatory factors, such as chemotactic factors and complement components (C3 and C5) from resident lung cells such as alveolar macrophages and type II cells. This theory is supported by our data demonstrating that isolated type II pneumocytes will synthesize and elaborate antigenically intact C3 and C5 when cultured in vitro (Fig. 2).

DISCUSSION

Whether diseases are caused by infectious agents, pollutants, or immunologic mechanisms, it has become apparent that much of the tissue damage in pulmonary disease is related to the consequences of the recruitment of inflammatory cells into the tissue by chemotactic factors with a resultant release of hydrolytic enzymes and oxygen metabolites from these cells. These hydrolytic enzymes of inflammatory cells, in particular, have the capacity to injure lung tissue and cause lung disease. Recently, oxygen metabolites (O_2 and H_2O_2) originating from leukocytes have been shown in vitro to be toxic to various cells including endothelial cells, lymphocytes and macrophages (1), and may be responsible for in vivo damage to the lung. Accordingly, it would be expected that the control of the accumulation of inflammatory cells into lung tissue plays a major role in both acute and chronic lung disease; and that this accumulation of inflammatory cells in lung tissue is dependent on both the generation and inactivation of chemotactic factors. Since these chemotactic factors may

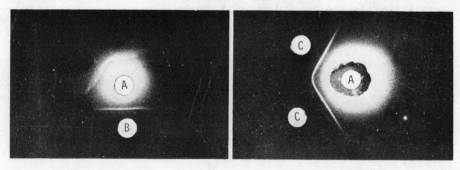

Fig. 2:   Radioautograph of the double immunoprecipitation of ^{14}C-
          labeled human fetal type II pneumocyte culture supernatants
          with specific anti-human C3 (Fig. 2A) or anti-human C5 (Fig.
          2B) antibody. Wells designated A contained ^{14}C-labeled human
          type II pneumocyte culture supernatants; B contained goat
          anti-human C3 antibody; and C contained goat anti-human C5
          antibody.

arise from humoral systems (such as complement) or from the lung itself (alveolar macrophages, type II cells or other lung cells), it
seems highly likely that understanding the basic mechanisms involved
in the production and control of chemotactic factors and chemotactic
factor precursors, such as the fifth component of complement, in the
lung and by the lung will provide important insights into the mechanisms of lung disease.

     Thus, our recent efforts have focused on a systematic investiga-
tion of the existence, role and control of lung-derived pro- and anti-
inflammatory activities, both in acute and chronic inflammatory reactions. To achieve this goal, we employ both in vivo and in vitro
techniques to determine the mechanisms by which chemotactic factors
and the fifth component of complement induce acute inflammatory reactions when instilled into the lungs of experimental animals; to
define and characterize potential sources of chemotactic factors and
complement components (C5) in the lung itself; and to determine the
cellular and molecular mechanisms that regulate the expression of
these pro- and anti-inflammatory activities in normal and inflamed
lung tissue, through the use of defined and isolated lung cells (type
II pneumocytes).

     Our recent in vivo and in vitro data clearly indicate that the
appearance of chemotactic factors (C5fr or F-Met-Leu-Phe) or intact
complement components in the alveoli of the lung will induce acute
inflammatory reactions in the lung (3,4). These mediator-induced

lung reactions are not blocked by complement depletion of the animals, suggesting that the initiation and amplification of these inflammatory reactions may be modulated in the lung itself, completely apart from the vascular compartment (15). The modulation and amplification of inflammatory reactions by the lung may be achieved by elaboration of pro-inflammatory factors, such as chemotactic factors and complement components (C3 and C5), from resident lung cells such as type II cells. This theory is supported by our data showing that in vitro type II cells elaborate complement components such as C3 and C5. Thus, the lung contains resident cells that can elaborate potent precursor or active inflammatory substances (complement components) could initiate or extend inflammation in normal and injured lungs. These data, coupled with our recent demonstration of the presence of a specific C5 cleaving activity in normal broncho-alveolar lavage fluids (15), suggest that the lung has a self-contained phlogistic apparatus of inflammation. That is, the lung itself has the capacity to initiate, amplify and/or suppress inflammatory reactions directly by the production and secretion of these pro-inflammatory activities in response to various immunologic, infectious or pollutant-induced injuries.

These studies are beginning to provide essential information on the basic biochemical and biological mechanisms by which acute inflammatory reactions are modulated in the lung and by the lung. This modulation by the lungs probably influences not only acute inflammation and lung injury, but also chronic inflammation and loss of lung function and architecture, e.g., sarcoidosis, idiopathic pulmonary fibrosis, emphysema or fibrosing lung diseases. By a rigorous and careful exploration of the biological and biochemical roles and sources of the chemotactic factors and complement components in lung tissue, we hope to obtain data that will have direct application to the problems of acute and chronic inflammatory lung disease in man.

REFERENCES

1.   Ward, P.A. In: Granulocyte Physiology Function and Dysfunction, ed. Beckman. American Association of Blood Banks (1979) 35.
2.   Kreutzer, D.L. et al. Clin Immunol Immunopathol 12 (1979) 162.
3.   Ward, P.A. et al. J Exp Med 122 (1965) 327.
4.   Showell, H.J. et al. J Exp Med 143 (1976) 1154.
5.   Fernandez, H.N. et al. J Immunol 120 (1978) 109.
6.   Schiffman, E. et al. Proc Natl Acad Sci USA 72 (1975) 1059.
7.   Kreutzer, D.L. et al. Immunopharmacol 1 (1979) 39.
8.   Tack, B.F.; Prahl, J.W. Biochemistry 15 (1976) 4513.
9.   Schreiber, R.D.; Müller-Eberhard, H.J. J Exp Med 140 (1974) 1324.
10. Krohn, K. et al. Biochem Biophys Acta 285 (1972) 404.
11. Kreutzer, D.L. et al. Chest 75 (1979) 259.
12. Desai, U. et al. Am J Pathol 96 (1979) 71.

13. Ward, P.A.; Hill, J.H. Proc Soc Exp Biol Med 141 (1972) 898.
14. Colten, H.R. Adv Immunol 22 (1976) 67.
15. Desai, U. et al. Am J Pathol (in press).

SECTION V

RESPONSES TO NON-VIRAL PATHOGENS

Chairpersons:

David A. Hart

John A. Shadduck

IMMUNE RESPONSE OF THE HAMSTER TO EXPERIMENTAL MYCOPLASMA PNEUMONIAE DISEASE

Wallace A. Clyde, Jr. and Gerald W. Fernald

Departments of Pediatrics and Bacteriology and
Immunology
University of North Carolina School of Medicine
Chapel Hill, NC   27514

INTRODUCTION

The Syrian hamster (Mesocricetus auratus) first was used for experimental Mycoplasma pneumoniae infections soon after the introduction of this species as a laboratory animal in the United States. Isolation of an infectious agent from patients with atypical pneumonia by intranasal inoculation of cotton rats (Sigmodon hispidus) with sputum samples was reported in 1942. Although unsuccessful for primary isolation of the agent, the hamster could be used for propagation of organisms recovered primarily in the cotton rat. Both animals developed pneumonitis in consequence of infection. Immune responses of patients and experimental hosts were demonstrated by the neutralization of sputum infectivity for animals following incubation of the inoculum with convalescent sera (2).

Identification of Eaton's agent as a mycoplasma (3-5), together with development of lifeless media for its propagation (6), provided the tools for further development of experimental models. Another report (7) explored use of the hamster in studies of infection produced with pure cultures grown in the laboratory. Delineation of the microbiologic and pathologic aspects of the experimental disease made possible a number of subsequent studies dealing with the immunologic responses of the hamster. This paper reviews and summarizes studies from our laboratories that form the basis of our current understanding of hamster immunity to experimental M. pneumoniae infection.

MATERIALS AND METHODS

Animals used were random-bred male Syrian hamsters obtained commercially. Unlike most small laboratory rodents, hamsters are not
known to harbor respiratory tract mycoplasmas, although we have encountered accidental M. pulmonis infection when animals were housed
in the same quarters with albino rats. The hamster appears susceptible to infection with a variety of M. pneumoniae strains. Representative organisms used in the studies to be summarized were strains
Bru (ATCC No. 15377), Mac (ATCC No. 15492), PI 104166 (8), M129-B7
(ATCC No. 29342) and M129-B169 (ATCC No. 29343). All strains were
propagated in Hayflick's medium (6), which consists of beef heart
infusion base (70%), horse serum (20%), aqueous extract of baker's
yeast (10%), and other additives including penicillin (1,000 U/ml),
dextrose (1%) and phenol red (0.002%). Solid media incorporated a
purified agar (0.85%) and omitted dextrose and phenol red.

Details of serologic methods employed have been described in
detail elsewhere. These include: the complement fixation test (8);
a chloroform-methanol extract of whole organisms used as antigen (9);
and a metabolic inhibition test (10) in which the ability of a set
dilution of antiserum to inhibit serially diluted organisms is
measured. Antibody classes reactive in the various serologic tests
were determined by separating whole serum on Sephadex G200 columns
or in sucrose gradients and testing fractions for their serologic reactions and characteristics by gel electrophoresis against rabbit
anti-hamster sera (8).

For special immuno-histologic studies, rabbit antisera to hamster IgG, IgA, and IgM were prepared and supplied by Dr. John Bienen-
stock (11). Antisera to hamster thymocytes were prepared in rabbits
as described elsewhere (12).

RESULTS AND DISCUSSION

The Hamster Model of M. pneumoniae Disease

After intranasal inoculation of anesthetized hamsters with virulent M. pneumoniae broth cultures, organisms replicate throughout the
respiratory tract. Maximum growth of the mycoplasma occurs by 10
days, but organisms persist in the lung tissue for four to six weeks.
Replication of the organisms is accompanied by the development of
histologic changes that reach their greatest intensity by 14 days
and usually clear before the lungs are sterilized. As in natural M.
pneumoniae disease, peribronchial cell infiltration occurs while the
periphery of the lung remains normal or is subject to subsegmental
areas of atelectasis. The peribronchial cells are predominantly mono-

nuclear, and endobronchial exudates are encountered frequently. The
exudate differs from the peribronchial infiltrates in that is consists of a mixture of polymorphonuclear cells and macrophages. The
bronchial epithelium at the interface of the cellular activity is the
site of infection. The mycoplasma, which in this instance is a 0.1
x 2 μm filament, can be visualized attached to the luminal borders of
both ciliated and non-ciliated epithelial cells as shown by electron
microscopy (13). The parasite is noninvasive, and determines the immunologic events to be described from this intimate, but superficial,
association with host cells.

Humoral Immune Response to Infection

      Various serologic techniques have been developed to measure anti-
bodies against M. pneumoniae. The most popular test in current clinical use is the complement fixation method, which employs a lipid antigen extracted from whole organisms with chloroform and methanol.
Another test with perhaps greater biologic significance is the metabolic inhibition reaction, in which the presence of antibody inhibits
glucose fermentation by the mycoplasma, resulting in prevention of an
acid pH shift in the growth medium. In the hamster, antibodies detectable by both procedures are generated beginning one week after
experimental infection, peaking at six to eight weeks, and persisting
at least six months.

      The immunoglobulins that constitute the hamster's antibody re-
sponse can be differentiated by conventional means. Serum globulin
fractions from Sephadex G200 columns can be tested for immunoglobulin
class by immunoelectrophoresis against hamster anti-globulin reagents
accompanied by tests of serologic reactivity. There is a transient
IgM response reflected by complement fixing activity between days 7
and 14 post-infection. The predominant response, however, is formation of IgG antibodies during the second and third weeks that mediate
both the complement fixing and metabolic inhibiting serologic reactions.

      Further delineation of the immunoglobulin response was obtained
by centrifugation of whole hamster sera through sucrose gradients and
serologic testing of fractions having various densities. Again, a
weak early IgM response that fixed complement was found. Globulin of
the 11S type, presumably IgA, failed to fix complement as expected
but produced metabolic inhibition. The prominence of IgG in complement fixation and metabolic inhibition was seen again in these experiments. When animals were hyper-immunized by vaccination followed by
a challenge infection, a more pronounced antibody response was produced, especially in the generation of IgM detectable by both serologic methods.

Immunopathologic Correlates in the Lung

Close inspection of the peribronchial infiltrates in infected hamster lungs reveals cells with the morphologic appearance of lymphocytes. Special stains, such as pyronin, indicate that many of the cells are rich in endoplasmic reticulum, suggesting that they are plasma cells. The cells were characterized further as to possible immunoglobulin content using the indirect immunofluorescence method with rabbit antisera specific for individual hamster immunoglobulins. The lymphocyte population reacted mainly with the anti-IgM and -IgG reagents. Scattered cells positive for IgA also were seen, although these were not increased in numbers or changed in distribution from those found in normal, uninfected hamsters.

These findings suggest that the peribronchial infiltrate constituting the pathologic changes of bronchopneumonia is, in fact, the morphologic evidence of host immune response to infection. This postulate was tested in another way by assessing the histologic changes occurring when animals were infected while receiving rabbit anti-hamster lymphocyte serum. In this case, the peribronchial lymphocytic response to infection was completely abrogated in comparison to infected control animals not given anti-thymocyte serum. Also, an associated difference occurred in the cellular composition of the endobronchial exudates. Only macrophages were seen in the bronchi of anti-lymphocyte serum-treated hamsters, while the control animals showed the expected polymorphonuclear leukocyte exudate. This could suggest that the serum used was not specifically suppressing only lymphocytes; however, since peripheral blood polymorphonuclear cells were present in normal numbers, while there was profound lymphopenia in treated animals, another explanation was needed.

Studies in vitro using guinea pig alveolar macrophages exposed to M. pneumoniae on glass coverslips have shown that phagocytosis of the mycoplasma is opsonin-dependent (14). Also, it has been shown that polymorphonuclear leukocytes require antibody and complement to interact with epithelial cells bearing mycoplasmas on their surfaces (15). The removal of the leukocytic part of the exudate by anti-lymphocyte serum thus could depend upon the absence of lymphocytes in the lung; this would eliminate or reduce production of antibody locally, and perhaps limit the role of lymphokines and activated complement as chemotactants to recruit leukocytes to the site of infection.

Nature of Protective Immunity

Humoral antibodies equivalent to those associated with experimental infection can be generated by injecting organisms into sites other than the respiratory tract, for example into the peritoneal cavity (16). With a series of injections, complement-fixing and

metabolic-inhibiting antibodies with titers of 32 to 64 can be
achieved with regularity in two to three weeks. There are marked differences, however, depending upon the strain of M. pneumoniae chosen
for immunization as well as use of different routes to introduce the
antigens. Intraperitoneal injections of fully virulent organisms
generally was more successful than injection via the subcutaneous,
footpad or intranasal routes. Use of attenuated (Mac strain) or
avirulent (M129-B169 strain) M. pneumoniae was found inferior in
stimulating antibodies when compared to fully virulent strains, such
as PI 104166.

The role of humoral antibody in protective immunity was assessed by first immunizing animals with the different methods described and then challenging them by intranasal inoculation of virulent organisms. The development of pneumonia was reduced by a third
to a half of that seen in non-immune control animals; the rate of infection was less affected by immunization. These results imply a protective effect of humoral antibody, but it is noteworthy that the
highest degree of protection was seen in hamsters immunized by prior
intranasal infection and allowed to recover before challenge inoculation.

While studies in humans have indicated that the presence of M.
pneumoniae-specific sIgA in nasal secretions is a better correlate
of protective immunity than is serum antibody (17), similar observations have not been made with hamsters. The results cited above on
the efficacy of prior infection in preventing re-infection suggest
that some mechanism local to the respiratory tract is important for
protection. Concentrated bronchial lavage fluid has been found to
be reactive in the metabolic inhibition test (18). The washings
failed to fix complement, suggesting that an immunoglobulin other
than IgM or IgG was involved. Absence of detectable albumin in the
lavage fluids suggests that the antibody was not derived by serum
transudation in the presence of inflammatory changes.

Other insights concerning protective immunity in the hamster
have been gleaned from comparison of infection and re-infection using
virulent and attenuated M. pneumoniae strains (15). The temporal
aspects of infection and pneumonia following virulent organism inoculation have been presented earlier. If inoculation of an avirulent
strain (M129-B169) is followed similarly, it can be shown that lung
infection persisting at least six weeks is produced, but this is not
accompanied by the development of peribronchial cellular infiltrates.
Further, avirulent organism infection fails to engender a serum antibody response, implying that the peribronchial cells could be a source
of the antibodies generated by virulent organisms. There are also no
endobronchial exudates of the type seen in virulent organism infection, although more macrophages are found in the airways than are
seen in normal animals.

After clearing avirulent M. pneumoniae infections, hamsters respond differently to virulent organism inoculation than do unprepared controls. The experienced animals could be re-infected readily with the same number of organisms to which normal animals were susceptible, but infection was cleared more rapidly (within two weeks). In contrast, it took 1,000-fold more organisms than expected to reproduce the pneumonia when the animals received virulent mycoplasma inoculation. Again, there is the implication that a protective mechanism local to the respiratory tract but not accompanied by any demonstrable host response has been stimulated by avirulent organism infection.

The foregoing suggests that the avirulent M. pneumoniae strain could provide a workable live vaccine candidate. Further studies on the infection-reinfection events, however, cast doubt on the wisdom of this approach. Hamsters were prepared as before by infection with avirulent organisms, which was allowed to clear. After challenge with the virulent strain, groups of animals then were killed at intervals up to 14 days, when maximal pulmonary lesions would be expected in inexperienced hamsters. The results showed that animals given avirulent organism infection prior to challenge developed the same pulmonary lesions as those not previously infected, but did so after three rather than 14 days. Thus, the initial avirulent organism infection appeared to promote rather than prevent the occurrence of pneumonia by accelerating the time of appearance of histologic changes. If, as suggested earlier, the pulmonary infiltrates are the morphologic aspects of host immune response, the accelerated pneumonia could be seen as the morphologic evidence of immune recall.

While it may seem difficult to synthesize the material that has been presented into a unified concept of the pathogenesis of M. pneumoniae disease, consideration should be given to the possibility that immunopathologic events are involved. Observations of natural human disease are compatible with this concept (19). Infections of infants and young children with M. pneumoniae have been documented repeatedly, but the peak incidence of pneumonia due to this organism is at age 10 years, by which time the opportunity for several reinfections has occurred. As discussed earlier, repeated infection in hamsters appears to hasten the time at which pulmonary lesions are seen. Several M. pneumoniae infections without demonstrable pulmonary infiltrates have been documented in immuno-deficient patients, providing a counterpart of the hamster response during anti-lymphocyte serum treatment. Further evidence of immunopathologic events is suggested by the occurrence of various non-respiratory tract complications of the disease; organisms are not recovered from these distant sites. The occurrence of what could be considered auto-antibodies in many patients adds other suggestive evidence.

The hamster as an experimental model of M. pneumoniae disease has provided many pieces of information concerning the interaction between host and parasite, especially in relation to the immunologic aspects. As with any experimental model, it is not possible to translate the results literally to the human condition; nevertheless, new hypotheses are generated that can be tested in clinical research. Notice should be taken of the major contribution the hamster has made to our current understanding of M. pneumoniae disease.

REFERENCES

1. Eaton, M.D. et al. Science 96 (1942) 518.
2. Eaton, M.D. et al. J Exp Med 79 (1944) 649.
3. Marmion, B.P.; Goodburn, G.M. Nature 189 (1961) 247.
4. Clyde, W.A., Jr. Proc Soc Exp Biol Med 107 (1961) 716.
5. Chanock, R.M. et al. Proc Natl Acad Sci USA 48 (1962) 41.
6. Hayflick, L. Tex Rep Biol Med 23 (1965) 285.
7. Dejani, A.S. et al. J Exp Med 121 (1965) 1071.
8. Fernald, G.W. J Infect Dis 119 (1969) 255.
9. Kenny, G.E.; Grayston, J.T. J Immunol 95 (1965) 19.
10. Fernald, G.W. et al. Proc Soc Exp Biol Med 126 (1967) 161.
11. Fernald, G.W. et al. J Immunol 98 (1972) 1028.
12. Taylor, G. et al. J Med Microbiol 7 (1974) 343.
13. Collier, A.M.; Clyde, W.A., Jr. Am Rev Respir Dis 110 (1974) 765.
14. Powell, D.A.; Clyde, W.A., Jr. Infect Immun 11 (1975) 540.
15. Clyde, W.A., Jr. Infect Immun 4 (1971) 757.
16. Fernald, G.W.; Clyde, W.A., Jr. Infect Immun 1 (1970) 559.
17. Brunner, H. et al. Infect Immun 9 (1973) 612.
18. Fernald, G.W. In: The Secretary Immunologic System. U.S. Dept. of Health, Education and Welfare, Washington, D.C. (1969) 215.
19. Fernald, G.W.; Clyde, W.A., Jr. In: Immunologic and Infectious Reactions in the Lung, ed. Kirkpatrick and Reynolds. Dekker, New York (1976) 101.

HEMADSORPTION AND VIRULENCE OF MYCOPLASMA PNEUMONIAE

Eric J. Hansen, Richard M. Wilson and Joel B. Baseman

Department of Microbiology, University of Texas Health
Science Center at Dallas, Dallas, TX 75235 and
Department of Bacteriology and Immunology,
University of North Carolina, Chapel Hill, NC 27514

INTRODUCTION

Mycoplasma pneumoniae is a prokaryotic respiratory tract pathogen of man which causes cold agglutinin-associated primary atypical
pneumonia. Although relatively little is known about the properties
of this organism that endow it with pathogenicity for man, the use
of a hamster model system established that the ability of M. pneumoniae
to adhere to respiratory tract epithelium is a critical virulence determinant for this pathogen (1,2). Virulent strains of M. pneumoniae,
in addition to being capable of adhering to respiratory epithelium,
also form colonies on solidified growth medium that readily adsorb
erythrocytes of many different species, in a process called hemadsorption (3). It has been established that trypsin treatment of virulent
M. pneumoniae colonies eliminated the hemadsorption ability of these
colonies (4). Previous studies from our own laboratory have established that trypsin-sensitive proteinaceous structures on the exter-
nal membrane surface of virulent strain cells of M. pneumoniae are involved in the attachment of this parasite to host respiratory epithelium (5). It has been shown further that a homologous avirulent strain
of M. pneumoniae that does not attach to respiratory epithelium in
vitro also forms hemadsorption-negative colonies (6). All of these
data taken together suggested that M. pneumoniae might utilize the
same mechanism(s) for both hemadsorption and attachment to respiratory
epithelium. In order to evaluate the relationship of the hemadsorption process to both respiratory epithelium attachment capability and
virulence of M. pneumoniae, we employed a mutant analysis approach in
conjunction with a hamster model system.

MATERIALS AND METHODS

The virulent wild-type M. pneumoniae strain used in this study was M129-B16, which has been thoroughly characterized and described previously (5,6). The homologous avirulent strain M129-B181 was derived from M129-B16 by 165 consecutive broth passages (6). Hemadsorption-negative mutants were produced by chemical mutagenesis and were identified by means of a hemadsorption test performed with chick erythrocytes (7). All mycoplasma cultures were grown at 37°C in liquid Hayflick medium (6) in 32-oz. prescription bottles or on solidified Hayflick medium containing 1.5% Noble agar (Difco). Two-dimensional non-equilibrium pH gradient gel electrophoresis of mycoplasma total cell proteins was performed as described (8).

Tracheal organ culture methods used in this study were described previously (5). Adherence of mycoplasmas to respiratory epithelium was quantitated by incubating [methyl-^{3}H]-thymidine-labelled mycoplasmas with hamster tracheal rings (2). Infection of hamsters with mycoplasmas was accomplished by instilling 10^6 mycoplasmas in 100 µl Hayflick medium into the anterior nares of anesthetized, supine animals (9). The severity of the resultant histologic pneumonia in these animals was scored by previously published methods (9).

RESULTS AND DISCUSSION

Hemadsorption-negative (HA$^-$) mutants of M. pneumoniae were isolated by the following protocol. Logarithmic phase cells of the virulent wild-type parent strain M129-B16 were mutagenized by a 30-minute exposure to N-methyl-N'-nitro-N-nitrosoguanidine at a final concentration of 25 µg/ml in pH 6.7 phosphate-buffered saline (PBS) (7). The surviving cells (5% of the original population) were washed thoroughly with PBS and then a portion of these cells was inoculated into Hayflick medium. After 96 hours of incubation of 37°C, the culture was diluted and plated on solidified Hayflick medium. The resultant colonies were screened for their hemadsorption characteristics, and HA$^-$ colonies were found to comprise about 1% of the total population (Fig. 1). Ten HA$^-$ colonies were cloned by four repeated single colony isolations (7), and four of the resultant purified clones were found to be still hemadsorption-negative, thus suggesting that the other six colonies were actually phenotypic variants. Two of the HA$^-$ clones (strains HA1 and HA2) were chosen for further study.

Analysis of the ability of these HA$^-$ mutants to attach to respiratory epithelium in vitro involved incubation of [methyl-^{3}H]-thymidine-labelled mycoplasmas with hamster tracheal rings (2). Neither mutant strain HA1 nor mutant strain HA2 could adhere to respiratory epithelium in vitro at as great a frequency as that exhibited by the wild-type parent strain M129-B16, although strain HA2 apparently possessed a greater attachment capability than strain HA1 (Table 1).

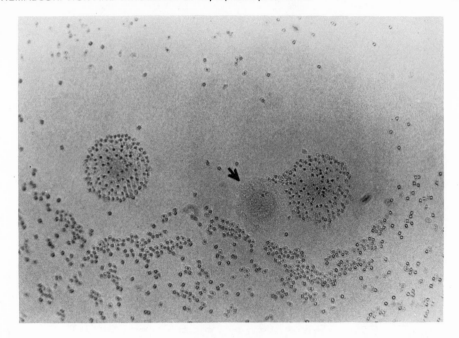

Fig. 1:   Photomicrograph of hemadsorption-positive and hemadsorption-
           negative colonies of M. pneumoniae in a hemadsorption test.
           The arrow indicates a hemadsorption-negative mutant colony
           devoid of adherent erythrocytes. The other two colonies
           are hemadsorption-positive colonies of the virulent wild-
           type parent strain, covered with adherent erythrocytes.

Both of these HA⁻ mutants, however, adhered to tracheal ring respiratory epithelium at frequencies higher than that exhibited by the avirulent M129-B181 strain, which is both hemadsorption-negative (6) and
incapable of attaching to respiratory epithelium in vitro at a frequency significantly greater than the "background level" of adherence
obtained when wild-type M. pneumoniae cells are incubated with tracheal rings at 4°C (Table 1). These data indicate that the loss of hemad
sorption capability adversely affects, but does not totally eliminate,
 the ability of M. pneumoniae to attach to respiratory epithelium in
vitro.

    Previous studies in this laboratory showed that two-dimensional
gel electrophoresis of mycoplasma total cell proteins is an exquisite-
ly sensitive method for resolving minor protein differences between
mycoplasma strains (8). Accordingly, we next employed two-dimensional
non-equilibrium pH gradient gel electrophoresis of total cell proteins

Table 1. Adherence of Wild-Type and Mutant Strains of M. pneumoniae to Tracheal Rings

Strain	CFU[1] added to ring	CPM added to ring	CFU attached to ring	CPM attached to ring	% attachment
M129-B16	4.1×10^7	21,251	3.8×10^6	1976	9.3
M129-B181	8.0×10^7	26,459	1.4×10^6	476	1.8
HA1	7.4×10^7	24,291	1.7×10^6	558	2.3
HA2	6.1×10^7	19,864	3.6×10^6	1191	6.0
HA1-R	6.2×10^7	22,426	5.0×10^6	1838	8.2
M129-B16/Incubated at 4°C	4.1×10^7	21,251	4.9×10^5	755	1.2

[1]Colony-forming units.

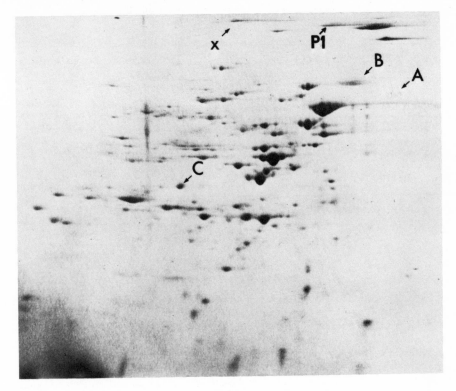

Fig. 2:   Two-dimensional non-equilibrium pH gradient gel of total
          cell proteins from the virulent wild-type parent strain
          (M129-B16) of M. pneumoniae. The acidic end of the gel is
          on the right, the basic end is on the left, and proteins of
          decreasing molecular weight run from the top to the bottom
          of the gel. Proteins A, B, and C are not synthesized by
          mutant strain HA1; protein X is not synthesized by mutant
          strain HA2. Protein P1 has been implicated in the adher-
          ence of M. pneumoniae to respiratory epithelium (5).

from the virulent wild-type strain M129-B16, the avirulent strain
M129-B181, and the HA⁻ mutant strains HA1 and HA2 to determine whether
the HA⁻ mutants differed from either the parent strain or one another
in terms of protein content. Fig. 2 depicts a two-dimensional non-
equilibrium pH gradient gel of total cell proteins from the virulent
wild-type parent strain M129-B16; the proteins of importance to this
investigation are labelled appropriately in this figure. The protein
content of the different strains, as determined by two-dimensional gel
electrophoresis, is summarized in Table 2. Mutant strain HA1 differed
from both the parent strain and mutant strain HA2 by its lack of the
virulent strain-specific proteins A, B and C (8) and in this regard

Table 2.   Protein Composition of Wild-Type and Mutant Strains of $\underline{M}$.
           pneumoniae

Strain	Protein A	Protein B	Protein C	Protein X	Protein P1
M129-B16	+[1]	+	+	+	+
M129-B181	-[2]	-	-	+	+
HA1	-	-	-	+	+
HA2	+	+	+	-	+
HA1-R	+	+	+	+	+

[1]Presence of protein.

[2]Absence of protein.

is apparently identical to the avirulent strain (Table 2). In contrast,
mutant strain HA2 differed from the wild-type parent strain by its
lack of a single high molecular weight protein, designated X in Fig. 2.
Mutant strains HA1 and HA2 thus represent two different classes of HA⁻
mutant, as defined by respiratory epithelium attachment ability (Table
1) and protein composition (Table 2). Neither of the HA⁻ mutant strains
lacked protein P1 (Table 2), which has been implicated previously in
the binding of $\underline{M}$. pneumoniae to respiratory epithelium (5).

In order to gain information about the potential relationship of
hemadsorption to the $\underline{M}$. pneumoniae infectious process, we next examined the HA⁻ mutants for their virulence potential and found that
these HA⁻ mutants did not survive well in vivo, relative to the virulent wild-type parent strain. When 10^6 colony-forming units each of
the virulent parent strain M129-B16, the homologous avirulent strain
M129-B181, and the HA⁻ mutant strains HA1 and HA2 were used to infect
hamsters via an intranasal inoculation method, the virulent parent
strain grew and persisted at relatively high levels in the lungs of
infected animals over the 28-day experimental period (Fig. 3). In contrast, colony-forming units of the HA⁻ mutant strains HA1 and HA2 were
not detectable within the lungs of infected hamsters at either 7, 14
21 or 28 days post-infection. It must be noted, however, that certain
substances in concentrated hamster lung homogenates drastically reduce
the plating efficiency of $\underline{M}$. pneumoniae, resulting in a lower limit of
detectability of 10^3 colony-forming units of $\underline{M}$. pneumoniae per gram of
lung tissue (10). The avirulent M129-B181 strain persisted at readily
detectable levels in the lungs of infected animals for at least seven
days post-infection, and was present just at the threshold of detection
in random infected animals up to 28 days post-infection.

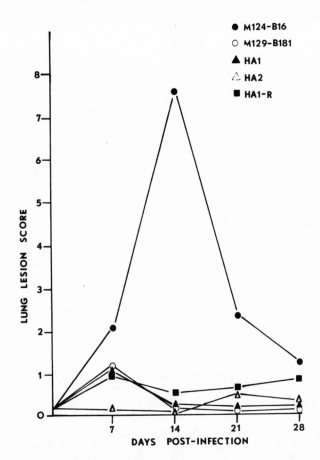

Fig. 3:   Survival and growth of wild-type and mutant M. pneumoniae
           strains in hamster lungs. 10^6 colony-forming units of each
           mycoplasma strain were used to infect twelve animals intra-
           nasally. Lungs were removed from the animals at the speci-
           fied times, homogenized with sand in Hayflick medium, and
           serial dilutions of the homogenates were plated on Hayflick
           agar plates. Each point on the graph represents the mean
           titer from three animals.

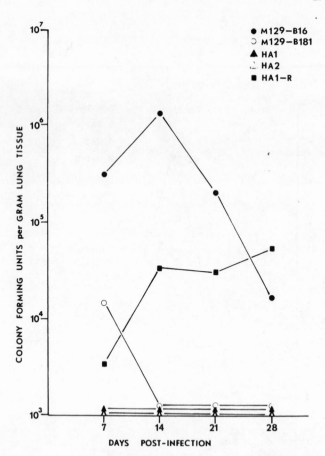

Fig. 4: Virulence of wild-type and mutant M. pneumoniae strains for
         hamsters. Histologic pneumonia was evaluated in sections
         prepared from formalin-fixed lung tissue obtained from the
         animals described in Fig. 3. Each point represents the
         mean lung lesion score from three animals.

This lack of extensive growth of the HA⁻ mutants in hamster lungs
was reflected by the occurrence of little or no histologic pneumonia
in the animals infected with these mutants (Fig. 4). Hamsters infected
with the virulent wild-type parent strain M129-B16 developed a histologic pneumonia, characterized by peribronchial round cell infiltration with or without an intraluminal polymorphonuclear exudate (9),
which peaked at two weeks post-infection and then gradually resolved
itself over the next two weeks (Fig. 4). In contrast, neither the
avirulent strain M129-B181 nor either of the HA⁻ mutant strains caused
any significant degree of histologic pneumonia over the course of the
experimental period.

The preceding data suggested, but did not prove, that the loss of hemadsorption capability resulted in significant alterations of both the physiology and virulence of M. pneumoniae. Elimination of the possibility that these changes were caused by an undetected secondary mutation required the isolation and characterization of a hemadsorption-positive revertant of a hemadsorption-negative mutant. Accordingly, a selective enrichment technique was devised for this purpose:

10^9 colony-forming units of the HA$^-$ mutant strains HA1 and HA2 were incubated independently with chick erythrocytes for 30 minutes at 37°C to allow adherence of any spontaneously-occurring hemadsorption-positive revertants in the mycoplasma populations. These cell suspensions then were layered onto 20% Hypaque/0.5% Methocel gradients and spun at 600 x g for 20 minutes to separate the erythrocytes and any adherent mycoplasmas from the hemadsorption-negative mycoplasmas. The resultant erythrocyte pellets were washed three times and were then inoculated into liquid Hayflick medium to permit growth of any mycoplasmas present in these pellets. This entire procedure, consisting of the adherence step followed by gradient centrifugation and subsequent growth of erythrocyte-adherent mycoplasmas in Hayflick medium, was repeated three more times in sequence, and the final mycoplasma cultures were plated on solidified Hayflick medium.

When mutant strain HA1 was employed in the above procedure, hemadsorption-positive colonies were found to comprise 50% of the resultant "selectively enriched" mycoplasma population. In contrast, no hemadsorption-positive revertants of mutant strain HA2 could be obtained by this method, suggesting that a single very stable genetic lesion or multiple genetic lesions are responsible for the HA$^-$ phenotype of strain HA2. Several of the hemadsorption-positive (HA$^+$) revertants derived from the HA$^-$ mutant strain HA1 were cloned by repeated single colony isolations, and one of these HA$^+$ revertants (strain HA1-R) was chosen randomly for characterization in the following experiments.

In contrast to the HA$^-$ mutant strain HA1, the HA$^+$ revertant strain HA1-R could adhere to respiratory epithelium in vitro at a frequency very similar to that shown by the virulent parent strain (Table 1). Autoradiographic studies have confirmed that, like the virulent parent strain, the HA$^+$ revertant strain HA1-R attaches to the luminal surface of the epithelial cells of the tracheal ring (data not shown). Therefore, in addition to regaining hemadsorption capability, this revertant strain also has regained the ability to adhere to respiratory epithelium in vitro at normal wild-type frequencies. Examination of the protein content of the HA$^+$ revertant strain HA1-R by two-dimensional non-equilibrium pH gradient gel electrophoresis showed that this HA$^+$ revertant also had regained the ability to synthesize the three virulent parent strain-specific proteins which are not synthesized by the hemadsorption-negative mutant strain HA1 (Table 2). Therefore, the genetic event(s) that resulted in the restoration of hemadsorption capability and respiratory epithelium attachment ability

in this HA$^+$ revertant also simultaneously conferred upon this strain
the ability to synthesize these three proteins normally found in the
virulent wild-type parent strain.   This finding implies that these
three proteins are structurally or functionally involved in both the
hemadsorption process and respiratory epithelium attachment by M.
pneumoniae. Although the exact cellular function(s) of these three
proteins is not known at this time, lactoperoxidase-catalyzed radioiodination experiments have established that protein B is exposed on
the mycoplasma cell surface (8).

Characterization of the virulence of the HA$^+$ revertant in the
hamster model system established that this revertant also had regained
the ability to survive and replicate in vivo. In contrast to the results obtained with the HA$^-$ mutant strain HA1, colony-forming units of
the HA$^-$ revertant strain HA1-R could be readily detected in the lungs
of infected animals at seven days post-infection, and these numbers
increased gradually over the course of the experimental period (Fig.
3). Despite the fact that this HA$^+$ revertant could survive and replicate in vivo, however, this revertant was still unable to cause significant histologic pneumonia in hamsters (Fig. 4).

The avirulence of this HA$^+$ revertant indicates that hemadsorption
capability and respiratory epithelium attachment ability can be separated genetically from virulence in M. pneumoniae. The actual basis
for the lack of virulence of the HA$^-$ revertant strain HA1-R is not
clear at this time. The fact that this HA$^+$ revertant persists in the
lungs of infected animals at somewhat lower levels than the virulent
wild-type parent strain suggests that this hemadsorption-positive revertant might carry a secondary mutation affecting the ability of
this revertant to survive and replicate in vivo. If this is true,
then this particular HA$^+$ revertant strain will be a valuable tool in
the analysis of the virulence mechanisms employed by M. pneumoniae in
the production of respiratory tract disease. In addition, this particular HA$^+$ revertant strain may be useful as an attenuated vaccine,
since the low level of growth of the avirulent organisms in the lung
would provide a sustained antigenic stimulus to the immune response
system. Animal protection experiments employing this HA$^+$ revertant
as a vaccinogen are currently in progress.

ACKNOWLEDGMENTS

The work was supported by the U.S. Army Medical Research and Development Command, under research contract DAD-17-73-C-3097; National
Heart, Lung and Blood Institute, Specialized Center of Research, under
grant no. HI-19171, and research career development award 1-KO4-AI-
00178 from the National Institute of Allergy and Infectious Diseases
to J.B. Baseman. The authors wish to thank Daisi Marcoulides for secretarial assistance in the preparation of this manuscript.

REFERENCES

1. Collier, A.M.; Baseman, J.B. Ann NY Acad Sci 225 (1973) 277.
2. Powell, D.A. et al. Infect Immun 13 (1976) 959.
3. Manchee, R.J.; Taylor-Robinson, D. J Gen Microbiol 50 (1968) 465.
4. Sobeslavsky, O. et al. J Bacteriol 96 (1968) 695.
5. Hu, P.C. et al. J Exp Med 145 (1977) 1328.
6. Lipman, R.P. et al. J Bacteriol 100 (1969) 1037.
7. Hansen, E.J. et al. Infect Immun 23 (1979) 903.
8. Hansen, E.J. et al. Infect Immun 24 (1979) 468.
9. Clyde, W.A., Jr. Infect Immun 4 (1971) 757.
10. Jemski, J.V. et al. Infect Immun 16 (1977) 93.

EXPERIMENTAL FILARIASIS IN THE SYRIAN HAMSTER; IMMUNOLOGICAL

ASPECTS OF COMPLEX HOST-PARASITE INTERACTIONS

Niklaus Weiss and Marcel Tanner

Swiss Tropical Institute, Department of Medicine,
Socinstrasse 53, CH-4051   Basel, Switzerland

INTRODUCTION

The Syrian hamster has been introduced as an experimental host
for a large number of infective agents such as viruses, bacteria, protozoa and helminths (1). Only a few researchers, however, have used
hamster models to study filarial infections. This is not surprising,
since filariae, tissue-dwelling nematodes, are known as highly host-
specific parasites of vertebrates and their life cycle can only be completed by selected arthropod vectors. A limited number of filarial
species develop in man; some can cause severe disease such as lymphatic filariasis, loiasis and onchocerciasis.

Dipetalonema viteae is a filarial parasite of gerbils and is cy-
clically transmitted by ticks (2). The Syrian hamster has been successfully infected with this parasite (3) and the course of infection
has been compared with the natural host (2). Other filarial species
such as Brugia pahangi or Litomosoides carinii are less easily adapted
to hamsters, as indicated by very low worm recovery rates (4,5).

The characteristics of D. viteae infection in the hamster are
summarized in Fig. 1 and Table 1. Infective third-stage larvae develop within six weeks, through a fourth larval stage, to fertile
adult male and female worms (= prepatent period). This development
includes two moults, processes during which the acellular "exoskele-
ton" of the worm, the cuticle, is shed and replaced by a newly synthesized one. The adult worms are found mainly in superficial connective
tissues. Female worms are viviparous. The first-stage larvae, the
microfilariae (MF), develop within the uterus, are subsequently released, and enter the bloodstream. Microfilaremia starts at about
seven weeks post-infection (PI) and in most hamsters, in contrast to
the natural host, is transient (= patent period). The susceptibility

253

Table 1. <u>Dipetalonema viteae</u> Infections in the Syrian Hamster

---

1. Larval development comparable to the natural host, but greater
   susceptibility with high individual variations.[1,2,4]
2. Adult worm size and duration of embryogenesis as in natural
   hosts. [1,2,3]
3. Life-long infection with no obvious, marked lesions.[1,2,6]
4. Transient microfilaremia.[2]
5. Duration of microfilaremia independent of the number of female
   worms.[4]
6. Adult worm recovery and duration of microfilaremia varies between
   different hamster strains (cf. Table 2).[4,5]

---

[1](3), [2](2), [3](32), [4](7), [5](6), [6](11).

to infection and the duration of microfilaremia show great individual
variability and depend on the hamster strain (6,7). For example, the
LSH strain (LSH/SsLak) is more susceptible to infection, as indicated
by a higher worm recovery and a significantly longer microfilaremia
when compared to the randomly-bred LAKZ strain (Table 2). Splenectomy
prior to infection has no influence on the recovery of adult worms nor
on the duration of microfilaremia (Table 2).

During a <u>D. viteae</u> infection, the hamster's immune system is con-
fronted with a great variety of antigens which can be classified
roughly into three groups (Table 3). Somatic antigens are released
from dying larvae and adult worms. Metabolites are excreted from the

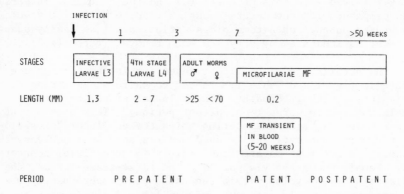

Fig. 1: Timing and course of a <u>D. viteae</u> infection in the Syrian
         hamster.

alimentary tract and from the excretory system of developing larvae and adult worms. Excretory/secretory products are known as especially potent antigens. This has been shown for uterine secretions of D. viteae (8). In addition, embryogenesis results not only in viable MF but also in a mass of highly antigenic egg-materials (egg sheathes, unfertilized eggs; [7]). Antibodies to all these antigens can be detected during early prepatency before oogenesis has started or after immunization with dead infective larvae. These results indicate that many antigens are similar or identical to the various life stages of D. viteae (= "common antigens"). But stage-specific antigens also can be detected in the cuticles of the different worm stages (9). Their role will be discussed below.

During the course of infection, the antigen load increases steadily because of larval development and reproduction. Each female worm releases several thousand MF daily. From week 20 PI on, the number of adult worms decreases (whether by natural death or immune reaction is unknown), and worms become calcified and disintegrate. This can be associated with nodule formation in hyperinfected hamsters (10,11).

Table 2. Adult Worm Recovery and Mean Duration of Microfilaremia in Relation to the Infection Dose and the Strain of Hamster (after [7]).

	LSH/SsLak		LAKZ	
	50 L3	150 L3	150 L3	150 L3 SPL
Adult worm recovery (%)[1]				
week 8-12 PI	60 ± 22	79 ± 10	46 ± 9	ND
week 30 PI	40 ± 4	17 ± 4	39 ± 7	42 ± 8
% postpatent at week 30 PI	75	66	96	88
Microfilaremia (weeks)[1]	14 ± 2	14 ± 2	9 ± 1	9 ± 1
Peak microfilaremia [2]	125	480	120	580
	(100/160)	(355/675)	(95/155)	(370/890)

[1]Arithmetic mean ± standard error.

[2]Geometric mean (± standard deviation).

L3 = infective third-stage larvae, SPL = splenectomized, PI = post infection, ND = not done.

IMMUNE RESPONSES TO FILARIAL INFECTION

For a first analysis of immune responses during filarial infection, whole phosphate-buffered-saline extracts from male or female
worms were used. These antigens allow the detection of specific cellular responses from week 1 PI, and of antibodies from week 2 PI on.
During early infection no antibodies against the surface of infective
larvae can be detected. Various serological methods such as passive
hemagglutination, gel diffusion, and immuno-electrophoresis revealed
increasing amounts of antibodies and more precipitating antibodies
during the first three months of infection. The indirect immunofluorescent antibody test (IFAT) on frozen sections of male or female
worms (Fig. 2) shows similar results. With all these techniques, however, we are unable to detect any differences between sera from patent
and postpatent hamsters.

D. viteae infections induce marked changes in the serum immunoglobulin levels: a 10- to 20-fold increase of IgG_1, a 2- to 3-fold increase of IgM, whereas there is no or only a slight increase in IgG_2
(C. Crandall, personal communication). IgG_1 hypergammaglobulinemia
is also seen in mice infected with helminths (12).

Homocytotropic antibodies are detected from week 4 PI on by early
footpad swelling reactions which become more prominent later in infection. Adult worm extracts also induce histamine release from peritoneal exudate cells, particularly in late infections (Weiss, unpublished observations). First evidence for the existence of the IgE immunoglobulin class in the hamster has been presented recently (13).
Whether such antibodies are produced during a D. viteae infection is
not yet known. Rats inoculated with D. viteae larvae produce highly
elevated (up to 200-fold) IgE serum levels from the third week PI on-
wards (14).

Table 3. Schematic Classification of Filarial Antigens Based on
          Investigations with the Dipetalonema viteae-Hamster Model[1-5]

	Filarial antigens		
	Somatic	Metabolic*	Cuticle
Common	+	+	−
Stage-specific	−	?	+

* Excretory/secretory antigens.

[1](33), [2](34), [3](7), [4](20), [5](9).

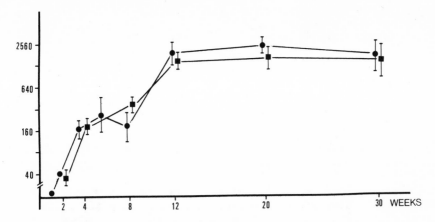

Fig. 2:   Humoral immune response during the course of a primary D.
          viteae infection with 150 larvae in LAKZ (●) and in LSH/
          SsLak hamsters (■). Reciprocal geometric mean titres ±
          standard deviation, indirect immunofluorescent antibody test
          on frozen sections of adult worms as antigen (after [7]).

    In vitro blastogenesis of spleen and lymph node cells to PHA and
filarial antigens has been analyzed intensively (15). Briefly, maximal lymphocyte responses are induced with soluble worm antigens during
the prepatent period (Fig. 3). Interestingly, no difference can be
detected between male and female worm extracts. Although these antigens are not mitogenic at the concentrations tested (1 and 5 µg), lymphocyte stimulation is almost as high as with PHA (1% to 2.5%). Whether
a polyclonal stimulation by these complex mixtures of antigens accounts for this phenomenon, or whether, in addition, unprimed cells
are trans-stimulated (16) during the five days of culture, cannot be
determined at the moment. Since the same filarial antigens do not
elicit delayed hypersensitivity reactions after foot-pad injections,
one wonders about the cell types involved in lymphocyte blastogenesis
in vitro. During patency, lymphocyte transformation to filarial antigens is highly variable, but cannot be correlated to parasitological parameters such as worm burden or intensity of microfilaremia.
At week 30 PI all lymphocyte cultures from LAKZ hamsters are unreactive to filarial antigens, whereas cultures from three out of eight
LSH hamsters can still be stimulated (Fig. 3). For both hamster
strains, however, lymphocyte reactivity cannot be correlated with the
ability to control circulating MF. Sera, but not lymph node cells,
from unreactive LAKZ hamsters (week 30 PI) can abolish the early
blastogenic response to filarial antigens. Further work is needed to
determine whether an antibody-mediated B suppressor modality is responsible for the observed unresponsiveness. Lymphocyte reactivity
is not restored after a challenge infection.

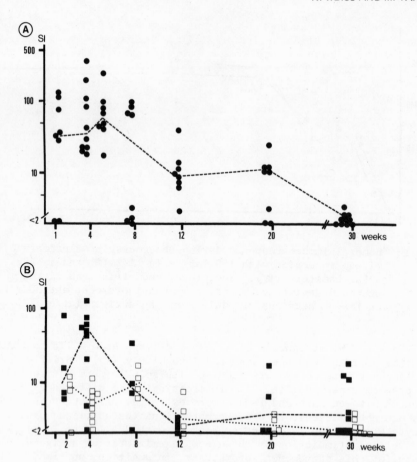

Fig. 3: Blastogenic responses of lymph node cells (●, ■) and spleen
         cells (□) to 5 µg female antigen per culture during the
         course of a primary <u>D. viteae</u> infection in LAKZ (A) and LSH/
         SsLak (B) hamsters. Symbols represent individual stimula-
         tion indexes (SI), and curves connect the medians of log SI
         of the different groups of hamsters (after [20]).

IMMUNOCOMPETENCE DURING INFECTION

    While the humoral immune response to filarial antigens remains
high during chronic infection (Fig. 2), the cellular response is obviously depressed (Fig. 3). The question arises whether chronic filariasis in the hamster leads to a generalized immunodepression. Analyzing our own results (summarized in Table 4), we can conclude that
cellular unresponsiveness is restricted to filarial antigens. A spe-

cific unresponsiveness to filarial antigens also was demonstrated in chronic lymphatic human filariasis (17) and in Brugia malayi-infected jirds (Kwa and Mak, personal communication). It is known that humoral immune responses are more often depressed in parasitized animals (18). When primary and secondary immune responses to sheep red blood cells (SRBC) are analyzed, however, no significant changes in hemagglutinin titres are detected in infected compared to normal hamsters (Fig. 4). This is in contrast to preliminary findings of other workers (19): after a single injection of SRBC, the mean number of plaque-forming cells (PFC) per 10^6 spleen cells was reduced significantly (44%) in D. viteae-infected hamsters (week 10 PI) compared to uninfected controls. No differences were found during the prepatent period. The marked splenomegaly, however, particularly associated with microfilaremia (20) was ignored by these authors. The absolute number of PFC in enlarged spleens might even be higher during microfilaremia. Humoral immune responses to certain antigens may be depressed, however (schistosomal antigens, see Table 4).

IMMUNITY TO MICROFILARIAE

When immune responses of D. viteae-infected hamsters are followed by use of common antigens, no correlation with parasitological findings becomes evident (Fig. 2,3). The transient microfilaremia observed in most hamsters (Table 1,2) has turned out to represent an acquired immunity to MF (cf. Table 5). Immunity to MF seems to be T-dependent, as neonatally thymectomized hamsters can also suppress microfilaremia and raise anti-cuticle antibodies to MF (7). Passive transfer experiments also have shown that spleen cell populations depleted of Ig$^+$ cells fail to induce immunity to MF (21). Researchers who worked with CBA/N mice recently supported the T-independent nature of the immunity to MF (22).

The appearance of serum antibodies to the cuticle of MF, as demonstrated by IFAT on intact MF in suspension, correlates with the suppression of microfilaremia (7; Table 5). This correlation raises questions concerning the effector mechanisms involved in the obvious ability of the host to overcome the daily MF output (several thousand MF per female per day). In vitro assays (23,24) and in vivo experiments using micropore chambers of 0.45-µm and 3.0-µm pore size (15) have clearly indicated that the killing and subsequent destruction of MF is initiated by an antibody-dependent cell-mediated mechanism (cf. Table 6). MF destruction occurs in less than 24 hours.

Antibodies along, or in combination with complement, do not affect MF in vitro or in vivo (in 0.45-µm micropore chambers), although the MF/antibody complex can activate complement (25).

Interestingly, the anti-cuticle antibody which collaborates with the various effector cells is of the IgM class, as evidenced by gel

Table 4. Immunocompetence of Syrian Hamsters During a Dipetalonema
          viteae Infection

LAKZ strain: 1. Blastogenic response of lymph node cells to
                          PHA unchanged during infection.[1]
                      2. One-way MLR to rabbit leukocytes unaffected
                          during patency and postpatency.[2]
                      3. Blastogenic response of lymph node cells to
                          soluble egg antigens of Schistosoma mansoni
                          unaffected in mixed infections.[1]
                      4. Humoral response to schistosomal antigens de-
                          pressed in mixed infections.[1]
                      5. Primary and secondary responses to SRBC
                          unaffected (Fig. 4).

LSH/SsLak strain: 1. Blastogenic responses of lymph node and
                          spleen cells to PHA unaffected during pre-
                          patency and early patency. In later infec-
                          tion some animals with depressed response,
                          but no correlation with parasitology
                          findings.[1]
                      2. One-way MLR to rabbit leukocytes unaffected
                          during patency and postpatency.[2]

[1] (20), [2] (35).

filtration, and by its 2-mercaptoethanol sensitivity and heat stability (Table 6). Even one year after infection, there is no switch
to the production of anti-cuticle antibodies of the IgG class. This
may be explained on the basis of the T-independent nature of cuticle
antigens rather than on the basis of the hamster's inability to switch
effectively from IgM to IgG synthesis (26). Unfortunately, biochemical data on cuticle antigens of MF are lacking.

Macrophages, neutrophils and eosinophils from mice, rats and
humans in collaboration with IgG and IgE are involved in the antibody-dependent cell-mediated killing of various helminths (e.g.
schistosomulae and Trichinella larvae). For the first time, in the
D. viteae-hamster model, there is clear evidence for an IgM-dependent
cell-mediated killing of helminths. The cuticle-specific IgM collaborates with polymorphonuclear, as well as with mononuclear, cells even
in the absence of complement (cf. Table 6). These latter findings
raise questions concerning the set of receptors displayed on the surface of these hamster cells.

IMMUNITY TO DEVELOPING LARVAL STAGES

Having realized the key role of anti-cuticle antibodies in the
phenomenon of immunity to MF, one is tempted to search for analogous

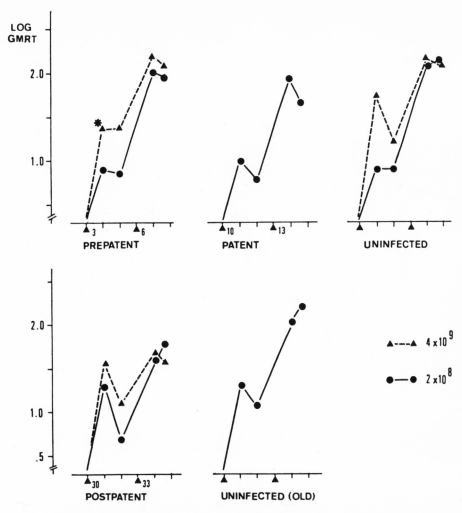

Fig. 4:   Primary and secondary immune responses to sheep red blood
          cells (SRBC) in uninfected, age-matched hamsters and in D.
          viteae-infected LAKZ hamsters. Reciprocal geometric mean
          hemagglutinin titres at different time of infection (weeks
          post-infection) following the injection (↑) of 4×10^9
          (▲ --- ▲) or 2×10^8 (●——●) SRBC.   * $2P < 0.01$.

mechanisms acting against the developing larval stages. D. viteae-
infected hamsters, however, do not produce any detectable antibodies
specific to the cuticle of infective third-stage larvae (L3), even if
the hamsters received trickle infections, freeze-thawed L3 or 34 krad
irradiated L3 (9). This phenomenon might explain the fact that no immunity to reinfection is observed (27).

Table 5.   Immunity to Microfilariae (MF)

1. Female worms from postpatent hamsters still produce MF when transferred to a clean host or when maintained in vitro.[1,2]

2. No recrudescence of microfilaremia after secondary and tertiary infections.[3]

3. Recrudescence of microfilaremia in postpatent hamsters after administration of immunosuppressive drugs.[4]

4. Detection of antibodies specific to the cuticle of MF correlates with the onset of postpatency.[5]

5. Repeated injections of MF into clean hamsters induce immunity to MF.[1]

6. Immunity to MF can be passively transferred with spleen cells from postpatent hamsters.[6]

[1](2), [2](36), [3](28), [4](37), [5](7), [6](20).

The view that hamsters are unable to recognize or process the cuticle of L3 is supported by the results from studies on the immunogenicity of L3 in other susceptible and unsusceptible hosts such as jirds, mice and rats (9). Jirds produce anti-cuticle antibodies to L3 during a D. viteae infection and after inoculation with irradiated L3. These anti-cuticle antibodies seem to be exclusively of the IgM class, as are anti-cuticle antibodies to MF. Dead larvae never elicit the production of anti-cuticle antibodies. The appearance of such anticuticle antibodies to L3 can be correlated with a significant larval growth inhibition (inability to moult L3 to L4) in micropore chambers (28). Larval growth inhibition is not associated with a cell adherence reaction. The significance of these results with respect to immunity to reinfection and to protection against infection is currently being investigated. A situation similar to that found with jirds is also found with C57/BL mice (29). In SIV rats, unsusceptible hosts, neither live nor dead L3 lead to the stimulation of anti-cuticle antibodies. In addition, L3 fail to develop and die in micropore chambers implanted into rats.

Summarizing our observations in relation to the humoral immune response specific against L3, we feel that the moulting process must be a crucial event. In this process, the L3 cuticle is shed and partly solubilized, and cuticle antigens might be recognized by the host. Consequently, whenever the moult of L3 can take place (live L3 in jirds and mice, irradiated L3 in jirds [28]), anti-cuticle antibodies may be expected. The comparative biochemical characterization of cuticles

Table 6. Characteristics of the Antibody-Dependent Cell-Mediated
          Destruction of Microfilariae (MF)

Serum activity: 1. Eluted in the first peak of a Sephadex G200
                        gel-filtration.[1,2]
                    2. Abolished by 2-mercaptoethanol treatment.[2]
                    3. Not sensitive to inactivation (3 hours at 56°C).
                    4. Opsonic for MF.[1,2]

Effector cells: 1. Hamster macrophages adhere to MF and mediate
                        killing in vitro.[1]
                    2. In vivo in micropore chambers: polymorphonuclear
                        and mononuclear cells adhere to MF and mediate
                        killing and disintegration of MF within 24
                        hours.[2,3]
                    3. Eosinophil-enriched cell populations from mice
                        adhere to MF and mediate killing and disinte-
                        gration of MF in vitro.[3]

---

[1](22), [2](24), [3](23).

from MF and L3 will probably help us to understand the host-specific
immunogenicity of cuticle components, and eventually to explain the
hamster's inability to recognize the L3 cuticle.

CONCLUSION

The D. viteae-hamster model represents a well-balanced host-parasite relationship. The infection does not elicit any immune responses
that can lead to severe lesions in the host. On the contrary, the
host is even able to control effectively the MF load released daily
by adult female worms. Thus, the model cannot at all serve to study
the pathogenesis of filarial infections with regard to a better understanding of the pathogenesis of human filariasis. The phenomenon of
immunity to MF, however, based upon an antibody-dependent cell-mediated effector mechanism(s), finds its analogy in occult human filariasis (30,31). In this connection, the present model provides a tool
to study the humoral responses to stage-specific cuticle antigens. It
therefore may also throw light upon basic mechanisms underlying the
immune system of the hamster: for example, the question of the T-independent cuticle antigens leading to an IgM which can finally collabo-
rate--even in the absence of complement--with both polymorphonuclear
and mononuclear cells to mediate killing of MF (see above). In addition, the phenomenon of a specific cellular unresponsiveness to filarial antigens during postpatency (Table 4) is along the same line and
offers a base to study mechanisms leading to antigen-specific immunodepression in the hamster. Fractionation and purification of the fi-

larial antigens could certainly facilitate such studies and might finally lead to the characterization of "protective antigens". At least
it helps us to learn more about the hamster's immune system, but not
necessarily about the dynamics of the host-parasite relationship or
the evolutionary and adaptive processes constituting the host's susceptibility to a parasite.

ACKNOWLEDGMENTS

        Supported by grants from the Swiss National Science Foundation
(Nr. 3.689.76 and 3.267.78).

REFERENCES

1.   Frenkel, J.K.   Prog Exp Tumor Res 16 (1972) 326.
2.   Weiss, N.   Acta Trop 27 (1970) 219.
3.   Worms, M.J. et al.   J Parasitol 47 (1961) 963.
4.   Malone, J.B.; Thomson, P.E.   Exp Parasitol 38 (1975) 279.
5.   Wenk, P.; Heimburger, L.   Z Parasitenkd 29 (1967) 282.
6.   Neilson, J.T.M.   J Parasitol 64 (1978) 378.
7.   Weiss, N.   Acta Trop 35 (1978) 137.
8.   Diesfeld, H.J.; Kirsten, C.   Tropenmed Parasitol 29 (1978) 27.
9.   Weiss, N.; Tanner, M.   Trans R Soc Trop Med Hyg (1980) in press.
10. Neilson, J.T.M.   Tropenmed Parasitol 27 (1976) 233.
11. Simpson, C.F.; Neilson, J.T.M.   Tropenmed Parasitol 27 (1976)
     349.
12. Chapman, C.B. et al.   Aust J Exp Biol Med Sci 57 (1979) 369.
13. Sullivan, T.J. et al.,   this volume.
14. Rousseaux, R. et al.   Clin Exp Immunol 38 (1979) 389.
15. Weiss, N.; Tanner, M.   Tropenmed Parasitol 30 (1979) 73.
16. Augustin, A.A. et al.   Eur J Immunol 9 (1979) 665.
17. Ottesen, E.A. et al.   Immunology 33 (1977) 413.
18. Terry, R.J.   In: Immunity in Parasitic Diseases, ed. INSERM,
     Paris (1978) 161.
19. Dalesandro, D.A.; Klei, T.R.   Trans R Soc Trop Med Hyg 70 (1976)
     534.
20. Weiss, N.   Exp Parasitol 46 (1978) 283.
21. Tanner, M.; Weiss, N.   Tropenmed Parasitol 30 (1979) 371.
22. Thompson, J.P. et al.   J Parasitol 65 (1979) 966.
23. Tanner, M.; Weiss, N.   Acta Trop 35 (1978) 151.
24. Rudin, W. et al.   Tropenmed Parasitol (1980) in press.
25. Kigoni, E.P.   M.Sc. Thesis, Dar-es-Salaam (1978).
26. Streilein, J.W. et al.   In: Immunoaspects of the Spleen, ed.
     Battisto and Streilein. Elsevier/North Holland, Amsterdam (1977)
     321.
27. Neilson, J.T.M.; Forrester, D.J.   Exp Parasitol 37 (1975) 367.
28. Tanner, M.; Weiss, N.   Trans R Soc Trop Med Hyg (1980) in press.
29. Gass, R.F. et al.   Z Parasitenkd 61 (1979) 73.

30. Wong, M.M.; Guest, M.F.   Trans R Soc Trop Med Hyg 63 (1969) 796.
31. Beaver, P.C.   Am J Trop Med Hyg 19 (1970) 181.
32. Johnson, M.H. et al.   J Parasitol 60 (1974) 302.
33. Neilson, J.T.M.   J Parasitol 61 (1975) 785.
34. Neilson, J.T.M.   Exp Parasitol 44 (1978) 225.
35. Weiss, N.; Tanner, M.   J Parasitol (1980) in press.
36. Haque, A. et al.   Parasitology 76 (1978) 61.
37. Neilson, J.T.M.   Acta Trop 35 (1978) 57.

TRANSMISSIBLE ILEAL HYPERPLASIA

Robert O. Jacoby and Elizabeth A. Johnson

Section of Comparative Medicine, Yale University School of
Medicine, 375 Congress Avenue, New Haven, CT 06510

INTRODUCTION

Transmissible ileal hyperplasia (TIH) is a common and devastating
infectious disease of young hamsters. It has been described by other
names (Table 1) that reflect different clinical and morphological interpretations. Unfortunately, the term "wet-tail" has been applied
frequently, but it is non-specific since other gastrointestinal disorders of hamsters cause wet tails (diarrhea).

The relevance of TIH for this symposium stems more from its potential for interfering with research involving hamsters than from
its importance to hamster immunobiology. Therefore this review is designed to increase investigator awareness of TIH as an undesirable
variable. Nevertheless, I hope it also stimulates interest in TIH
as a model for deciphering proliferative responses of intestinal
mucosa to infection. Much of the work to be presented comes from our
laboratory and has already been published. Results of more recent experiments, especially on the causes of TIH, are given in preliminary
form since they soon will be reported separately.

CLINICAL SIGNS AND EPIZOOTIOLOGY

Clinical Signs

TIH is a disease principally of weanling and young adult hamsters
(1-5). Typical signs include diarrhea, rapid weight loss and dehy-
dration, anorexia, hunched posture, ruffled hair, lethargy and death.
The incidence and severity of signs can vary considerably and the
course of disease can range from several days to several weeks. Ap-

Table 1.   Synonyms for Transmissible Ileal Hyperplasia of Hamsters

	Ref. No.
Atypical ileal hyperplasia	2
Enzootic intestinal adenocarcinoma	1
Hamster enteritis	5
Hamster ileitis	42
Proliferative ileitis	3
Regional ileitis	43
Terminal ileitis	5
Wet-tail	41

parently healthy animals occasionally die from TIH without premonitory
signs. In most animals, ropelike intra-abdominal masses indicative
of proliferative intestinal lesions are palpable before clinical signs
begin. Studies of experimentally infected animals have shown that
clinical disease generally commences at about three weeks after exposure, but that ileal hyperplasia is detectable by palpation within
two weeks (2,6).

Epizootiology

     TIH usually occurs as an explosive outbreak with high morbidity
and high death rates. It is not unusual for mortality to exceed
ninety percent. Susceptibility to TIH appears to be age-related (3).
The incidence of clinical signs and lesions begins to decline in ham-

Table 2.   Effect of Age at Time of Infection on the Incidence of
           Experimentally-Induced TIH[1].

Age (weeks)	No. animals	% Lesions	% Anti-TIH antibody
4	8	100	100
6	8	80	100
8	8	50	100
10	8	0	100

[1]Inoculated orally with a homogenate of ileal tissues from hamsters
  with TIH.

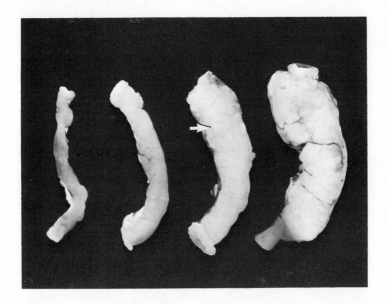

Fig. 1: Distal ileums from hamsters with experimental TIH. Specimens
         taken just proximal to the ileocecal junction (top). From
         left to right: ileums collected on days 0, 15, 25, and 35.
         The ileum at the left is normal. The other three specimens
         demonstrate progressive enlargement. The 25-day specimen
         has small granulomas visible through the serosal surface
         (arrow). The 35-day specimen has extensive granulomatous
         inflammation and a sharp demarcation between affected and
         normal ileum. From Jacoby (6) with permission of The Ameri-
         can Journal of Pathology.

sters infected experimentally after 6 weeks of age and animals infected at 10 weeks are highly resistant (Table 2). Occasionally, animals
that appear to have weathered the acute stages of TIH die suddenly
several months later from ileal stenosis secondary to scarring at the
ileocecal junction.

     TIH seems to spread by oral infection, and it is reasonable to
assume that the hamster's penchant for cannibalism contributes to morbidity. Transmission by aerosol is not a major factor, but the influence of environmental contamination with feces or soiled bedding
has not been adequately studied.

     Hamsters are thought to be the only natural host for TIH. Inbred
strains (LSH, LHC, MHA) and outbred stocks (LVG) are susceptible.
Natural infection of other rodents has not been reported, but mice,

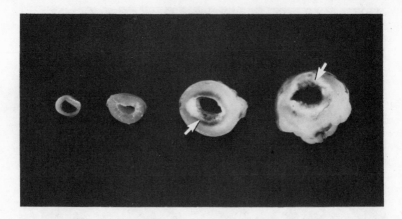

Fig. 2: Transverse sections of the ileums shown in Fig. 1. There is
         progressive thickening of walls due to mucosal hyperplasia.
         The specimens taken at 25 and 35 days have gray-white
         mottling of mucosa from necrosis and hemorrhage (arrows) and
         the 35-day ileum has extensive granulomatous thickening of
         ileal wall. From Jacoby (6) with permission of The American
         Journal of Pathology.

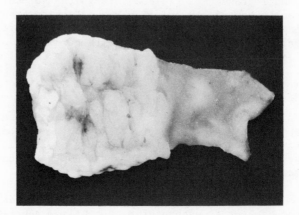

Fig. 3: Mucosa of distal ileum from a hamster with experimental TIH
         30 days after infection. The mucosal surface is raised,
         there is distortion of surface texture due to fusion of hy-
         perplastic villi, and there are foci of mucosal necrosis and
         hemorrhage. From Jacoby (6) with permission of The American
         Journal of Pathology.

rats and guinea pigs develop anti-TIH antibody after experimental infection (11). This finding suggests that transient infections can
occur in these species.

PATHOLOGY AND PATHOGENESIS

     TIH is characterized by segmental mucosal hyperplasia and pyo-
granulomatous inflammation of the distal ileum. The lesion has stirred
controversy; it has been called neoplastic by some ("enzootic intestinal adenocarcinoma") because the hyperplastic epithelium often pene-
trates subjacent muscle tunicae (1), whereas others have stressed its
inflammatory aspects ("proliferative ileitis") (3). These contrasting
interpretations were based on studies of naturally-occurring lesions.
Recent studies of experimentally-induced TIH have confirmed that a hyperplastic phase precedes an inflammatory phase (2,6,7).

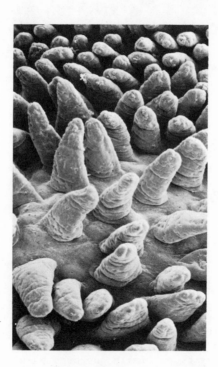

Fig. 4: Scanning micrograph of ileal mucosa from a normal hamster.
         Villi are slightly flattened and taper toward the tips.
         Narrow crypt openings punctuate intervillus spaces, and
         transverse infoldings occur along villus surfaces (X 117).
         From Johnson and Jacoby (7) with permission of The American
         Journal of Pathology.

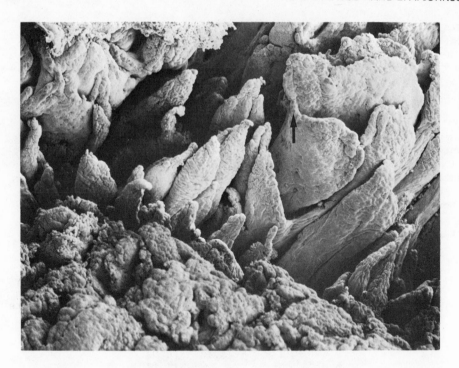

Fig. 5:   TIH lesion at 26 days. There is a sharp demarcation between
          plateaus that have formed by fusion of villus apices (lower
          left) and areas composed of large, overlapping, leaf-like
          villus structures interconnected by cellular bridges (X 123).
          From Johnson and Jacoby (7) with permission of The American
          Journal of Pathology.

Gross Lesions

        The primary lesion is progressive thickening and dilatation of
the distal ileum with occasional involvement of more proximal segments
of the small intestine or even the proximal colon (Fig. 1,2). The
transition from hyperplastic to normal mucosa is relatively abrupt
(Fig. 3) especially at the ileocecal junction, but the cecum is often
flaccid and filled with abnormally liquified contents. The thickened
mucosa has a slightly textured hyperemic surface during early stages
of the disease, but may be partially obscured by necrotic grey-yellow
plaques or hemorrhage in advanced lesions. The severity of mucosal
hyperplasia is revealed dramatically by scanning electron microscopy.
Villi elongate (four to five times) and become leaf-like. Plateaus
are formed by fusion of distorted villi (Fig. 4,5). The serosa is
initially smooth and grey-red, but it eventually becomes grey-white
and nodular from pyogranulomatous inflammation (Fig. 1). Advanced

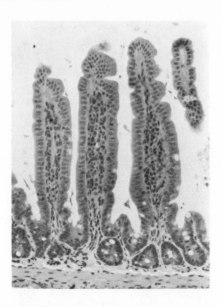

Fig. 6:   Ileum from a normal hamster showing crypts with crowded,
          mitotically active cells and villi covered by mature colum-
          nar epithelium. The lamina propria contains some mononuc-
          lear cells (H and E, X 175). From Jacoby (6) with permis-
          sion of The American Journal of Pathology.

lesions also provoke focal adhesions among adjacent loops of intestine,
mesentery and parietal peritoneum. Colonic intussusception is a common
agonal lesion.

Histology and Ultrastructure

The hyperplastic phase of TIH develops by expansion of crypt epithelium onto villus walls and begins within 10 days of infection (Fig.
6,7). These changes are reflected in an increase in the number of
cells per crypt-villus unit (Fig. 8). As villi elongate they become
tortuous and fuse. Ascending columns of immature, pseudostratified
crypt-type epithelium with a high mitotic index eventually replace
mature villus epithelium completely (Fig. 9).

The luminal movement of hyperplastic epithelium is often followed
by penetration of proliferating crypts into Peyer's patches and supporting tissue layers of the ileal wall (Fig. 10). Downward expansion of dilated or tortuous hyperplastic crypts had been interpreted
by some investigators as a neoplastic change. It is more likely, how-

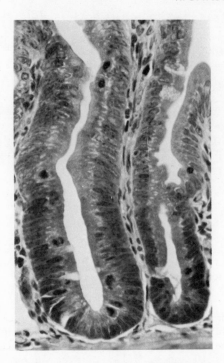

Fig. 7: Distal ileum from a hamster with TIH. Day 10 after inocula-
         tion. Crypt-type epithelium extends onto lower portions of
         villus walls. Cells are pseudostratified and mitotic figures
         are common (H and E, X 440). From Jacoby (6) with permission
         of The American Journal of Pathology.

ever, that penetration results from the pressures of proliferating
crypt epithelium against ileal walls rendered turgid by preceding
villus expansion than from invasion by neoplastic epithelium. As in-
trusion proceeds, crypt epithelium begins to die and inflammation begins. The submucosa and hypertrophied muscular tunicae fill with
macrophages and neutrophils (Fig. 11). Crypt abscesses form and vio-
lation of serosal integrity by pyogranulomatous inflammation causes
focal peritonitis. Concomitant necrosis and hemorrhage of hyperplastic mucosa often occurs and thick collars of pyogranulomatous inflammation complete their encirclement of the partially devitalized
mucosa. These advanced lesions are often fatal, but animals that survive are at risk from scarring and secondary ileal stenosis.

    Despite the intrusive behavior of mucosal hyperplasia, signs of
neoplasia such as cellular pleomorphism and anaplasia, breaching of
basement membranes and metastasis do not occur. The chronology of
TIH is outlined in Table 3.

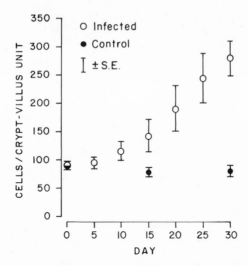

Fig. 8: Average number of mucosal epithelial cells per crypt-villus unit among hamsters with TIH (open circles) compared with control hamsters (closed circles). Bars indicate + SE. From Jacoby (6) with permission of The American Journal of Pathology.

ETIOLOGY

The cause of TIH has been sought intermittently and with limited success for about 20 years. The search has focused on infectious agents, and recent studies have revealed that bacteria parasitize the cytoplasm of hyperplastic epithelial cells in naturally-occurring lesions (8). Morphologically identical organisms are found in experimentally-induced TIH (7,9). The ability to transmit TIH by gavage with homogenates of ileal lesions (2,10) has permitted temporal studies of the relationship between the intracellular organisms and hyperplasia (6,7). To summarize briefly, the intracellular organisms are rod-shaped, slightly curved gram-negative bacteria with crenulated cell walls. They measure approximately 0.3 x 2.0 μm (Fig. 12). They are detectable in ileal mucosal epithelium as early as five days after infection, which is several days before hyperplasia begins (Table 3). They replicate and accumulate in apical regions of the cytoplasm, but they are not separated from the cytoplasm by cell membranes (Fig. 13). They appear first in crypt epithelium, but they also replicate in mature villus cells. They are never seen in unaffected segments of intestine from hamsters with TIH or in intestines from normal hamsters. Their mode of cell penetration as well as the mechanisms by which they may provoke cell proliferation are unknown. It is worth noting that other intracellular infectious agents such as protozoa and viruses

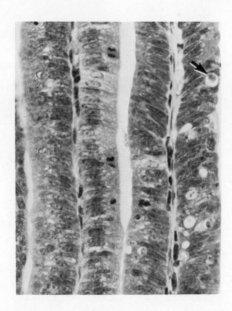

Fig. 9:   Upper third of two villi showing typical changes of TIH. Day
          20 after inoculation. Mature villus epithelium has been re-
          placed by hyperplastic crypt-type epithelium with numerous
          dividing cells. Many cells contain tinctorially heterogen-
          eous intracytoplasmic inclusions (arrow). The lamina prop-
          ria is compressed so that no mononuclear cells remain (H and
          E, X 440). From Jacoby (6) with permission of The American
          Journal of Pathology.

have not been found. Mucosal hyperplasia subsides in chronic lesions
and new mature villus epithelium is free of intracytoplasmic bacteria.

     Another association between TIH and intracellular bacteria was
uncovered during attempts to develop a serodiagnostic test (2,6).
Serum from infected hamsters reacted strongly by indirect immunofluorescence with an intracytoplasmic particulate antigen found only in
ileal lesions. The antigen was localized to the apical cytoplasm of
hyperplastic epithelial cells in early stages of TIH, but was also
found in inflammatory cells that infiltrated more advanced lesions.
Therefore the distribution of "TIH-associated antigen" coincides with
that of the intracellular bacteria (Fig. 14). "Anti-TIH" antibody can
be detected by indirect immunofluorescence as early as 10 days after
infection. The antibody appears to be specific for TIH since: 1. it
reacts only with affected segments of hamster intestine; 2. it does
not react with intestine from normal hamsters; 3. it develops shortly

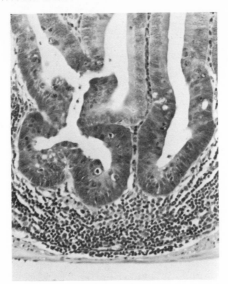

Fig. 10: Ileal Peyer's patch compressed by downward expansion of tortuous hyperplastic crypts. The subjacent segment of muscle tunicae is thin. Day 20 after inoculation (H and E, X 175). From Jacoby (6) with permission of The American Journal of Pathology.

after bacterial invasion of ileal mucosa; and 4. it neither reacts with nor is absorbed by bacteria recovered by conventional methods from normal or affected hamsters (Table 4). The role of anti-TIH antibody in host immunity to TIH is obscure. We have made several attempts to protect hamsters from TIH by passive immunization, but they were unsuccessful, and we have not been able to abrogate disease by pre-incubating immune serum with infectious inocula. Anti-TIH serum has immediate value as a diagnostic reagent, however (see below).

Several years ago we found that TIH can be easily transmitted by oral inoculation of weanling hamsters with saline homogenates of ileal lesions (2). Transmission studies have shown that the infectivity and antigenicity of ileal homogenates is abrogated by heating, by exposure to chloroform and by passage through bacteria-retaining filters (Table 5). Nevertheless, attempts by us and by others (2,10, 11) to transmit TIH or to induce seroconversion with bacteria isolated from infectious ileal lesions have not been fruitful (Table 6). Selective inhibition of intestinal flora in infected donors by neomycin (neomycin sulfate in drinking water at 2 mg/ml for three days followed by neomycin sulfate per os at 10 mg b.i.d. for two days) did not re-

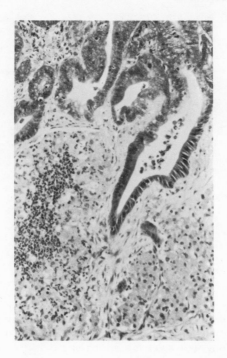

Fig. 11: Typical advanced lesion of TIH.   Day 35 after inoculation.
Fronds of hyperplastic epithelium are penetrating underlying
supporting tissues distorted by severe pyogranulomatous inflammation (H and E, X 175).   From Jacoby (6) with permission of The American Journal of Pathology.

duce the incidence of lesions or inhibit the ability to transmit TIH.
Because neomycin is not readily absorbed from the intestine, the data
were consistent with a causal role for the intracellular bacteria. A
curious sidelight to this work was that hamsters treated prophylactically with neomycin developed cecal hyperplasia rather than ileal
hyperplasia.

These transmission trials increased our suspicion that the causative agent could not be cultured by conventional methods. Therefore,
we turned to the possibility that the intracytoplasmic organism pre-
fers or requires living cells to survive and replicate. Trypsinized
mucosal cell suspensions were prepared from affected hamsters pretreated with neomycin to "sterilize" the intestinal tract.   The suspensions were inoculated into several continuous cell lines and into
primary hamster embryo (PHE) cells grown in 30-mm plastic dishes in
5% CO_2 at $37^{\circ}C$.   The medium was minimum essential Earle's medium
without antibiotics, supplemented with fetal calf serum (10%).   By

Table 3. Summary of the Typical Course of TIH in Experimentally-
          Inoculated Weanling Hamsters

Day	Clinical signs	Ileal lesions	Intracellular bacteria	TIH-associate antigen	Anti-TIH antibody
5			+	+	
10		Hyperplasia	+	+	+
15	Palpable ileums	Penetration	+	+	+
20	Diarrhea, etc., some dead	Mild necrosis and inflammation	+	+	+
25	Many dead	Severe necrosis and inflammation	+	+	+

one week post-inoculation cells contained intracytoplasmic rod-shaped
bacteria that reacted with anti-TIH serum, but not with normal serum
or hyperimmune serum to conventional intestinal organisms (Table 7).
The heaviest concentrations of bacteria developed in CER cells (Fig.
15). Infected cultures remained viable for up to three weeks, and conventional bacteria were not detected. After the second week, however,
the intracytoplasmic bacteria began to degenerate and clump. Infected
cells also were passaged at weekly intervals, but they ceased to be infectious for new CER cultures after two passages. Therefore, culture
conditions for serial propagation of the bacteria must be improved.
We have made two attempts to transmit TIH with organisms grown in CER
cells for a week. Weanling hamsters inoculated either orally or intra-
cecally or both failed to develop TIH or to produce anti-TIH antibody.
There are many possible explanations for these negative results, including the chance that transmission of TIH requires more than one
agent (9). Nonetheless, it seems likely from current evidence that
the unidentified intracellular organism has a causal link to TIH.

DIAGNOSIS

    TIH can be easily diagnosed from the pattern of clinical disease
and by demonstrating the pathognomonic intestinal lesions. Reliance
on clinical signs alone should be avoided, for there are other causes
of diarrhea in hamsters, such as Tyzzer's disease (12) and cecal hyperplasia (13). Anti-TIH antibody as detected by indirect immunofluorescence is a useful marker for the presence of TIH. The value
of the immunofluorescence test stems from the fact that virtually all
hamsters exposed to TIH seroconvert whether or not they develop active
disease. The test is usually performed on cryostat sections of ileal

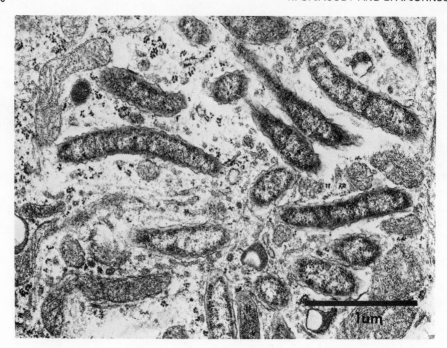

Fig. 12: Bacteria in villus cell at five days. The bacteria are
         slightly curved rods surrounded by a double crenulated cell
         wall and are in intimate contact with host cytoplasm. Gran-
         ules which resemble lysosomes lie near the bacteria, but
         fusion and secondary lysosomes are not seen (uranyl ace-
         tate and lead citrate, X 35,800). From Johnson and Jacoby
         (7) with permission of The American Journal of Pathology.

lesions that contain TIH-associated antigens. Our laboratory will provide an antigen source for interested colleagues.

CONTROL

    Strict quarantine, culling and husbandry procedures will reduce
the spread of infection. Animal technicians should wash their hands
between cage changes, water bottles and feed should not be exchanged
between cages, and caging should be thoroughly sanitized before being
reused. Filter bonnets may be placed over cages to help control possible cage-to-cage transmission by scattered food and bedding. There
is no known effective therapy for TIH, but antibacterial drugs have
been used prophylactically with moderate success (11,14,15) (Table 8).

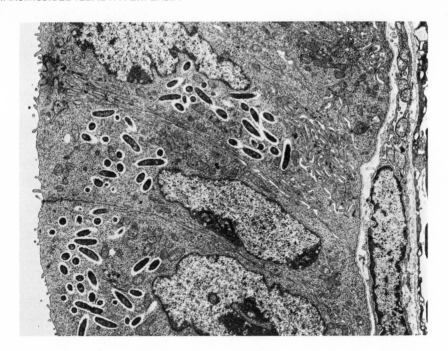

Fig. 13: Hyperplastic villus epithelium at 14 days. Columnar cells
with interdigitating lateral membranes abut a continuous
basement membrane. Numerous bacteria occupy the apical cytoplasm which is otherwise composed almost entirely of free
ribosomes and scattered mitochondria. Only a few rudimentary
microvilli are seen at the luminal surface (uranyl acetate
and lead citrate, X 6480). From Johnson and Jacoby (7) with
permission of The American Journal of Pathology.

The use of antibacterial prophylaxis should be coupled with elimination of all animals in cages where TIH has occurred. Severe outbreaks
may require depopulation of animal rooms followed by thorough decontamination. The prevention and control of TIH requires that hamsters
be purchased from TIH-free colonies, since newly-received, infected
animals are a major source of fresh outbreaks. Vendors should have a
monitoring program to detect and eliminate TIH from their production
rooms.

The severity of a TIH outbreak may be influenced by environmental and husbandry factors. Stress from overcrowding, excess noise,
and experiment-related treatments have, in our experience, exacerbated
morbidity and mortality. Commercial diets can also modulate the severity of disease (Table 9). The dietary component(s) responsible
for this effect have not been determined.

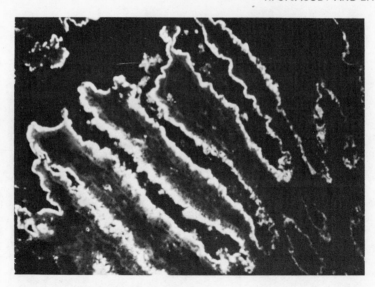

Fig. 14: Typical ribbon-like pattern of TIH-associated antigen demonstrated by indirect immunofluorescence staining of hyperplastic ileal villi. Antigen has accumulated in the apical cytoplasm of epithelial cells. A few fluorescing exfoliated cells
occupy intervillus spaces. Day 15 after inoculation (X 110).
From Jacoby (6) with permission of The American Journal of
Pathology.

COMMENTS

It is not clear how bacteria infect epithelial cells in TIH. Bacteria have not been seen invading cells or in close association with
the brush border as reported for enteric pathogens such as Salmonella
typhimurium, Shigella flexneri, or Escherichia coli (16-18). TIH-
associated bacteria are not enclosed in host-cell membranes unless
secondary lysosomes develop, whereas intracellular enteric bacteria
are often in phagocytic vacuoles. In addition, bacteria are always observed in rows of infected cells, and have a predilection for crypt
cells. These observations speak against a random distribution of penetration by intraluminal organisms. A more likely possibility is that
the bacteria enter a few crypt cells, e.g., by phagocytosis, soon after
hamsters are inoculated, so the chance of observing penetration is
small. Intracellular replication of organisms may rupture the phagocytic vacuoles, leaving the bacteria in intimate contact with the cytoplasm. If bacterial replication proceeds in undifferentiated di-
viding crypt cells, a pool of infected cells would be available to migrate onto villus walls.

Table 4. Reactivity of Immune Sera with Bacterial Isolates and with TIH-Associated Antigen[1].

	Reacts with	
Immune serum to:	Autologous isolate	TIH-associated intracytoplasmic antigen
B. fragilis	+	-
F. varium	+	-
C. sordelli	+	-
E. coli	+	-
TIH	B. fragilis (-)	+
	F. varium (-)	
	C. sordelli (-)	
	C. innocuum (-)	
	Enterococcus spp. (-)	
	E. coli (-)	

[1]As determined by indirect immunofluorescence. From Jacoby and Onderdonk, manuscript in preparation.

Enteric bacteria which penetrate mucosal epithelium commonly produce cytolytic changes (16-19), whereas the bacteria found in TIH are associated primarily with hyperplastic changes. Cell necrosis in TIH is variable and usually follows development of hyperplasia. Nevertheless, large secondary lysosomes containing bacteria and cell debris form in epithelial cells. They probably correspond to intracytoplasmic bodies or inclusions observed in histologic sections (see Fig. 9).

The inflammatory phase of TIH is characterized by severe pyogranulomatous infiltration of ileal wall. It is usually preceded by dilatation of crypts with crypt abscess formation and necrosis of flattened crypt epithelium. Inflammation probably is caused in some areas by preexisting tissue necrosis, but the role of TIH-associated bacteria must be considered.

Proliferative lesions of the small intestine have been reported in several species. Of particular interest is a syndrome in swine called "intestinal adenomatosis," which resembles TIH morphologically (20). Hyperplastic segments of intestinal mucosal epithelium contained intracytoplasmic bacteria which were identified as Campylobacter sputorum mucosalis by immunofluorescence techniques. Campylobacter

Table 5. Effect of Various Treatments on the Ability of Ileal
          Tissues from Affected Hamsters to Transmit TIH to Suscep-
          tibility Weanling Hamsters[1].

Inoculum	Cumulative experiments	Hamsters with lesions / Hamsters inoculated
Ileal homogenate	4	28/28
F/T homogenate[2]	2	15/15
Whole-cell free supernatant	6	30/30
5.0μm filtrate	3	18/23
1.2 μm filtrate	1	6/6
0.65 μm filtrate	1	5/5
0.45 μm filtrate	4	3/30
0.22 μm filtrate	3	0/21
Chloroform-treated homogenate[3-6]	1	0/6
Heated homogenate[4]	1	0/6
Normal ileal homogenate[5]	3	0/15
Sentinel controls[6]	2	0/8

[1-6]Cumulative results of several experiments are presented. Positive
controls, consisting of animals inoculated with untreated segments
or homogenates of ileal lesions which subsequently developed TIH,
were included in each experiment.

[2]Freeze-thawed five times.

[3]10% chloroform (v/v) for 10 minutes.

[4]56°C for 30 minutes.

[5]Homogenized ileum from uninoculated weanlings.

[6]Uninoculated weanlings housed on racks with inoculated weanlings
(modified from refs. 2 and 1, and with permission of Lab Anim Sci).

was isolated from ileums of infected swine but not from normal swine
(21,22). Experimental induction of lesions in swine has not been reported. Campylobacter has not been detected in hamsters with TIH.

     TIH does not mimic any disease of man. Proliferative lesions of
the human small intestine are rare. Granulomatous lesions are characteristic of Crohn's disease (23,24) and Whipple's disease (25). PAS-
positive macrophages with intracellular bacteria are found in both

Table 6.   Attempts to Induce TIH with Bacteria Isolated from Ileal
           Lesions[1,2]

Organism	Route Oral	Route Intracecal	Lesions	Anti–TIH Antibody
Bacteriodes fragilis				
Isolate A	+		0/20	0/20
B	+		0/16	0/16
C		+	0/8	0/8
Fusobacterium varium	+		0/18	0/18
Fusobacterium spp.		+	0/8	0/8
Clostridium sordelli	+		0/10	0/10
Escherichia coli	+		0/10	0/10
Pooled Bacteria	+		0/8	0/8
(E. coli, F. varium, B. fragilis, Cl. sordelli, Cl. innocuum)		+	0/9	0/9
Brain-heart infusion broth	+		0/8	0/8
TIH ileal homogenate	+		19/19	19/19
		+	9/13	13/13

[1]For most experiments, 1.0 ml of 18-hour broth cultures were inoculated into weanling hamsters. Pooled bacteria consisted of 5 x
0.2-ml aliquots of each culture. Intracecal inoculation was made
with a 25-gauge needle after laparotomy under anesthesia.

[2]From Jacoby and Onderdonk, manuscript in preparation.

Whipple's disease and TIH. In Whipple's disease, however, mucosal
epithelium is not hyperplastic and intracellular bacteria are found
primarily in inflammatory cells of the lamina propria. Bacteria have
been suspected of playing a role in causing Whipple's disease. A cell-
wall-deficient Streptococcus from a patient with Whipple's disease has
been isolated recently, and organisms in granulomatous ileal lesions
have been demonstrated by immunofluorescence (26).

TIH may be an excellent model to study regulation of mucosal proliferation. Mucosal hyperplasia in TIH begins in the crypt cell compartment. Crypt hyperplasia is a common response to mucosal injury.

Table 7. Culture of TIH-Associated Bacteria in vitro

Cell culture	Type	Source	Infection rate[1]
CER	Established	(Chicken + hamster)	Excellent
NCTC 1469	Established	Mouse liver	Good
PHE	Primary	Hamster embryo	Fair
L	Established	Mouse fibroblast	Fair
BHK-21	Established	Hamster kidney	Poor

[1]Cultures were examined by immunofluorescence one week after primary inoculation. Ratings based on estimates of the number of cells with organisms and the concentration of organisms per cell. Heavily infected CER cultures usually have more than 75 percent of cells infected with intracytoplasmic organisms.

From Jacoby and Onderdonk, manuscript in preparation.

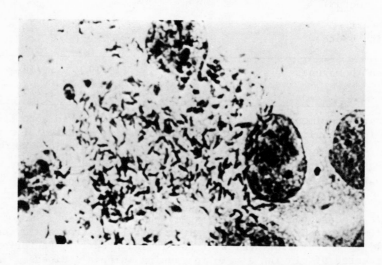

Fig. 15: Rod-shaped bacteria in the cytoplasm of CER cells nine days after culture was inoculated with trypsinized mucosal scrapings from neomycin pretreated hamsters with TIH.

Table 8. The Effect of Antibacterial Drugs on the Incidence of Experimentally Induced TIH

Drug	Treatment	No. with TIH / No. inoculated[1]	Ref.
Neomycin	2 mg/ml in drinking water for 2 weeks beginning with day of inoculation	14/16	(11)
	125 mg/liter in drinking water for 10 days beginning by three days post-inoculation	38/45	(15)
Metronidazole	2 mg/ml in drinking water for two weeks beginning with day of inoculation	3/13	(11)
Dimetridazole	500 mg/liter in drinking water for 10 days beginning by three days post-inoculation	25/46	(15)
Tetracycline	400 mg/liter in drinking water for 10 days beginning by three days post-inoculation	9/47	(15)

[1]Control animals for these experiments had $\sim$ 80% incidence of TIH.

It occurs following infection of the mucosa by cytolytic agents (27, 28), after radiation injury (29), and in diseases such as tropical and celiac sprue (30,31). Mechanisms initiating mucosal hyperplasia, however, are not well understood. Recent work indicates that the proliferation and differentiation of crypt-villus epithelium may be controlled by a feedback regulatory system (32-34). It has been hypothesized that such a feedback mechanism might stimulate proliferation of cells in the critical decision zone in response to reductions in the size of the mature villus cell compartment (33,34). It has been suggested that hormones, chalones, other humoral factors, and nutritional factors also help regulate the kinetics of epithelial turnover (35-40). The role of putative feedback regulatory systems in the initiation of TIH and the potential influence of the causal agent on feedback regulation are speculative, but pose interesting questions for future research.

ACKNOWLEDGMENTS

The authors gratefully acknowledge the collaboration of Dr. Andrew Onderdonk in portions of the studies reviewed in this report. Mrs. Katharine White has contributed her skills to the expert preparation of the manuscript. This work was supported by Grants RR00945, RR00393 and RR05358 from the Public Health Service.

Table 9. Effect of Four Commercially Prepared Closed Formula Diets on the Incidence of TIH in Weanling Hamsters Inoculated per os with 1.0 ml of Homogenate of Ileal Lesions Two days after Diet was Initiated[1]

Diet	No. of animals	% with lesions	Infected[2]
A	12	100	100
B	10	0	100
C	10	90	100
D	10	0	100

[1]Animals were observed for 30 days. Animals given diets plus homogenates of normal ileum did not become infected.

[2]Sum of hamsters with lesions and hamsters with anti-TIH antibody.

REFERENCES

1.   Jonas, A.M. et al. J Am Vet Med Assoc 147 (1965) 1102.
2.   Jacoby, R.O. et al. Lab Anim Sci 25 (1975) 465.
3.   Boothe, A.D.; Cheville, N.F. Pathol Vet 4 (1967) 31.
4.   Jackson, S.T.; Wagner, J.E. Lab Anim Digest 6 (1970) 12.
5.   Frisk, C.S.; Wagner, J.E. Lab Anim 11 (1977) 79.
6.   Jacoby, R.O. Am J Pathol 91 (1978) 433.
7.   Johnson, E.A.; Jacoby, R.O. Am J Pathol 91 (1978) 451.
8.   Wagner, J.E. et al. Am J Vet Res 34 (1973) 249.
9.   Frisk, C.S.; Wagner, J.E. Am J Vet Res 38 (1977) 1861.
10. Amend, N.K. et al. Lab Anim Sci 26 (1976) 566.
11. Jacoby, R.O.; Onderdonk, A. In preparation, 1980.
12. Zook, B.C. et al. J Am Vet Med Assoc 171 (1977) 833.
13. Barthold, S.W. et al. Lab Anim Sci 28 (1978) 723.
14. Frenkel, J.K. Prog Exp Tumor Res 16 (1972) 326.
15. La Regina, M. et al. Lab Anim Sci 30 (1980) 38.
16. Takeuchi, A. Am J Pathol 50 (1967) 109.
17. Takeuchi, A. et al. Am J Pathol 52 (1968) 503.
18. Staley, T.E. et al. Am J Pathol 56 (1969) 371.
19. Takeuchi, A. Curr Top Pathol 54 (1971) 1.
20. Dodd, D.C. Pathol Vet 5 (1968) 333.
21. Rowland, A.C.; Lawson, G.H.K. Res Vet Sci 17 (1974) 323.
22. Lawson, G.H.K.; Rowland, A.C. Res Vet Sci 17 (1974) 331.
23. Morson, B.S. Proc R Soc Med 61 (1968) 79.
24. Saltzstein, S.L.; Rosenberg, B.F. Am J Clin Pathol 40 (1963)
     610.
25. Trier, J.S. et al. Gastroenterology 48 (1965) 684.
26. Clancy, R.L. et al. Br Med J 3 (1975) 568.
27. Abrams, G.D. et al. Lab Invest 12 (1963) 1241.
28. Takeuchi, A. et al. Am J Pathol 47 (1965) 1011.
29. Withers, H.R. Cancer 28 (1971) 75.
30. Perera, D.R. et al. Hum Pathol 6 (1975) 157.
31. Paduka, H.A. Gasteroenterology 21 (1962) 873.
32. Galjaard, H. et al. Exp Cell Res 73 (1972) 197.
33. Rijke, R.P.C. et al. Cell Tissue Kinet 7 (1974) 586.
34. Rijke, R.P.C. et al. Cell Tissue Kinet 8 (1975) 441.
35. Loran, M.R.; Carbone, I.V. Nuclear Medicine and Biology Mono-
     graph No. 1, ed. Sullivan. Excerpta Medica Foundation,
     Amsterdam (1968).
36. Tilson, M.D.; Wright, H.K. Surgery 67 (1970) 687.
37. Gleeson, M.H. et al. Clin Sci Mol Med 43 (1972) 731.
38. Feldman, E.J. et al. Gastroenterology 66 (1974) 691.
39. Brugel, G. Stem Cells: Renewing Cell Population, ed. Cairnie.
     Academic Press, Inc., New York (1976).
40. Tutton, P.J.M. Cell Tissue Kinet 6 (1973) 211.
41. Sheffield, F.W.; Beveridge, E. Nature 196 (1962) 294.
42. Christensen, L.R.; Matanic, B. Proc 13th Annu Meet Anim Care
     Panel, Chicago (1962).
43. Gans, J.H. et al. Proc 16th Annu Meet Anim Care Panel,
     Philadelphia (1965).

LSH HAMSTER MODEL OF SYPHILITIC INFECTION AND TRANSFER OF RESISTANCE WITH IMMUNE T CELLS

Ronald F. Schell, Jack L. LeFrock,
John K. Chan and Omar Bagasra

Department of Medicine (Infectious Diseases)
Hahnemann Medical College and Hospital
Philadelphia, PA   19102

INTRODUCTION

The immunologic basis of host defense in syphilis has not been elucidated. The humoral immune response appears to afford only negligible protection. The disease progresses from a local lesion to secondary syphilis with 24% of patients developing relapsing secondary lesions despite the development of a vigorous antibody response. Passive immunization of rabbits or hamsters with immune serum (1-5) or immunoglobulin (6) has failed to prevent infection of animals with Treponema pallidum.

A role for cell-mediated immunity in the pathogenesis of syphilis is recognized (7); its contribution to the host's defense against infection, however, is unclear. One study (8) showed that lymphocytes from outbred rabbits previously exposed to T. pallidum and treated with penicillin conferred resistance on recipient rabbits. The evidence was the occurrence of fewer lesions and the delayed incubation period of the lesions, as compared to those in the control groups. In contrast, in another study (9), using inbred rabbits resistant to syphilitic rechallenge, resistance could not be transferred passively with syngeneic immune spleen cells and the authors concluded that cell-mediated immunity may not be involved in resistance to treponemal infection.

Attempts to elucidate the mechanism by which animals respond to syphilitic infection have been hindered by the unavailability of suitable inbred animals. In this paper we present evidence that the LSH/Ss LAK (LSH) strain of inbred hamster responds to syphilitic infection, develops pathologic changes that can be quantitated readily, and acquires resistance dependent upon T cells.

MATERIALS AND METHODS

LSH hamsters were obtained from Charles River Breeding Laboratories, Inc., Wilmington, Mass. Hamsters weighing 80-100 g were housed five or six per cage at an ambient temperature of 18°C, a condition which facilitates the development of cutaneous lesions (10).

T. pallidum strain Bosnia A was maintained by passage in hamsters. The inguinal lymph nodes were removed aseptically five to six weeks after intradermal infection, teased apart in sterile saline, and filtered through 60-mesh steel wire. After centrifugation at 270 x g for three minutes to remove cellular debris, the number of treponemes in the supernatant was determined by dark-field microscopy.

The approximate number of treponemes per lymph node was determined as described (11). Briefly, duplicate slides of each homogenized lymph node were prepared and 120 fields per slide were examined for treponemes by dark-field microscopy.

The protocol for this study has been described in detail (12,13). In a double-blind experiment, 35 hamsters were infected intradermally in the inguinal region with 7×10^5 treponemes. Sixteen weeks after infection they were treated with penicillin to terminate infection. Sixteen days after treatment, 30 of the hamsters were killed and single-cell suspensions of their splenic and lymph node cells were prepared. The other five animals, when reinfected with T. pallidum, did not develop lesions.

Pooled immune or normal (spleen and lymph node) cells were filtered through glass-wool and then nylon-wool columns, as described (14), to obtain enriched T cell suspensions. From 15% to 20% of the cells were recovered.

Four groups of normal hamsters then were irradiated (900 rads) and inoculated intravenously with either fractionated immune, unfractionated immune, fractionated normal, or unfractionated normal lymphoid cells. All animals were reconstituted with normal bone-marrow cells. As an additional control, a fifth group was irradiated and reconstituted but received no lymphoid cells. Each animal then was challenged with 10^5 T. pallidum and monitored for the development of cutaneous lesions. All animals were killed on day 24 after infection, and their lymph node weights and the number of treponemes in their nodes were determined.

To confirm that the fractionated immune cell suspensions were rich in T cells and depleted of B cells, they were assayed by four procedures:

1.   Five syphilitic hamsters that had been treated with penicillin were inoculated intravenously with sheep red blood cells.
Their pooled immune cells, fractionated and unfractionated, were
tested by Dresser's (15) modified hemolytic plaque technique.

2.   Fractionated or unfractionated lymphoid cells from five peni-
cillin-treated hamsters were incubated with rabbit anti-hamster gamma-
globulin serum, washed with fetal calf serum, and then incubated with
fluorescein-conjugated goat anti-rabbit immunoglobulin serum. All
three reagents had been heat-inactivated. The cells were examined for
speckled, ringed, or crescent fluorescence.

3.   Fractionated or unfractionated lymphoid cells were incubated
with complement plus either normal rabbit serum (NRS) or rabbit anti-
hamster thymocyte serum (ATS). Both sera had been absorbed with sheep
red blood cells, hamster bone-marrow cells, or cells from a GD-36 B
cell lymphoma (16). The cytotoxic activity of the absorbed ATS was
high against thymoyctes ($94 \pm 3\%$), moderate against pooled immune
cells ($56 \pm 2\%$), and virtually undetectable ($2 \pm 2\%$) against hamster
bone-marrow or lymphoma cells. The cytotoxicity index (CI) for the
lymphoid cells was calculated as $CI = 1 - (N_{ATS}/N_{NRS}) \times 100$, where
N_{ATS} and N_{NRS} are the number of viable cells remaining after incubation with ATS or NRS, respectively.

4.   Single-cell suspensions of fractionated or unfractionated
lymphoid cells were cultured with a B cell mitogen (either lipopolysaccharide from Escherichia coli or dextran sulfate) or a T-cell mitogen (either concanavalin A or phytohemagglutinin P). Each culture was
incubated further with ^{3}H-thymidine, harvested, and counted for radioactivity. The results are given as the geometric means of quadruplicate cultures.

Fischer's least significant difference test was used to examine
pairs of means when a significant F ratio indicated reliable mean differences. The alpha level was set at 0.05 before the experiments
started.

RESULTS

Thirty-six hamsters were infected with 4×10^5 T. pallidum and
examined daily for inflammation. Each week for 12 weeks three of these
syphilitic hamsters were killed, along with three age-matched, non-in-
fected hamsters as controls. Each site of inoculation became erythe-
matous three weeks after infection in all hamsters. The intensity of
erythema increased until day 26 after infection, at which time the
skin appeared roughened and scaly. Within 24 to 48 hours thereafter,
the skin ulcerated and became either a larger crusted lesion or an
open lesion, while the periphery of the lesion continued to expand.

Table 1:   The Weight and Approximate Number of Treponemes
           in Inguinal Lymph Node after Infection with T.
           pallidum Bosnia A

Weeks after infection	Weight (mg)	Treponemes x 10^3 [1]
1	10 ± 1[2]	7
2	19 ± 2	16
3	23 ± 1	85
4	30 ± 4	440
5	40 ± 2	2500
6	59 ± 3	3500
7	73 ± 5	3300
8	80 ± 4	2500
9	100 ± 6	2000
10	120 ± 6	750
11	105 ± 3	500
12	95 ± 2	200

[1]Three hamsters per week.

[2]Geometric mean ± SE.

Central healing of the lesions began four months after infection,
while the margin of the lesion still showed marked erythema. The lesions were not resolved until six to nine months after infection.

The inguinal nodes from syphilitic hamsters gradually increased
in weight, reaching a peak 10 weeks after infection. The number of
treponemes detected in the lymph nodes increased concomitantly until
six weeks (Table 1). After 10 weeks both the node weights and the
number of treponemes had begun to decrease.

Infections with 4×10^5 T. pallidum were timed so that three
groups of experimental hamsters could be studied simultaneously 8,10,
and 16 weeks after infection. For each time period there were six
hamsters for each group. Six normal hamsters also were included as
controls.

Each animal in the four groups was given 4000 units of penicillin.
Ten days later, each was challenged with 1×10^5 T. pallidum. Reinfection produced lesions after 21 ± 4 days in controls and 31 ± 3

Table 2.   Development of Resistance in Hamsters Infected with T. pallidum Bosnia A to Reinfection with the Same Strain

Week after initial infection	Reinfected with T. pallidum Bosnia A	
	Lesions/sites[1]	Treponemes x 10^3/node
6	12/12	10.1
8	8/12	2.0
10	0/12	2
16	0/12	0
Controls	12/12	423

[1]Six animals per group. Each animal was inoculated at two sites.

Table 3.   Ability of B Cell-Depleted Immune Cells to Confer Resistance[1] against T. pallidum in X-Irradiated Bone-Marrow-Reconstituted Hamsters

Recipients of[2]	Lesions/sites[3]	Lymph nodes	
		weight (mg)	Treponemes x 10^3 node
Normal cells			
Unfractionated	6/6	27±2	168
Fractionated	6/6	41±5	133
Immune cells			
Unfractionated	0/6	13±5	6
Fractionated	0/6	16±6	20
Control (received only bone marrow cells)	6/6	38±6	130

[1]At 24 days after infection.

[2]Three hamsters per group.

[3]Each hamster was inoculated at two sites.

Table 4. The Effect of Column Fractionation on the Number of Ig-
          Bearing and Anti-thymocyte Serum-(ATS) Sensitive Cells
          Obtained from Syphilitic Hamsters

Treatment with:	Before fraction-ation	After fraction-ation	% depletion of fluores-cent positive cells after fractionation	% enrichment of ATS-sensi-tive cells after frac-tionation
Rabbit anti-hamster Ig + labelled goat anti-rabbit Ig[1]	36±3%	3±1%	94%	----
ATS + complement	37±9%	87±4%	----	135%

[1]Mean (%) ± SE of fluorescent-positive cells per 200 cells counted.
No fluorescent-positive cells were detected for unfractionated and
fractionated cells treated with either rabbit anti-hamster Ig or
labelled goat anti-rabbit Ig.

days in most animals that had been infected previously for only eight·
weeks. In contrast, hamsters that had been infected for 10 to 16
weeks developed no lesions (Table 2).

Twenty-eight days after reinfection, three hamsters from each experimental group and three control hamsters were sacrificed. Very few
treponemes were detected in the lymph nodes of hamsters previously infected for 8 or 10 weeks, compared to controls (Table 2). No treponemes were found in hamsters previously infected for 16 weeks.

Thus after 10 weeks of infection with T. pallidum, the hamsters
had acquired an effective immune response.

To determine whether syphilitic-immune cell suspensions depleted
of B cells could confer resistance, fractionated or unfractionated
normal or immune lymphoid cells were transferred to X-irradiated,
bone-marrow-reconstituted hamsters, which subsequently were infected
intradermally with T. pallidum. Within 12 days, all hamsters developed cutaneous lesions. In animals that had received normal cells,
the lesions gradually enlarged and became necrotic. In animals that
had received fractionated or unfractionated immune cells, the lesions
regressed and were completely healed by day 24 after infection (Table
3). As a corollary, the lymph nodes of animals that had received
immune cells, whether fractionated or unfractionated, weighed less
and had significantly fewer treponemes. Thus immune cell suspensions
depleted of B cells closely resembled the unfractionated suspensions
in their ability to confer resistance to challenge with T. pallidum.

Table 6. Effect of Column Fractionation on Number of Plaque-Forming Cells (PFC) Recovered from Immune Hamsters Sensitized with Sheep Erythrocytes[1]

Assay	No. PFC (geometric mean $\pm$ SE/10^6 viable cells)		
	Before fractionation	After fractionation	Reduction (%)
Direct	5861 $\pm$ 123	348 $\pm$ 16	94.0
Indirect	4132 $\pm$ 523	411 $\pm$ 19	90.0

[1]No PFC were detected before or after fractionation in cultures treated with only anti-hamster IgG or RPMI 1640.

DISCUSSION

A major obstacle in delineating the mechanism by which experimental animals acquire resistance to syphilitic infection has been the unavailability of a suitable inbred animal model. Syphilitic disease is not induced regularly in guinea pigs (17) or mice (18-20). Inbred rabbits can regularly develop clinical manifestations of syphilis (9), but are difficult to obtain commercially. LSH inbred hamsters, however, are available and can be infected readily with T. pallidum Bosnia A, the causative agent of endemic syphilis. When infected, this strain developed cutaneous lesions that lasted for six to nine months. The infected hamsters' lymph nodes increased significantly in weight and teemed with treponemes for several weeks. Animals infected for 10 or 16 weeks were resistant to reinfection.

The ability to acquire resistance to reinfection makes this strain an appropriate one for studies of passive transfer of resistance. The results of our present study show that resistance to syphilitic infection can be conferred by suspensions of immune cells significantly depleted of B cells. No significant differences were detected between recipients of suspensions of fractionated or unfractionated immune cells. These two groups had no cutaneous lesions 24 days after infection, significantly lower lymph node weights, and significantly fewer treponemes in the nodes, compared with recipients of suspensions of fractionated or unfractionated lymphoid cells or only the normal bone-marrow cells.

Cell preparations were depleted of B cells by passage through glass and nylon-wool columns. This procedure has been shown to separate hamster T and B cells (14). To verify that our eluents were enriched in T cells, they were characterized by serological and functional assays indicating the number of immunoglobulin-bearing cells, response to treatment with ATS, and stimulation by T and B cell mitogens. The ability of the glass and nylon-wool columns to remove cells

Table 5.   Effect of Column Fractionation on Mitogenic Responses of
Lymphocytes from Syphilitic Hamsters

| Mitogen (per 0.2 ml) | ^{3}H-thymidine incorporated (cpm)[1] | |
	Before fractionation	After fractionation
Concanavalin A 1 µg	186,391±4591	98,911±2271
Phytohemagglutinin 10µl	43,189±4877	1,399±143
Lipopolysaccharide 50µg	16,276±738	2,805±201
Dextran sulfate 10µg	12,956±5469	1,439±196
Unstimulated	6,871±938	1,119±89

[1]Geometric mean ± SE of quadruplicate cultures.

     To verify that our fractionated lymphocyte suspensions were
highly enriched in T cells, we incubated the unfractionated or fractionated immune cells with ATS in the presence of complement, anti-
hamster immunoglobulin, or classical T- or B-cell mitogens.

     For cells treated with both rabbit anti-hamster immunoglobulin
and fluorescein-labeled goat anti-rabbit immunoglobulin, fractionation
reduced the proportion of cells bearing immunoglobulins from 36 ± 3%
to only 3 ± 1% (mean ± standard error, SE), a reduction of 94% (Table
4). No fluorescent cells were detected after treatment with either
immunoglobulin alone. In contrast, the proportion of cells susceptible to ATS plus complement increased from 37 ± 9% to 87 ± 4% (mean
± SE), an increase of 135%. The response of syphilitic lymphocytes
to the four classical T- or B-cell mitogens, concanavalin A, phytohemagglutinin, lipopolysaccharide and dextran sulfate, was decreased
significantly by fractionation. The minimal decrease, however, was
seen with the T cell mitogen concanavalin A (Table 5). As an additional measure of the proportion of B cells in the fractionated cells,
immune hamsters were inoculated with sheep erythrocytes. After five
days the number of direct and indirect plaque-forming cells in the
fractionated and unfractionated cell populations was determined. Fractionation reduced the number of direct and indirect plaques by 94%
and 90%, respectively (Table 6).

producing functional antibody to sheep erythrocytes also was determined.

Fractionation removed approximately 90% of the functional anti-
body-producing cells and 94% of the immunoglobulin-bearing cells. The
fractionated cell suspensions were less responsive to stimulation by
B cell mitogens, but were enriched with ATS-sensitive cells and were
more responsive to stimulation by the T cell mitogen concanavalin A
than by two B cell mitogens. These results indicate that the suspensions of fractionated immune cells were indeed depleted of B cells
and enriched for T cells.

We have shown earlier that cells from hamsters immune to infection with T. pallidum Bosnia A conferred protection on recipients
against challenge by the same strain (5,13). Our new results confirm
our previous findings (13) and provide direct evidence that T cells
are involved in resistance to challenge with T. pallidum. The mechanism by which these T cells confer protection is not yet clearly understood. Since T cells have not been shown to exert a direct trepone-
micidal effect on T. pallidum, the effect of other cells or cellular
products on the destruction of the treponemes needs to be defined.

In summary, experimental studies of immune reactions to syphilitic infection in hamsters have several distinct advantages:

1.   Inbred LSH hamsters are readily available.
2.   Infection of inbred hamsters with T. pallidum produces extensive, chronic skin lesions that can be measured easily.
3.   Syphilitic lymph nodes increase in weight, a useful measure
of pathogenicity and infectivity.
4.   The number of treponemes in the lymph nodes can be estimated
readily by dark-field microscopy.
5.   The hamster has no known treponemal disease that might influence an experimental infection.
6.   Infection of hamsters with T. pallidum Bosnia A induces
cross-resistance to T. pallidum Nichols and T.pertenue, the causative
agents of venereal syphilis and frambesia, respectively (21).
7.   The inbred hamster is relatively inexpensive and does not
require elaborate animal facilities.

ACKNOWLEDGMENTS

This investigation was supported by the World Health Organization and Public Health Service research grant AI-13307 from the National Institute of Allergy and Infectious Diseases.

REFERENCES

1. Perine, P.L. et al. Infect Immun 8 (1973) 787.
2. Turner, T.B. et al. Johns Hopkins Med J 133 (1973) 241.
3. Sepetjian, M. et al. Br J Vener Dis 49 (1973) 241.
4. Bishop, N.H.; Miller, J.N. J Immunol 117 (1976) 191.
5. Schell, R.F. et al. J Infect Dis 140 (1979) 378.
6. Titus, R.G.; Weiser, R.S. J Infect Dis 140 (1979) 904.
7. Pavia, C.S. et al. Br J Vener Dis 54 (1978) 144.
8. Metzger, M.; Smogor, W. Arch Immunol Ther Exp (Warsz) 23 (1975)
    625.
9. Baughn, R.E. et al. Infect Immun 17 (1977) 535.
10. Hollander, D.H.; Turner, T.B. Am J Syph 38 (1954) 489.
11. Miller, J.N. Spirochetes in Body Fluids and Tissues. Charles
    C. Thomas, Springfield, Illinois (1971).
12. Chan, J.K. et al. Infect Immun 26 (1979) 448.
13. Schell, R.F. et al. J Infect Dis (1980) in press.
14. Blasecki, J.W.; Houston, K.J. Immunology 35 (1977) 1.
15. Dresser, D.W. In: Assays for Immunoglobulin-Secreting Cells,
    ed. Weir, pp. 28.1 - 28.25. Blackwell Scientific Publications,
    Oxford (1978).
16. Coe, J.E.; Green, I. J Natl Cancer Inst 54 (1975) 269.
17. Wicher, K.; Jakubowski, A. Br J Vener Dis 40 (1964) 213.
18. Bessemans, A.; DeMoor, A. Ann Inst Pasteur (Paris) 63 (1939)
    569.
19. Gueft, B.; Rosahn, P.D. Am J Syph 32 (1948) 59.
20. Schell, R.F. et al. Br J Vener Dis 51 (1975) 19.
21. Schell, R.F. et al. Infect Immun (1980) in press.

SECTION VI

RESPONSES TO VIRAL INFECTIONS

Chairpersons:

John A. Shadduck

Kenneth P. Johnson

EXPERIMENTAL SUBACUTE SCLEROSING PANENCEPHALITIS (SSPE)

IN THE HAMSTER

Kenneth P. Johnson

Neurology Service, Veterans Administration Medical Center
and the University of California
San Francisco, CA   94121

Experimental animal models that faithfully duplicate most aspects of a significant human disease have contributed greatly to the understanding of the condition in man. Experimental diseases produced in small animals also allow more comprehensive studies at less cost in that many more individuals can be investigated and significant variations in populations can be assessed. This is of major value in infectious diseases in which only a few animals may manifest significant changes. Experimental diseases, especially infectious ones, in animals are highly useful because a disease state can be studied in all its complexity only in the intact mammal. Thus, although important information can be gained from in vitro studies, ultimately the essential combination of genetic, immunological, dosage, and cell specificity factors can be assayed only in the intact animal, allowing a more complete understanding of the disease process to be unraveled.

Most of the clinical, pathological, serological, and virological characteristics of human SSPE have been duplicated in an experimental model of the disease in outbred Syrian golden hamsters. This research effort has developed over the past decade and has now reached the stage where the essentials and elements necessary for viral persistence are becoming clear. The broad outlines of the pathogenesis of this experimental infection are described here, along with a brief description of the natural disease in man, to allow meaningful comparisons.

In man, SSPE is clearly the most significant central nervous system (CNS) slow virus infection produced by a conventional virus (1). The number of individuals affected with the disease throughout the world is still considerable, and the disease is caused by a common human pathogen. In areas of the world where vaccination practices

303

are inadequate, SSPE occurs at a rate of one to three per million people each year. Measles virus, the infectious agent of SSPE, has been linked serologically to a much more serious and common neurological disease of man, multiple sclerosis (2). The clinical signs of SSPE appear most commonly between the ages of 6 and 16, often following exposure to measles virus in the first two years of life (3). Thus there is indirect evidence of an "incubation period" between initial infection and onset of disease of from four to over 10 years. The clinical condition can be divided roughly into three phases: (a) a period of intellectual decline when psychological changes and failure in school are common; (b) a period when various types of epileptic seizures and neurologic malfunction appear, usually heralded by unpredictable diffuse myoclonus; and (c) a period of coma or inattention to the surrounding environment, leading finally to death. The clinical disease may last from three months to over 10 years, during which time evidence of virus is always present in the CNS. Some cases show marked variability in symptoms over time, with periods of semi-recovery. Approximately 50% of cases show a progressive retinitis, which is a useful diagnostic sign (4).

Diagnostic criteria are a peculiar type of suppression burst abnormality in the electroencephalogram and markedly elevated titers of antibodies to measles virus in the serum and cerebral spinal fluid (3). Pathologically, children with SSPE show evidence of progressive focal cerebral necrosis with inflammatory cells in perivascular cuffs and in the tissues. Such cells are usually lymphocytes and plasma cells. Neurons, oligodendrogliocytes, ependymal cells and possibly astrocytes may show both intranuclear and cytoplasmic eosinophilic inclusions which, by their ultrastructure, are collections of measles virus nucleocapsids. Measles antigens can be demonstrated in affected areas by immunofluorescence techniques. The pathogenesis of the human condition is still poorly understood, however; heroic efforts to define a genetic or immunologic defect have failed (5). In many instances it has been possible to recover measles virus from brains of children with SSPE; this has always required co-cultivation of trypsinized brain cells with a permissive cell type, however, indicating that the virus in brain is cell-associated or defective (1). The importance of the defective character of the virus in SSPE is unknown, but may be significant in understanding the pathogenesis of this chronic infection. No known therapy has been defined for human SSPE. The number of cases in the United States has fallen dramatically over the last decade, however, probably as a result of widespread use of live measles virus vaccine (6). A few cases clearly seem related to the vaccine strain of virus. In other parts of the world, such as Latin America, where vaccination is not readily available, numerous cases of SSPE still are recognized yearly.

Three experimental models of SSPE have been developed in the hamster; all are different and thus will be useful for comparative studies. The first, described in 1971 (7), employed a laboratory strain

of measles virus inoculated intracerebrally into newborn hamsters
born to measles-immune mothers. The newborn hamsters therefore had
passively-transferred antibody to measles virus antigens. Persistent
infection was demonstrated and clinical symptoms such as myoclonus
appeared when animals were given immunosuppression drugs more than 60
days after inoculation. This interesting model has not been studied
further; it does suggest, however, that antibodies may play a role in
promoting viral persistence.

More recently, a persistent infection of hamsters has been described (8,9), with delayed onset of clinical disease produced by intracerebral inoculation of newborn hamsters with LU-106 cells persis-
sistently infected with measles virus. Such animals show no acute
disease but do develop several types of seizure, months after inoculation. During the prolonged incubation period, only minor pathologic changes are noted, such as occasional perivascular lymphocytic
cuffs, although immunofluorescence studies show focal collections of
cells containing viral antigen. Such foci may number only 10 to 50
cells. In this model, late disease occurs spontaneously without immunosuppression. All animals with evidence of persistent infection develop serum measles antibodies. In both this and the preceding model,
laboratory strains of measles virus, rather than SSPE isolates, were
used, indicating that human SSPE probably is not caused by a different
and unique virus strain.

The most extensively studied hamster model of SSPE (10) employs
the HBS strain of virus, a hamster-adapted agent derived from the Man-
tooth strain of SSPE virus isolated from a human brain biopsy (11).
While most investigation has been done after intracerebral inoculation of HBS, recent studies indicate that inoculation of the lung of
suckling animals produces CNS invasion and clinical encephalitis in
approximately 5% to 15% of animals (Johnson, unpublished data).
Whether a persistent CNS infection will result from this type of CNS
invasion is as yet unknown. Additional recent work shows that following both CNS and peripheral inoculation, several strains of virus
may invade the hamster retina and produce acute giant cells and necrosis followed by a variety of static abnormalities, including multi-
layered rosette formation (12). In some cases, persistence of virus
in the retina has been demonstrated months after initial exposure.
This experimental model of virus-induced retinal changes may be useful
to ophthalmologists in the future.

Studies of the pathogenesis of SSPE in the HBS-hamster model indicated that age at time of initial exposure to virus may be important,
and that the host immune response probably plays a significant role
in the development of viral persistence. Inoculation of HBS into
suckling hamsters produces a rapidly fatal acute giant cell encephalitis (13). During such encephalitis, large amounts of cell-free complete virus are produced, and budding virions can be observed in brain
tissue (14). Alternatively, intracerebral inoculation of HBS into

adults produces a self-limited subclinical cerebral disease lasting
10 to 15 days. Persistence occurs only in the weanling (21-day-old)
animal, however. After intracerebral exposure, approximately one-
third to one-half of such animals die of acute encephalitis, and perhaps one-half of survivors show evidence of persistent infection (10).
During the first seven to 10 days after inoculation, increasing titers
of free virus can be isolated from brain, and budding virions can be
observed in cerebral tissue. Abruptly, in a two to four day period,
the CNS virus becomes cell-associated or defective and can be rescued
only by primary brain cell culture or by co-cultivation techniques
(15). Persistent virus can be demonstrated by histologic studies,
which show chronic inflammatory cells, primarily lymphocytes and
plasma cells, along with typical measles inclusion-bearing cells. Ul-
trastructural studies of such cells show masses of smooth paramyxo-
virus nucleocapsids in the nucleus and multiple collections of fuzzy
nucleocapsids in the cytoplasm. No budding of virions has been observed, however (16). Immunofluorescence studies show evidence of
viral antigens within infected cells. Immunoperoxidase ultrastructu-
ral investigation indicates insertion of measles antigens into the cytoplasmic membranes of infected cells (17). Why such cells are not detected and destroyed by some immunologic mechanism is unknown.

The influence of the host immune response on the development of
persistence has been studied in several ways. First, it was observed
that the conversion from a complete, infectious form to a cell-associated type of CNS virus in the hamster appeared to be coincident
with the first appearance of measles antibodies in serum (10). The
first antibodies to appear usually are directed against the hemagglutinin antigen. This was studied further with a variety of dosage
schedules of anti-lymphocyte serum given intraperitoneally prior to
and following virus inoculation into adults. These experiments indicated that the appearance of serum antibodies as an indicator of host
immunity could be delayed, and that the conversion from complete infectious to defective virus also could be retarded so that the conversion still coincided with the first appearance of serum antibodies
(18). In another series, hamsters were thymectomized neonatally and
then, as adults, exposed intracerebrally to HBS virus. In such animals, a subacute, rapidly fatal disease developed and it was found
that no serum antibodies had appeared and that large amounts of cell-
free virus were present in the brain (19). Such studies clearly indicate that it was an immune effect, rather than some intrinsic CNS cell
maturation effect, that was operative in producing the cell-associated
type of virus.

Recent human and hamster studies have shed light on the mechanism by which the defective viral state develops and how specific
viral proteins with discrete functions may be involved in the defective, persistent state of measles infection in the mammalian CNS.
Measles virus contains six well-defined structural proteins ranging
in size from 200,000 to 37,000 daltons (20). Of these, the smallest,

the matrix or "M" protein, has been the subject of most interest. The function of measles M protein has not been firmly established experimentally; by analogy with other paramyxoviruses, however, it probably is required for alignment of the RNA-containing nucleocapsid beneath the cytoplasmic membrane prior to bud formation and maturation of complete measles virions (21). Several recent studies of the immune response to individual measles proteins show that sera of SSPE patients contain little or no antibody to M protein, whereas serologic activity to the other viral proteins is readily demonstrated (22-24). The suggestion has been made that this absence of antibody to M protein reflects a relative lack of the protein, which in turn may explain the defective nature of the virus and the lack of budding virions in SSPE. All such studies have been serological and thus provide only indirect evidence of events occurring in the brain. In such a situation, availability of a faithful animal model may prove invaluable.

In collaboration with Dr. Erling Norrby, Karolinska Institute, Stockholm, Sweden, we have studied the development of CNS HBS infection in weanling hamsters through the acute into the chronic phases with immunofluorescence techniques employing antibodies monospecific for individual measles virus polypeptides. The two most useful antisera have been the nucleocapsid protein (NP) antiserum and the matrix protein (M) antiserum.

During the initial phase of infection, when the complete virus can be readily isolated from brain, both NP and M proteins are present in hamster brain sections that were rapidly frozen, cryostat sectioned, and fixed with acetone. Between days 12 and 17, however, when titers of serum antibodies rise rapidly, considerable amounts of NP antigen remain, whereas the M protein completely disappears. The rapid disappearance of M protein over a five-day period coincident with both the appearance of serum antibodies and the conversion of virus from a complete to a defective state strongly suggests that this viral protein alteration is related to the defective state of the chronic virus infection, and may be necessary for the virus to persist in the mammalian brain. Thus, a significant advance in understanding the pathogenesis of SSPE may come from ongoing hamster studies.

The Syrian hamster has been highly useful in the development of faithful models of the human prototype slow virus infection, SSPE. Most of the clinical, pathological, serological, and virological characteristics of the human condition have been duplicated in one or more hamster models, and now the availability of at least three different models will allow for comparative studies to determine just how molecular virologic events lead to the capacity of a conventional virus to remain in the CNS of an immune host. Further immunologic studies are also necessary to obtain a complete picture of the disease process. Sequential hamster studies in which one or more controlled variables can be analyzed exclusively have allowed a better understanding of SSPE pathogenesis to evolve.

Based on presently available human and hamster data, a hypothesis of events leading to measles virus persistence in the CNS of SSPE patients can be developed. Invasion of the CNS during acute infection is required; this may be related to as yet undefined genetic factors, viral dose, age at initial measles virus infection, and perhaps other, as yet unrecognized, factors. Based on the LU-106 and HBS-hamster models, it is evident that subclinical CNS measles infection may remain for prolonged periods in small focal groups of brain cells, probably neurons. Such persistent cells harbor a defective or cell-associated type of virus which nevertheless is able to insert some viral antigens into the cytoplasmic membrane of infected cells. Why such cells are not recognized and destroyed by the host immune system is as yet unknown. The presently postulated reason for the cell-associated or defective nature of the persistent virus is a lack of M protein, which is necessary for maturation and budding of virus. This is consistent with recent studies of SSPE in man. It is also consistent with work cited above indicating that M protein rapidly disappears shortly after initiation of infection, as the host immune system first becomes evident. A possible explanation for the disappearance of M protein could be a process of selective degradation, possibly by some intracellular enzyme mechanism triggered by cell-surface events involving the host immune system. Other possibilities include selective suppression of M protein synthesis, or a mutation involving M protein, although the latter possibility seems highly unlikely. This hypothesis, interestingly, relies on both human and hamster-derived data and is strengthened by the consistence of findings in both the natural human infection and in the experimental hamster study.

ACKNOWLEDGMENTS

Supported by the Research Service of the Veterans Administration and by NIH Grant NS 14069. The excellent technical aid of Mrs. Peggy Swoveland is gratefully acknowledged.

REFERENCES

1.   Agnarsdotter, G. In: Recent Advances in Clinical Virology, ed. Waterson. Churchhill Livingston Inc. London   (1977) 21.
2.   Norrby, E. Prog Med Virol 24 (1978) 1.
3.   Johnson, K.P. et al. In: Advances in Neurology, ed. Thompson and Green, Vol. 6. Raven Press, New York (1974) 77.
4.   Andriola, M.; Karlsberg, R.O. Am J Dis Child 124 (1972) 187.
5.   Lennette, E.H. Arch Neurol 32 (1975) 488.
6.   Modlin, J.F. et al.   J Ped 94 (1979) 231.
7.   Wear, D.; Rapp, F. J Immunol 107 (1971) 1593.
8.   Norrby, E.; Kristensson, K. J Med Virol 2 (1978) 305.
9.   Norrby, E. et al. J Med Virol 5 (1980) 109.
10. Byington, D.P.; Johnson, K.P. J Infect Dis 126 (1972) 18.

11. Byington, D.P. et al. Nature 225 (1970) 551.
12. Parhad, I.M. et al.   Lab Invest, in press.
13. Johnson, K.P.; Byington, D.P. Exp Mol Pathol 15 (1971) 373.
14. Raine, C.S. et al. Lab Invest 33 (1975) 108.
15. Johnson, K.P.; Norrby, E. Exp Mol Pathol 21 (1974) 166.
16. Raine, E.S. et al. Lab Invest 31 (1974) 355.
17. Johnson, K.P.; Swoveland, P. Lab Invest 37 (1977) 459.
18. Byington, D.P.; Johnson, K.P. Lab Invest 32 (1975) 91.
19. Johnson, K.P. et al. Infect Immun 12 (1975) 1464.
20. Morgan, E.M.; Rapp, F.   Bacteriol Rev 41 (1977) 636.
21. Yoshida, T. et al. Virology 71 (1976) 143.
22. Hall, W.W. et al. Proc Natl Acad Sci USA 76 (1979) 2047.
23. Wechsler, S.L. et al. J Immunol 123 (1979) 884.
24. Machamer, C.E. et al. Infect Immun 27 (1980) 817.

ENHANCED INTRAUTERINE TRANSMISSION OF HERPES SIMPLEX VIRUS INFECTION

IN IMMUNOSUPPRESSED HAMSTERS

T. Kurata, K. Kurata, and Y. Aoyama

Institute of Medical Science, University of Tokyo
Shirokanedai 4-6-1, Minato-ku, Tokyo 108, JAPAN

INTRODUCTION

Herpes simplex virus (HSV) infection during pregnancy in man may result in abortion, fetal death, perinatal infection and malformations (1-6). The source of infection in the newborns is obscure; it is unknown whether they are infected in utero transplacentally or their infection is acquired during delivery through the birth canal. There is some evidence suggesting vertical transmission of HSV infection in the mother (7-9). In animal experiments, vertical transmission of HSV infection has been demonstrated in rabbit, mouse, hamster and cat (10-14). We have documented elsewhere (15) that type 1 and 2 HSV caused placental lesions and vertical transmission of the infection in the mother into the fetus when the virus was inoculated intravenously (IV) at the middle and late stage of pregnancy.

Immunosuppression with cyclophosphamide (CP) has been shown to increase significantly the lethality and susceptibility of animals infected with various viruses (16-18). This paper presents the increased incidence of vertical transmission of HSV infection in pregnant hamsters by immunosuppression procedure with CP.

MATERIALS AND METHODS

Female 8- to 12-week-old golden hamsters were obtained from the Experimental Animal Center of our Institute and were placed with the male animals in the evening. The following day was considered to be the first day of gestation as determined by the vaginal smear test.

The pregnant animals were placed in separate cages during the experiment. The gestation period of hamsters is 17 days.

Two types of HSV were used. Strain Mori, isolated from the vesicle of a newborn baby, was used as the type 2 virus. Strain HF, kindly supplied by Dr. K. Yoshino of our Institute, was used as the type 1. The viral stocks were prepared in human embryonic fibroblasts; their titers were 8.5×10^5 and 1.86×10^6 plaque-forming units (PFU) per ml strain Mori, and 7.6×10^6 PFU/ml for strain HF by the plaque counting method with primary chick embryonic fibroblasts.

For the immunosuppression procedure, CP (Endoxan, Shionogi Pharmaceutical Co. Ltd.) was used. The drug was rehydrated with sterile distilled water immediately before use and injected intraperitoneally (IP) as a single dose of 100 mg/kg body weight one day before virus inoculation.

Anti-HSV antibodies were prepared in New Zealand white rabbits using type 2 Mori strain and type 1 Takaichi strain, originally isolated from a patient with acute herpetic dendritic keratitis, as described (19). The IgG fraction of the antisera was separated and conjugated with fluorescein isothiocyanate (FITC; BBL, USA), and absorbed two times with acetone-treated powder of hamster liver and brain to eliminate the nonspecific fluorescence. The staining titers of labeled anti-HSV type 2 and type 1 IgG were 256 and 128, respectively. Cryostat sections of organs removed at the time indicated in tables were fixed in acetone for five minutes at room temperature and stained for one hour at $37^\circ C$ or overnight at $4^\circ C$ with FITC-labeled antibody. After repeated washings with phosphate buffered saline (pH 7.2), they were mounted in carbonate-bicarbonate-buffered glycerol (pH 9.5) and observed under a fluorescence microscope (Olympus Co. Ltd., Tokyo).

To compare the infectivity between type 1 and 2 viruses, the hamsters were divided into eight groups each according to the day of injection as shown in Table 1. Each hamster was given a single injection of 0.1 to 0.5 ml of diluted tissue culture medium containing 10^5 PFU of HSV, IP or IV through a vein of the upper extremity under light anesthesia with Nembuthal (Abbot Laboratories, USA). For immunosuppression, one day before virus inoculation, CP was administered IP as a single dose of 100 mg/kg body weight. In the CP treatment experiment, only type 2 HSV was used. The hamsters were observed daily to check the signs of illness. At various intervals after infection, hamsters were killed and various organs as well as whole fetuses, placentas, uteri and brains removed. The tissues were quickly frozen in N-hexan immersed in dry ice-acetone mixture at $-70^\circ C$. Frozen sections were examined to detect viral antigen by direct immunofluorescence. Some pieces of the organs were fixed in 10% formalin solution, embedded in paraffin, sectioned and stained with hematoxylin and eosin.

RESULTS

Clinical Signs

During experiments, type 1 virus caused no clinical signs in any infected hamsters, but some type 2 virus-infected animals showed paralysis of the lower extremities and general weakness. No signs were seen in the hamsters receiving the virus IP.

Macroscopic Changes

Macroscopic lesions were not clear in placentas, except for a few cases with small necrotic foci, by surface examination or on section. Fetuses dead and autolyzed in utero were found in two hamsters given the type 1 virus on the ninth day of gestation. In the type 2 virus infection, even severe placental lesions at the 16th day of gestation were not associated with dead fetuses. Abortion or congenital malformation was not found.

Table 1. Distribution of Viral Antigen in Placenta and Fetus after Type I and Type 2 Herpes Simplex Virus Infection

Day of gestation	Type 1 mother	Type 1 fetus	Type 1 fetus(+)[1]	Type 1 placenta(+)	Type 2 mother	Type 2 fetus	Type 2 fetus(+)	Type 2 placenta(+)
V[2] (day 1) ———— X[2] (day 16)	5	43	0	0	5	44	0	0
V (day 3) ———— X	5	53	0	0	5	69	0	0
V (day 4) ———— X	5	48	5	28	5	72	2	15
V (day 6) ———— X	5	39	0	4	5	47	3	23
V (day 8) ———— X	5	38	5	28	5	65	5	27
V (day 10) ———— X	5	38	5	5	5	69	0	35
V (day 12) —— X	5	44	2	19	5	50	0	12
V (day 15) X	5	47	9	16	5	43	0	0

[1]Number with positive immunofluorescence.

[2]Virus was inoculated intravenously (10^6 PFU) on the day indicated.

[3]The hamsters were killed on the final day of pregnancy.

Table 2.   Effect of Cyclophosphamide on the Vertical Transmission
of Herpes Simplex Virus Infection in the Early Stage of
Pregnancy

Day of gestation 0 1 2 3 4 5 6 . . . . .15 16	No.[1]	No. of placentas	Fetal	Placenta (+)[2]	Fetus (+)
C[3] V[4] X[5]	1	14	0	0	0
C V X	1	18	0	0	0
C V X	3	48	7	15	0
C V X	1	13	0	0	0
C V X	1	9	0	0	0
C V X	3	36	8	13	0
C V X	1	7	0	0	0
C V X	1	16	0	0	0
C V X	3	44	12	16	0

[1]Number of pregnant hamsters used.

[2]Number positive by immunofluorescence.

[3]Intraperitoneal inoculation of cyclophosphamide (100 mg/kg body
weight).

[4]Herpes simplex virus (type 2) inoculation via vein.

[5]Hamsters were killed on the day indicated.

Type 2 HSV infection in CP-treated hamsters was very different
from that in non-treated infected animals.   CP-treated hamsters were
associated with high incidence of fetal death, especially when the
drug and virus were given at the middle and late stage of pregnancy.
(Table 2, 3).   On section, the placenta associated with fetal death
showed extensive necrosis and the fetuses were autolyzed in utero.
Abortion or congenital malformation was not found, at least at the
time of death.   As is clear in Table 4, there was neither fetal death
nor placental lesions in the hamsters treated with CP alone.

Table 3. Effect of Cyclophosphamide on the Vertical Transmission of Herpes Simplex Virus Infection in the Middle and Late Stage of Pregnancy

Day of gestation 0 1 .....7 8 9 10 11 12 13 14 15 16	No.[1]	No. of placentas	Fetal death	Placentas (+)[2]	Fetuses (+)
C^3 V^4 X^5	3	35	8	22	0
C V X	3	27	10	26	0
C V X	3	35	5	32	8
C V X	3	32	17	31	6
C V X	3	29	13	24	8
C V X	3	31	23	28	9
C V X	1	12	4	5	0
C V X	1	16	7	12	0
C V X	1	13	9	10	0
C V X	1	13	13	13	0
C V X	1	16	14	14	6
C V X	3	35	28	33	11
C V X	1	15	0	6	0
C V X	1	14	0	10	0
C V X	1	17	0	17	0
C V X	1	16	0	16	1
C V X	3	42	0	40	12

See footnotes for Table 2.

Histology

There were no marked differences between both types of HSV infection without CP treatment. Numerous tissue blocks from the CP-treated placentas had essentially the same appearance as found in the previous experiments. Similar but more severe changes were found, such as coagulative necrosis in the placental labyrinth, thrombosis of ma-

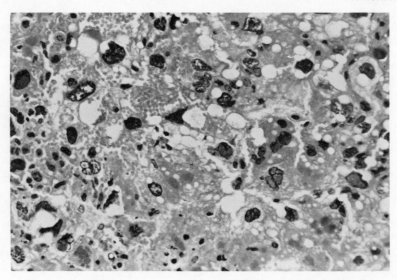

Fig. 1: Hemorrhagic necrosis of the placenta showing single or multiple eosinophilic intranuclear inclusion bodies (HSV type
2) (400 X). (Reduced 14% for reproduction.)

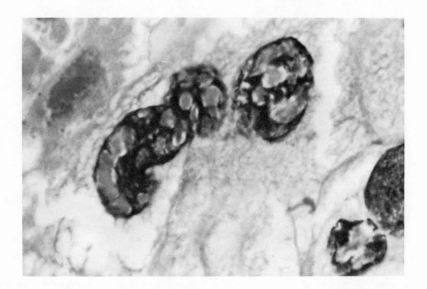

Fig. 2: Intranuclear inclusion bodies (Cowdry type A) in the multi-
nuclear giant cells derived from trophoblast (type 2)
(1000 X). (Reduced 14% for reproduction.)

ternal vessels in the placenta, and degenerative necrosis characteristic of HSV infection in the trophoblasts, that formed giant cells
(Fig. 1,2). None of these responses contained an inflammatory component. All deceased fetuses of mothers killed at the end of pregnancy
showed various stages of mummification. In spite of these lesions,
the pregnancy was maintained up to the final day of pregnancy. No
changes were noted in the fetal side of the placenta and uterine
muscle layer.

In some mothers infected IV, there was moderate to severe focal
destruction of the adrenal cortex. Maternal livers showed small necrotic changes with a few inclusion bodies. In the fetuses, typical
herpetic lesions with intranuclear inclusion bodies (Cowdry type A)
were found in brain, spinal cord, dorsal root ganglion, skin, liver,
adrenal gland, and lung (Fig. 3,4).

In hamsters given the virus IP without CP treatment, no microscopic lesions were detected in the mothers or fetuses.

The hamsters with CP treatment without virus inoculation showed
no lesions such as destruction of placental structure or abnormal
findings in the fetuses (Table 4). Spleen size decreased slightly at
two or three days after CP treatment. Follicles within periarteriolar
sheaths were depleted of cells compared to the non-treated ones.

Immunofluorescence

Intraperitoneal injection of both types of HSV into the pregnant
hamsters at different times between the 1st and 15th day of gestation
failed to produce any specific immunofluorescence in placentas or fetuses. In several organs of the mother, viral antigens were not detected. Briefly, vertical transmission of both types of HSV was not
demonstrated.

In the kinetic study with type 2 HSV (15), the viral antigen was
found in placentas only when the hamsters were infected in the middle
and late stage of pregnancy. In the present experiment, the infectivity of type 1 and type 2 viruses was compared by intravenous administration of the virus. All animals were killed on the 16th day of
gestation regardless of the day of virus inoculation. Distribution of
viral antigen detected in organs by immunofluorescence is summarized
in Table 1. With both viruses, injection on the fifth day of gestation caused specific fluorescence for the first time in placentas and
in fetuses. The proportion of virus-positive tissues was different
at every stage, depending upon the day of inoculation. Vertical transmission of infection was demonstrated in the hamsters that received
the virus from the fifth to ninth day of gestation in the type 2, and
from the fifth to 15th day in the type 1, as shown in Table 1.

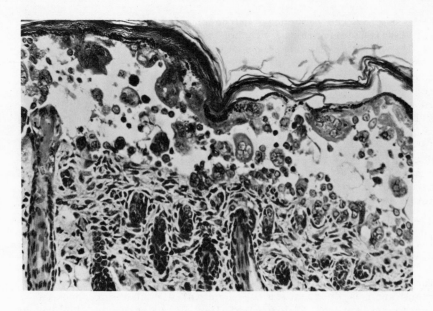

Fig. 3:   Vesicle of the skin showing herpetic inclusion bodies(type
          2) (200 X). (Reduced 14% for reproduction.)

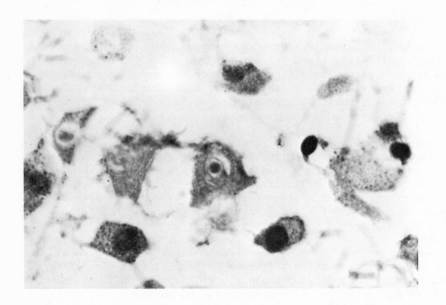

Fig. 4:   Nerve cells with inclusion body in dorsal root ganglion
          (type 2) (1000 X). (Reduced 14% for reproduction.)

Table 4.   Effect of Cyclophosphamide on Pregnant Hamsters Without
           Virus Infection

Day of gestation 0 1 2 3 4 . . . . . 8 9 10 . . . . . 15 16	No.[1]	No. of placentas	Lesions in placenta	Fetal death
C[3] . . . . X[5]	3	33	0	0
C X	3	42	0	0
C X	3	37	0	0
C X	3	48	0	0
C X	3	42	0	0
C X	3	39	0	0

See footnotes for Table 2.

In fetuses, the viral antigens were localized in the skin,
forming clear vesicles (Fig. 5) in the epidermal layer, dorsal root
ganglion (Fig. 6), liver, spinal cord (Fig. 7), adrenal gland, brain,
tongue, lip (Fig. 8), and bone marrow. In placentas, focal fluorescence was detected especially in the multinucleated giant cells derived from trophoblasts on the maternal surface (Fig. 9). Multiple or
extensive foci of specific fluorescence also were present in the trophoblasts and the chorionic plates of the placenta, and sometimes the
chorioallantois. Viral antigen was rarely present, however, in the
uterine blood vessels and uterine muscle layer. Maternal livers,
brains and adrenal glands in some cases showed positive fluorescence
regardless of the day of injection or death. It seems that the infectivity in the mother's organs depends upon the varied individual susceptibility to the virus (Table 5). No marked difference of distribution of viral antigens between types 1 and 2 HSV was found.

Effect of CP Treatment

The times of CP and HSV inoculation into hamsters and their
deaths are shown in Tables 2 and 3. To test the effect of CP on the
early stage of pregnancy, CP was administered IP on day 1, 2, or 3,
and the HSV was inoculated IV on day 2, 3, or 4 of gestation, respectively. Hamsters were killed on day 5, 6, or 16 of gestation. Immunofluorescence revealed the presence of viral antigen of HSV in the placentas and adrenal glands of the mother, while no specific fluores-

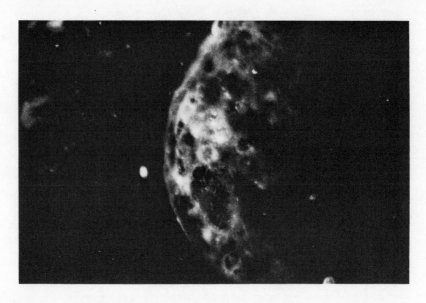

Fig. 5: Viral antigen in the vesicle of fetal skin (type 2) (200 X).
         (Reduced 14% for reproduction.)

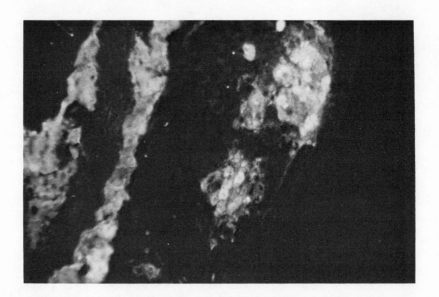

Fig. 6: Specific fluorescence shows the viral antigen in the dorsal
         root ganglion of the fetus (type 2) (400 X).
         (Reduced 14% for reproduction.)

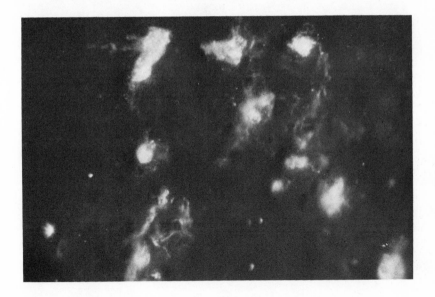

Fig. 7: Viral antigen in the spinal cord of the fetus (type 1)
         (400 X). (Reduced 14% for reproduction.)

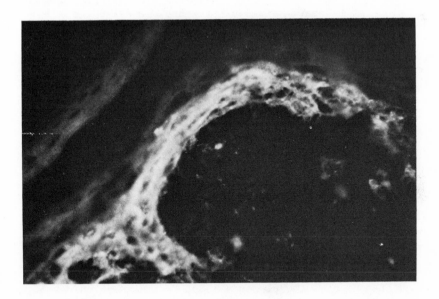

Fig. 8: Viral antigen in the lip of the fetus (type 1) (200 X).
         (Reduced 14% for reproduction.)

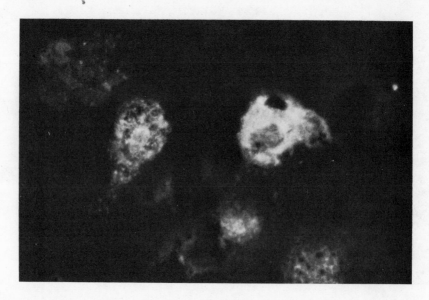

Fig. 9: Viral antigen in a multinucleated giant cell derived from
         trophoblast (type 2) (400 X). (Reduced 14% for reproduction.)

cence was detected in the fetuses. In the previous experiments, virus
inoculation alone at the early stage of pregnancy revealed specific
fluorescence neither in placentas nor in fetuses. After CP treatment,
the hamsters maintained till the final day of pregnancy showed a few
fetal deaths, but not the presence of viral antigen in the fetuses
(Table 2). All placentas associated with fetal death showed wide distribution of the viral antigens.

To test the effect of CP on the middle and late stages of pregnancy, the drug was administered IP on day 8, 9, or 10 and the virus
was inoculated IV on day 9, 10, or 11 of gestation, respectively. The
hamsters were killed according to the schedule in Table 3. In the previous experiments, virus inoculation on day 9 resulted in the highest
incidence of vertical transmission, and so more animals were used in
this group. It is quite clear from Table 3 that CP treatment and HSV
infection at the eighth to 11th day of gestation produced positive evidence of viral antigen in placenta in a high proportion of animals.
The hamsters that maintained pregnancy more than three days after infection showed viral antigen in at least 82.7% of placentas. With
reference to fetal death, CP treatment on day 8 or 9, and HSV infection on day 9 or 10, resulted in high incidence of fetal death associated with destruction of the placenta. But CP treatment on day 10,
late stage of pregnancy, and HSV inoculation on the following day,
brought no death in 103 fetuses, suggesting that fetal death is re-

Table 5. Distribution of Viral Antigen in Mother's Organs

	No.[1]	Adrenal gl.	Brain	Liver	Uterus
Without cyclophosphamide					
HSV type 1	40	5	0	3	4
HSV type 2	40	8	7	4	4
With cyclophosphamide[2]					
HSV type 2					
Early[3]	15	8	0	3	0
Late	33	20	3	9	8

[1]Number of hamsters used.

[2]Cyclophosphamide was administered intraperitoneally one day before virus inoculation (100 mg/kg body weight).

[3]Stage of pregnancy.

lated to the stage of embryogenesis. There was no fetal death without severe destruction of placenta and the presence of viral antigen in the placenta. In live and dead fetuses, the viral antigen was detected in the liver, spinal cord, brain, skin, lips, dorsal root ganglion and sometimes in indistinguishable tissues of autolysed bodies. In the mother, 53.3% of adrenal glands showed specific fluorescence in the early stage, and 61.2% were similarly positive in the late stage infection; only 20% were positive without CP treatment. The viral antigen also was seen in the liver and rarely in the brain (Table 5).

DISCUSSION

The studies were done to define more clearly the mechanism by which HSV deleteriously influences pregnancy under immunosuppressed conditions with CP treatment. The results shown in this report indicate that both types of HSV cause placental lesions and vertical transmission in fetuses when the virus is inoculated IV into a pregnant hamster at the middle and late period of pregnancy and that CP can enhance the severity of infection in pregnant hamsters and in their fetuses. There were no clear differences in infectivity between type 1 and type 2 HSV, such as in placental lesions examined histologically or in antigen distribution detected by immunofluorescence. Histological and immunofluorescent studies showed that focal placental lesions in decidua basalis spread diffusely up to the chorionic plate in the late stage of pregnancy, and these findings indicated the possibility of fetal death, spontaneous abortion, or premature birth under appropriate conditions of suitable virus growth or infectious period.

In some human cases, possible intrauterine infection was suggested by early onset of disease after delivery or by some other clinical evidences (7-9,20). The presence of inclusion bodies in endome-
trium infected with HSV has been shown in man (21). The evidence of
the increase of primary infection in adult humans (22) has serious significance, considering the primary infection before or during pregnancy with respect to the effect on embryogenesis, resulting in abortion
or congenital HSV infection of the fetus.

Animals treated with CP are more susceptible than the ones without
CP to infectivity and to lethality from the virus infection by suppressed antibody production or interferon activity (23,24). In the
present experiments, it is apparent in Tables 2 and 3 that CP treatment one day prior to HSV inoculation produces severe lesions both in
placentas and fetuses. The results of immunofluorescence studies
showed viral antigen in 90.3% of placentas and 29% of fetuses in the
hamsters treated with CP on day 8, followed by HSV infection on day 9
and death on the final day of pregnancy. Without CP, in the same
stage specific fluorescence was detected in 41.5% of placentas and 7.7%
of fetuses. CP caused specific fluorescence in the placentas infected
at the early stage of pregnancy, but without the drug no viral antigen
was seen. The present investigation demonstrated that slight suppression of immune mechanisms by CP influences the barrier function of placenta, increasing susceptibility to the virus and resulting in vertical
transmission. The direct cause of fetal death was presumably the
blockade of nutritional supply by severe infection of the placenta,
and another cause was infection of HSV in the fetus itself, considering
the presence of viral antigen in dead fetuses. There seem to be two
steps in the vertical transmission of the HSV infection from mother
into fetus. The first is the proliferation of the virus in placenta
after viremia and growth there, and the next is the transmission of
the virus from placenta into fetus. Each step seems to have a separate defense mechanism. Our experiments reveal that the first defense
step is easily destroyed by CP treatment. Taking into account the
fact that CP treatment alone with 100 mg/kg body weight caused no
changes in placenta or fetus, this dose of the drug might be effective
only after HSV infection results in suppression of the barrier activity
of the placenta. The failure to detect viral antigen in fetuses without its existence in the placenta suggests that a "barrier" is formed
in the placental membrane, probably related to the placental macrophages, which may inhibit virus passage.

Some organs of the mother were infected, too, as shown in Table
5. Compared to the results of infectivity in nonpregnant hamsters,
pregnant animals are significantly more liable to be infected. This
tendency is accelerated by CP administration.

It is known that CP has a depressant effect on the reticuloendothelial systems. In our experiments, the drug reduced slightly the
number of mononuclear cells in lymph follicles of the spleen compared

to the non-treated controls. It seems likely, therefore, that virus elimination in the placenta is at least partly mediated by these mononuclear cells.

Further experiments, in which host defense mechanisms are suppressed more selectively, and in which the interaction of HSV with placental structure and function is defined more precisely, may lead to a clear understanding of the determinants for vertical transmission of HSV infection.

REFERENCES

1. Florman, A.L. et al. JAMA 225 (1973) 129.
2. Cibis, A.; Burde, R.M. Arch Ophthalmol 85 (1971) 220.
3. Golden, B. et al. JAMA 209 (1969) 1219.
4. South, M.A. et al. J Pediatr 75 (1969) 13.
5. Naib, Z.M. et al. Obstet Gynecol 35 (1970) 260.
6. McCallum, F.O. Proc R Soc Exp Biol Med 65 (1972) 585.
7. Mitchell, J.E.; McColl, F.C. Am J Dis Child 106 (1963) 207.
8. Sieber, O.F. et al. J Pediatr 69 (1966) 30.
9. Witzleben, C.L.; Driscoll, S.G. Pediatrics 36 (1965) 192.
10. Biegeleisen, J.Z., Jr.; Scott, L.V. Proc Soc Exp Biol Med 95 (1958) 411.
11. Biegeleisen, J.Z., Jr., et al. Am J Clin Pathol 37 (1962) 289.
12. Hoover, E.A.; Griesemer, R.A. Am J Pathol 65 (1971) 173.
13. Middelkamp, J.N. et al. Proc Soc Exp Biol Med 125 (1967) 757.
14. Munk, K.; Radsak, K. Arch Gesamte Virusforsch 25 (1968) 263.
15. Kurata, K. et al. Jpn J Exp Med 46 (1976) 187.
16. Albrecht, P. et al. J Infect Dis 126 (1972) 154.
17. Hough, V.; Robinson, T.W.E. Arch Virol 48 (1975) 75.
18. Weiner, L.P. et al. J Immunol 106 (1971) 427.
19. Aoyama, Y. et al. In: Fluorescent Antibody Techniques and their Applications, ed. Kawamura. University Park Press (1977) 144.
20. Strawn, E.Y.; Scrimenti, R.J. Am J Obstet Gynecol 115 (1973) 581.
21. Goldman, R.L. Obstet Gynecol 36 (1970) 603.
22. Hondo, R. Jpn J Med Sci Biol 27 (1974) 205.
23. Lagrange, P.H. et al. J Exp Med 139 (1973) 1529.
24. Hoffsten, P.E.; Dixon, F.J. J Immunol 112 (1974) 564.

SUSCEPTIBILITY TO FATAL PICHINDE VIRUS INFECTION IN THE SYRIAN HAMSTER

Sydney R. Gee, Marcia A. Chan, David A. Clark and
William E. Rawls

McMaster University Health Sciences Centre
1200 Main St. W., Hamilton, Ontario,
Canada L8S 3Z5

INTRODUCTION

Pichinde virus, an arenavirus, causes a fatal infection in the inbred MHA strain of Syrian hamsters within 10 to 20 days of an intraperitoneal inoculation (1). High titres of virus are present, and death appears to be a direct consequence of the virus-induced necrosis in cells of the liver and spleen (2). Other strains of hamsters, including the inbred LSH strain and the random-bred LVG line, survive the infection. Resistance to the fatal virus infection is associated with an ability to limit Pichinde virus replication to low levels. The phenotypes of survival and the ability to limit viremia are each controlled by a single dominant gene (3, 4); it is not known whether the same gene controls both properties. Since the pathogenesis of Pichinde virus infection in Syrian hamsters resembles the pathogenesis of human arenavirus infections in several respects (5), an understanding of the events leading to the recovery of hamsters from Pichinde virus disease may contribute some insight into the factors controlling the human diseases. In this paper, early events of Pichinde virus infection and the immune response to the virus in the resistant and susceptible hamster strains are described.

MATERIALS AND METHODS

The MHA, LSH and LVG strains of Syrian hamsters were purchased from Charles River/Lakeview, Lakefield, N.J. (LSH X MHA)F_1 animals and back-cross progeny were bred in our animal quarters. Hamsters aged 5 to 10 weeks were inoculated intraperitoneally (IP) with 2000 plaque-forming units (PFU) of Pichinde virus, strain AN3739, in a volume of 0.2 ml diluent. The virus was inoculated subcutaneously into the foodpad (FP) using 2000 PFU in 0.05 ml diluent. Pichinde virus was assayed by plaque formation on monolayers of Vero cells as described previously (6); infectious centers of Pichinde virus-producing cells were enumerated by inoculating dilutions of infected cells on mono-layers of Vero cells and observing for plaques as detailed elsewhere (3).

Natural killer (NK) activity was determined in a ^{51}Cr-release assay. A line of cells derived from an adenovirus type-12-induced tumour in an MHA hamster (MAD) was used as targets (3). A constant number of targets (10^4) was mixed with different numbers of effectors to give effector: target cell ratios of 100:1, 50:1, 25:1, 12.4:1 and 6.25:1 in 96 well microtiter plates, and the mixtures were incubated for 16 hours. The supernatants then were aspirated and counted in a gamma counter as reported previously (3). Mean per cent specific release was calculated from four replicates, where

$$\% \text{ specific } {}^{51}\text{Cr release} = \frac{\text{test cpm } - \text{ spontaneous cpm}}{\text{maximum releasable cpm } - \text{ spontaneous cpm}} \times 100\%.$$

Spontaneous release was determined by incubating the labelled target cells in medium alone, and values for maximum release were obtained by adding 1% (v/v) NP-40 to 10^4 target cells.

Spleen cells were separated into adherent and non-adherent fractions by incubating 4×10^7 cells on 150 mm^2 plastic dishes for 1 hour at 37°C, as described previously (3). A further separation according to size was performed by allowing the cells to sediment at unit gravity in a bovine serum albumin (BSA) gradient for 3 1/2 hours at 4°C. This procedure has been described in detail (3).

Footpad swelling was assessed in two ways. Spring-loaded calipers were used to measure the thickness of hind footpads of animals that had received an inoculation of Pichinde virus. The mean difference in measurements between the virus-infected test foot and the control foot was calculated. An inoculation of supernatant from BHK cells, in which Pichinde virus is propagated, failed to elicit a footpad swelling response. In a second assay for footpad swelling, the radioisotopic assay of Paranjpe and Boone (7) was employed. In this assay, ^{125}I-labelled hamster serum albumin was injected IP 24 hours before assay, and the hind feet were amputated and counted in a gamma counter. These results were expressed as the ratio of the cpm-test foot/cpm-control foot.

RESULTS AND DISCUSSION

Death following Pichinde virus infection of the susceptible MHA strain of hamsters appears to be a result of the tropism of the virus

for cells of the reticuloendothelial system (2). The high levels of
viremia, which peak eight to 11 days after the IP injection, presumably reflect the earlier proliferation of the virus in suitable target
cells. Indeed, marked histological changes are apparent in the spleen
within four days of the IP injection of Pichinde virus (2). Virus
titres at four to eight days after infection are greater in the spleen
than in any other site in both the susceptible and resistant hamsters
(1), raising the possibility that early viral proliferation in the
spleen is an important step in the spread of the virus. To test this
idea, a kinetic study of the appearance of virus-producing cells in
the spleens of IP-inoculated hamsters was performed. The results of
this study are illustrated in Fig. 1.

A difference in the number of virus-producing spleen cells between susceptible and resistant hamster strains is manifested early
in infection. As early as two days after IP injection, susceptible
MHA hamster spleens contained about 10-fold more infectious centers
of virus per 10^6 cells than in the resistant LSH strain. Peak titers
were attained on day 3 in both strains. In contrast to the MHA strain,
LSH hamster spleens subsequently showed a decline in the number of infected cells, and almost no virus-producing cells were found in spleens
taken eight days after injection. Two points can be made from these
findings: first, spleen cells in the susceptible MHA strain are subjected to a rapid viral proliferation two to three days after infection, and second, the resistant strain is able to curtail virus replication in the spleen within eight days of infection.

Studies were then initiated to characterize the target cell for
Pichinde virus growth in spleens of susceptible and resistant hamsters. Previous work had suggested that the MHA target cell was associated with an NK-like cell. NK cells have the property of being
non-adherent to plastic and sediment under unit gravity at a rate
typical of medium-sized cells. Therefore, spleen cells from MHA and
LSH hamsters injected IP with Pichinde virus three days previously
were separated into plastic-adherent and non-adherent populations,
and then further separated according to size by sedimentation through
a BSA gradient at unit gravity. Fractions of cells were pooled,
counted and assayed for infectious centers of Pichinde virus. The
data are shown in Table 1. There was essentially no difference in
the number of infectious centers in the adherent fractions of spleen
cells from MHA and LSH hamsters. There were, however, 6.7 times more
infectious centers in the non-adherent spleen cells of MHA hamsters
compared to those of LSH hamsters. When the non-adherent cells were
separated by sedimentation through a BSA gradient, substantial differences were found in the medium fraction, with 5.2 times more infectious centers detected in MHA than LSH spleens. No difference was apparent in the large non-adherent fraction. These results strongly suggest that susceptible hamsters have greater numbers of a population
of spleen target cells for Pichinde virus replication than the resistant strain. The presence of this additional spleen target cell may

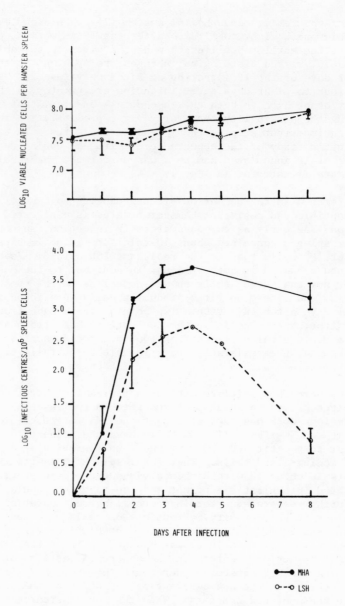

Fig. 1:   Kinetics of appearance of infectious center in the spleens
          of MHA (●---●) and LSH (o---o) hamsters that had received
          an IP inoculation of 2000 PFU Pichinde virus. Spleens
          were excised on the days indicated, and dilutions of cells
          were plated on monolayers of Vero cells to quantitate virus-
          producing cells. Bars represent the standard deviation.

Table 1. Infectious Centers in Spleen Cells Separated by Plastic Adherence and Size

| | | Infectious centers[2] | | | | |
| | | LSH | | MHA | | |
Sample[1]	Fraction	Per 10^5 cells	Per fraction	Per 10^5 cells	Per fraction	MHA/LSH[3]
Adherent	—	74.7	3.1×10^4	341.0	4.9×10^4	1.6
Non-adherent	—	108.0	5.7×10^4	355.0	3.8×10^5	6.7
Adherent	Large	125.0	3.6×10^3	171.0	9.1×10^2	0.3
	Small	29.5	3.5×10^3	39.7	2.0×10^3	0.6
Non-adherent	Large	153.0	1.7×10^3	142.0	2.3×10^3	1.4
	Medium	20.2	2.1×10^3	91.3	1.1×10^4	5.2

[1]Spleen cells were obtained from LSH and MHA hamsters that had been inoculated with 2000 PFU Pichinde virus IP three days previously. Populations of adherent and non-adherent cells were obtained by incubating on plastic dishes (3). These cell populations were allowed to sediment through a gradient of BSA in a STA-PUT apparatus for 3½ hours at 4°C, as previously described (3). Fractions were collected, and the cells were counted. Fractions were then pooled as indicated.

[2]Ten-fold dilutions of spleen cells were tested for infectious centers by plaquing on Vero cells.

[3]Ratio of infectious centers per fraction of MHA compared to LSH.

result in an early, overwhelming virus proliferation in the susceptible strain when the virus is inoculated intraperitoneally.

An interesting possibility was raised by the finding that hamster spleen NK activity also co-purified with the non-adherent,
medium-sized population of cells (data not presented). It has been
reported previously that endogenous spleen NK activity is greater in
MHA hamsters than in LSH hamsters, and that Pichinde virus infection
augments this lytic activity to a greater extent in the MHA strain
compared to the LSH strain (3, 4). This difference appears to be genetically controlled, since (LSH X MHA)F_1 progeny have levels of NK
activity comparable to that of their LSH parent (3, 4). Furthermore,
the kinetics of appearance of NK activity parallel the appearance of
infectious centers of Pichinde virus in the spleen (data not shown).
Taken together, these observations suggest that the MHA hamster activated NK cell may be the additional target cell for Pichinde virus
replication. In agreement with this idea, it has been reported (8)
that poly(ICLC) treatment aggravates the severity of infection of the
arenavirus Machupo in Rhesus monkeys and increases titers of Machupo
virus in the blood. Since poly(ICLC) is an inducer of NK activity,
this report is consistent with the idea that certain arenaviruses may
be able to replicate in NK cells. Such a tropism for cells involved in
the immune response has been reported for several other viruses, including measles, VSV and LCMV (review, 9).

The observation that LSH hamster spleens contained almost no
virus-producing cells eight days after infection in contrast to the
continued infection observed in susceptible MHA hamster spleens (Fig.
1) suggested that the anti-viral immune response may be important in
clearing the virus later in the infection. Indeed, other evidence supports this suggestion. Resistance to Pichinde virus infection is age-
acquired; LVG hamsters infected before eight days of age are fully susceptible (1), the assumption here being that this age-acquired resistance reflects the maturation of the immune response. Also, treatment
of the resistant strain with cyclophosphamide, an immunosuppressant,
abrogates resistance; the treated animals are unable to limit Pichinde
virus replication and die (1). Thus, the immune response against the
virus does appear to play a role in recovery from Pichinde virus infection. No difference could be demonstrated, however, in the ability
of susceptible and resistant hamsters to produce antibodies against
an internal structural Pichinde virus antigen or against virus antigens present on the surface of infected cells (1). These findings
imply that the humoral immune response, as measured by antibody production, is adequate in the susceptible hamster strain.

As a measure of cell-mediated immunity, the footpad swelling response to a primary footpad inoculation of Pichinde virus was assessed. This response correlates with the appearance of other parameters of cell-mediated immunity in mice and rats (10) and seems to
be a manifestation of delayed-type hypersensitivity. An inoculation

Table 2. Comparison of the Effect of IP and FP Routes of Inoculation on the Pathogenesis of Pichinde Virus Infection in MHA and LSH Hamsters

Strain	MHA			LSH		
Route of immunization	IP	FP	FP-IP	IP	FP	FP-IP
Survival (%)	25%	100%	100%	100%	100%	100%
Viremia at 8 days; ($\log_{10}$ PFU/ML)	5.91 ± 0.10	3.90 ± 0.80	<2.70	3.53	<2.0	<2.70
Anti-viral antibodies (mean titre)						
3 days	<1:4	<1:4	1:646	<1:4	<1:4	1:631
8 days	1:38	1:34	<1:646	1:53	<1:16	NT

Animals received an inoculation of 2×10^3 PFU Pichinde virus intraperitoneally (IP) or sub-cutaneously into the footpad (FP). Footpad-immunized animals were challenged via the IP route within 4-6 weeks of the first inoculation. Animals were bled by cardiac puncture, and the sera were assayed for Pichinde virus, and for antiviral antibodies by the complement fixation test.

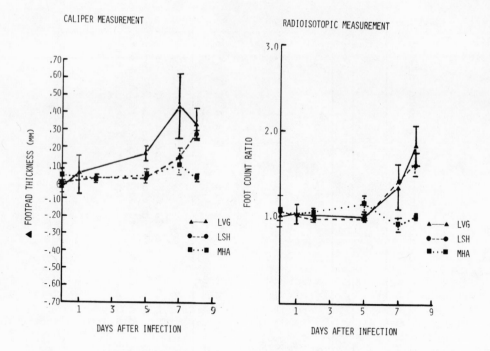

Fig. 2:   The footpad swelling response to Pichinde virus MHA
          (●---●), LSH (▲---▲) and LVG (■——■) hamsters were in-
          oculated with 2000 PFU Pichinde virus in the right rear
          footpad and with control antigen from uninfected cells in
          the left rear footpad. At various times after injection,
          the hind feet were measured with spring-loaded calipers,
          and the difference in thickness was plotted (A-caliper
          measurements). Other hamsters received an IP inoculation
          of ^{125}I-hamster serum albumin, and the feet were amputated
          and counted in a gamma counter (B-radioisotopic measure-
          ment).

of Pichinde virus into the footpads of resistant LSH or LVG hamsters
elicited a swelling response that peaked eight days after the injection (Fig. 2). In contrast, no swelling was detectable in the susceptible MHA strain at this time. The lack of response was not at-
tributable to a failure of Pichinde virus to infect the MHA animals
when inoculated by the footpad route, since high titres of complement-
fixing anti-viral antibodies could be demonstrated (Table 2). This
unresponsiveness was not limited to Pichinde virus; an inoculation of
herpes simplex virus type 1 also failed to elicit footpad swelling in
MHA hamsters, but produced a vigorous response in the resistant strain
(data not presented). These observations suggest that the MHA hamster strain may have a defective delayed-type hypersensitivity response.

Table 3. Genetics of the Footpad Swelling Response in Syrian Hamsters

Background	No.	Phenotype	Mean foot-count ratio $\pm$ SD $(\frac{\text{Test CPM}}{\text{Control CPM}})$
LSH	19		1.83 ± 0.43
MHA	21		1.20 ± 0.15
F_1	8	8 LSH	$2.00 \pm .16$
F_1 X LSH	18	17 LSH	$1.87 \pm .31$
		1 MHA	1.31
F_1 X MHA	36	19 LSH	$1.72 \pm .27$
		16 MHA	$1.16 \pm .12$

Animals received an inoculation of 2000 PFU Pichinde virus in
25 µl in the right rear footpad, and 25 µl of supernatant from uninfected cells in their left rear footpad on day 0. On day 7, 106 CPM
^{125}I-labelled hamster serum albumin was injected IP. Animals were
killed eight days after infection, and the hind feet were amputated
and counted in a gamma counter. Animals were then divided into phenotypic classes using the mean foot-count ratio $\pm$ SD of the parents as
a criterion. Means of the phenotypic groups were then calculated.

It should be noted that MHA hamsters survived the footpad inoculation of Pichinde virus, and were able to limit virus replication
to low levels (Table 2). The response was independent of the amount
of virus inoculated, over a range of 10^3 to 10^6 PFU (data not presented). In addition, footpad-immunized MHA hamsters were protected
against a normally·lethal IP challenge of Pichinde virus. We interpret these findings to indicate that the susceptible MHA hamster strain
is able to develop a protective immune response against Pichinde
virus when the virus is inoculated by the footpad route.

In order to determine whether the lack of footpad swelling response in MHA hamsters was genetically acquired, individual (LSH X
MHA)F_1 and back-cross progeny were inoculated with Pichinde virus in
the right hind footpads, and the radioisotopic method was used to
assess swelling eight days later. The data presented in Table 3 indicate that the footpad swelling response to Pichinde virus is a dominant trait controlled by a single gene. No sex linkage was apparent
(data not presented). In a preliminary experiment, the popliteal
lymph nodes were excised from these footpad-infected hamsters, and
the titres of Pichinde virus were determined for each animal (Table
4). Popliteal lymph nodes from MHA hamsters contained 3.80 ± 0.62 $\log_{10}$
PFU Pichinde virus, compared to 2.64 ± 0.53 $\log_{10}$ PFU in the popliteal

lymph nodes of footpad-inoculated LSH hamsters. Using the range of
mean +1 SD as a criterion, virus titres in back-cross progeny were
classified as LSH-like or MHA-like. All (LSH X MHA)F_1 progeny and
16/18 F_1 X LSH progeny had titres comparable to their LSH parent. Of
20 F_1 X MHA animals, ten had titres comparable to their LSH parent
and ten had MHA-like titres; no influence of gender of the animal was
noted. These results are consistent with the idea that a single autosomal dominant gene controls Pichinde virus replication in the popliteal lymph node. This gene does not appear to be the same gene that
controls the footpad swelling response; of the 10 F_1 X MHA hamsters
which showed the LSH footpad swelling phenotype, six had LSH-like
titres of Pichinde virus and four had MHA-like titres. Of the nine
F_1 X MHA animals that manifested the MHA footpad swelling phenotype,
four had LSH-like titres of Pichinde virus and five had MHA-like
titres. The single animal that demonstrated an intermediate footpad
swelling response had MHA-like titres of Pichinde virus in its popliteal lymph node. These preliminary results suggest that two independently segregating autosomal dominant genes control the footpad swelling response and Pichinde virus replication in the popliteal lymph
node. The relationship of these genes to those responsible for survival and levels of viremia is unknown.

The influence of the route of injection on the susceptibility of
MHA hamsters to a lethal Pichinde virus infection suggests that the
outcome of infection depends upon virus replication and immune reactivity. Survival may result from either minimal virus replication
early in infection, or an effective cell-mediated immune response
against Pichinde virus, or a combination of both. We have studied
the kinetics of virus replication in hamsters inoculated in the footpad and found that peak titres of infectious centers and NK activity
in the popliteal lymph node occur three days after infection in both
susceptible and resistant strains. Interestingly, the rise in splenic
NK activity and infectious centers is delayed and peak levels are observed on day 5 after a footpad inoculation (data not shown). Since
the hamster spleen appears to be a major reservoir of NK cells (11;
unpublished observations), a footpad inoculation of Pichinde virus may
retard virus replication in a crucial target organ sufficiently to
permit the host to generate a protective immune response. When the
antigenic challenge is a replicating agent such as a virus, a delay
of one to two days in spread of the virus infection could mean the
difference between survival and death.

The failure of a footpad inoculation of Pichinde virus to elicit
footpad swelling in MHA hamsters could have several explanations.
Lack of immune recognition is one possibility; this seems unlikely,
however, since footpad-immunized MHA hamsters developed an antibody
response to the virus and were protected against an IP infection.
This protection is not mediated by antibody, suggesting that a cell-
mediated immune reaction can develop in these hamsters. A second possibility is that the cell-mediated immune response is delayed in MHA

Table 4. Number of Genes Controlling Footpad Swelling and Pichinde Virus Replication

Background	No.	Footpad swelling phenotype	Virus Replication phenotype[1]	Mean Virus titre per lymph node[2] $\log_{10}$ PFU $\pm$ SD
LSH	13	13 LSH	13 LSH	2.64 $\pm$ .53
MHA	13	13 MHA	13 MHA	3.80 $\pm$ .62
F_1	8	8 LSH	8 LSH	2.24 $\pm$ .27
F_1 X LSH	18	17 LSH	16 LSH	2.59 $\pm$ .45
			1 MHA	3.22
		1 MHA	0 LSH	
			1 MHA	3.29
F_1 X MHA	20	10 LSH	6 LSH	2.59 $\pm$ .53
			4 MHA	3.58 $\pm$ .15
		9 MHA	4 LSH	2.61 $\pm$ .40
			5 MHA	3.69 $\pm$ .31
		Intermediate	1 MHA	3.28

[1] Immunization and assay as in Table 3. Animals were classified as showing the LSH or MHA phenotype using the criterion of mean foot-count ratio $\pm$ SD.

[2] Popliteal lymph node cells were excised eight days after infection from individual animals and assayed for Pichinde virus. Animals were classified as LSH-like or MHA-like using the criterion of mean virus titre $\pm$ SD; the means of the resulting phenotypic groups were then calculated.

hamsters due to a lack of helper function or to enhanced suppressor activity. Finally, accessory cells involved in the delayed-type hypersensitivity response may be defective or may not traffic properly. While we cannot presently distinguish between these possibilities, results of preliminary experiments suggest that the inhibition of footpad swelling in MHA hamsters may be due to a suppressor activity.

SUMMARY

The data presented in this paper suggest that the susceptible MHA hamster strain possesses a spleen target cell for Pichinde virus replication which is minimally expressed in the resistant strain. This target cell co-purifies with cells mediating NK activity, raising the possibility that the NK cell itself may be the additional target cell for Pichinde virus replication in the susceptible hamster strain. We hypothesize that early virus replication in the spleens of IP-inoculated hamsters leads to an overwhelming proliferation of virus. In contrast, a footpad inoculation of Pichinde virus retards virus spread into the spleen, and the host's immune response can effectively clear the relatively low amount of virus.

In addition, data have been presented that show that a footpad inoculation of Pichinde virus elicits swelling in resistant hamster strains at eight days after infection, but fails to evoke a response in the susceptible MHA hamster strain. The response is controlled by a single autosomal dominant gene, and suggests that the MHA hamster strain has a defective delayed-type hypersensitivity response. The gene responsible for footpad swelling appears to be distinct from the single autosomal dominant gene that controls virus replication in the popliteal lymph nodes of footpad-injected hamsters. The phenotype of survival, then, may be the result of either limited virus replication early in infection, or an effective anti-viral cell-mediated immune response, or both.

ACKNOWLEDGMENTS

This work was supported in part by a grant from the Eastburn Fund of the Hamilton Foundation and by a grant from The National Cancer Institute of Canada.

REFERENCES

1.   Buchmeier, M.J.; Rawls, W.E.   Infect Immun 16 (1977) 413.
2.   Murphy, F.A. et al. Lab Invest 37 (1977) 502.
3.   Gee, S.R. et al. J Immunol 123 (1979) 2618.
4.   Gee, S.R. et al. Academic Press (1980) in press.
5.   Rawls, W.E.; Leung, W.-C. Comprehensive Virol 14 (1979) 157.
6.   Mifune, K. et al. Proc Soc Exp Biol Med 136 (1971) 637.
7.   Paranjpe, M.S.; Boone, C.W. J Natl Cancer Inst 48 (1972) 563.
8.   Stephen, E.L. et al. Texas Rep Biol Med 35 (1977) 449.
9.   Oldstone, M.B.A. Comprehensive Virol 15 (1979) 1.
10. Zinkernagel, R.M. et al. J Immunol 119 (1977) 1242.
11. Datta, S.K. et al. Int J Cancer 23 (1979) 728.

GENETICALLY DETERMINED RESISTANCE TO LETHAL VESICULAR STOMATITIS

VIRUS IN SYRIAN HAMSTERS

Patricia N. Fultz, J. Wayne Streilein, John A. Shadduck,
and C. Yong Kang

Departments of Cell Biology, Pathology and Microbiology
University of Texas Health Science Center at Dallas
Dallas, TX   75235

INTRODUCTION

Vesicular stomatitis virus (VSV), the prototype for the Rhabdo-
virus group of single-stranded RNA viruses, is indigenous to and
pathogenic for cattle and horses. Under most conditions VSV is non-
pathogenic for adult members of other mammalian species; if the virus
is administered intracerebrally, however, death will usually follow;
e.g., intracerebral injection of 25 plaque-forming units (PFU) of VSV
will result in the death of an adult mouse within two days (1), whereas intraperitoneal (IP) or intravenous (IV) injection of as many as
10^8 PFU of VSV is not lethal (2,3). In contrast, we have found that
adult animals of certain inbred strains of Syrian hamsters are extremely susceptible to infections of VSV and succumb between 48 and
72 hours after IP injection of as few as 10 PFU per animal. We also
found that one inbred strain is resistant to relatively high doses of
VSV (10^6 PFU), which implies that the susceptibility/resistance to
lethal infections of VSV is genetically determined.

Studies on genetically determined susceptibility/resistance to
different viruses have revealed no common pattern either in the number of genes involved or in gene linkage. Resistance of mice to fla-
viviruses (4,5) and to certain myxoviruses (6) as well as susceptibility of mice to mouse hepatitis virus 2 (MHV-2) (7) have been shown to
be inherited as a single-gene dominant characteristic. Polygenic control of resistance to viruses also has been described; resistance of
SJL mice to a neurotropic strain of MHV is under control of one dominant and one recessive gene, neither of which is linked to the major
histocompatibility complex (MHC) (8), whereas resistance of chickens
to Marek's disease virus is associated with two loci, one linked and

one not linked to that species' MHC (9). Sex linkage has been demonstrated in the resistance of mice to herpes simplex virus 2 (10).

Furthermore, no one mechanism appears to be operative in rendering a host resistant to a particular virus. Important factors in sus-
ceptibility/resistance have been shown to include the ability of the
host or target cell to replicate the virus (4,7,11), to respond to interferon (12), to be transformed by tumor viruses (9), and to produce
defective interfering (DI) particles (13,14).

VSV is one of many animal viruses that produce DI particles--
defined as truncated versions of the standard virus that contain all
of the viral proteins but only a fraction of the viral genome. In
addition, VSV is highly cytopathic to most, if not all, animal cells
in culture; however, if cells in culture are co-infected with the
standard virus and DI particles, they are protected from the cytopathic effects of VSV (15-17), since DI particles are produced at the
expense of the standard virions (18). This observation led to the
suggestion that DI particles may be important as a host defense mechanism against viral infections (19).

It was first shown in 1973 that DI particles could protect a host
from the lethal effects of a virus. This was accomplished using VSV
and rigorously purified homologous DI particles, injected simultaneously into the brains of mice. DI particle-mediated protection has
since been shown with DI particles of influenza A virus (20,21), reovirus (22), and lymphocytic choriomeningitis virus (LCMV) (23). (In
the above cases protection was shown not to be mediated by interferon.)
In addition, DI particles have been demonstrated in adult and neonatal mice acutely and persistently infected with LCMV (24), in the
brains of newborn mice infected with rabies and VSV (25), and in 2-
day-old rats acutely and chronically infected with reovirus (21).

This paper describes the lesions of the genetically determined
lethal disease induced by VSV in Syrian hamsters as well as the results of experiments directed towards elucidating the mechanism(s)
by which some strains are rendered resistant.

MATERIALS AND METHODS

All inbred lines of Syrian hamsters were obtained from our
breeding facility at UTHSCD and ranged in age from 3 to 10 months.
Strains designated MHA, LSH, and CB are isogenic lines established
from three littermates captured in Syria 50 years ago. Strains designated MIT, UT1, and UT2 are partially inbred lines (having reached 14,
11, and 11 filial generations, respectively) derived from more recently captured wild Syrian hamsters. As shown by several assays of
alloimmune reactivity (26), MHA, LSH, and UT1 strains possess the hamster MHC haplotype $\underline{Hm-1}^a$, the haplotype present in virtually all ran-

dom-bred LVG hamsters tested. CB, MIT, and UT2 each possess unique
Hm-1 haplotypes, designated 1^b, 1^c, and 1^d, respectively. Animals of
the random-bred LVG strain were purchased from Lakeview Hamster Colony,
Charles River, Inc., and were 3 months old.

VSV of the Indiana serotype was described previously (27). Virus
stocks were prepared by infecting confluent R(B77) cells (avian sarcoma virus-transformed non-producer rat cells [28]) with virus from a
plaque-purified clone. After incubation at 37°C for 45 minutes to
allow for virus adsorption, Dulbecco's minimal essential medium (DMEM)
was added to the culture dishes and these were incubated at 37°C for
16 hours to allow for virus production. Cellular debris was removed
from the culture fluid by centrifugation and the supernatant containing VSV was stored at -70°C. The titer of the VSV stock was determined by the plaque assay method on L-cell monolayers using an agar
overlay.

The DI-2 and DI-LT stocks were prepared by co-infecting confluent
R(B77) cells with either a mixture of wild-type VSV and DI particles
obtained after four undiluted serial passages (described below) of
VSV on R(B77) cells, or a mixture of a heat resistant strain of VSV
(HR-LT) and the single DI particle it produces. After 16 hours of
growth, the resulting viral particles were harvested, concentrated by
high-speed centrifugation, and layered on a 5% to 30% sucrose gradient.
Centrifugation at 30,000 rpm in an SW41 rotor for 45 minutes resulted
in separation of the standard virus from the DI particles, which then
were collected from the top of the gradient with a pasteur pipet;
stocks were maintained at -70°C. The number of DI particles in the
stock preparations was calculated using the size of the DI particles
relative to that of a standard virion, the percentage of protein in
a standard virion, the weight of the virion, and the amount of protein
in the DI preparations (29). The number of physical particles present
in the DI-2 and DI-LT stocks was determined to be 1.3×10^{13} and $1.1
\times 10^{13}$ particles per ml, respectively; this method can only give an
upper limit to the actual number of biologically active DI particles,
the number of which is probably ten- to 100-fold lower. Since these
stocks were gradient purified one time only, they contained contaminating standard virions, the number of which was determined to be approximately one PFU of VSV per 10^7 physical DI particles.

Primary fibroblast cultures were prepared from lung explants of
3-week-old hamsters of each of the six strains. The cells were maintained in RPMI 1640 containing 10% fetal calf serum (FCS) and 0.1%
lactoalbumin hydrolysate, and were designated HL-CB, HL-MHA, HL-LSH,
HL-MIT, HL-UT1, and HL-UT2. DI-free VSV was titrated on each of these
fibroblast cell strains; plaques were picked, resuspended in DMEM,
and used as the initial inoculum for ten serial undiluted passages
of the virus on the respective cell cultures. Briefly, a 100-mm culture dish was seeded with 5×10^6 fibroblast cells two days prior to
infection. The confluent monolayer was infected with 0.5 ml of the

virus harvested from the previous passage, incubated for 45 minutes at 37°C to allow for virus adsorption, covered with 7 ml DMEM containing 10% FCS, and reincubated for 15 hours, at which time the viral progeny were harvested and stored at -70°C until titrated. All ten passages of VSV on a single fibroblast strain were titrated at the same time. To analyze a particular passage for the presence of DI particles, confluent monolayers on three culture dishes were infected as above with the appropriate virus, the media pooled, and the virus purified in the same manner as were the DI particles for the stock preparations. Sucrose gradients were collected from the top using a Buchler Auto-Densi-Flow IIC with continuous scanning at 280nm on an LKB Uvicord II and Fisher Recordall 5000.

Tissues for light microscopic examination were taken from animals at the time of death or from animals killed at given times after VSV injection, fixed in formalin, sectioned in paraffin, and stained with hematoxylin and eosin. Tissue homogenates were prepared as 10% (wt/vol) suspensions in Hank's balanced salt solution, clarified by centrifugation, and stored at -70°C until titrated on L-cell monolayers.

The presence of neutralizing antibodies in serum from infected hamsters was ascertained by mixing serial dilutions of heat-inactivated serum with equal volumes of DMEM containing approximately 100 PFU of VSV. After incubation at 37°C for one hour, all mixtures were titrated on L-cell monolayers. Controls contained VSV plus DMEM and VSV plus 1:10-diluted non-immune hamster serum. Neutralizing anti-VSV titers are expressed as the reciprocal of the dilution of immune serum which gave a 50% reduction in the number of plaques (PR_{50}).

RESULTS AND DISCUSSION

Adult hamsters from the six inbred strains described above were infected IP with either 10 or 100 PFU of VSV. Based on the number of deaths occurring within seven days post-injection, the strains were grouped into three categories (Table 1): 1. highly susceptible, LSH MHA, and CB; 2. intermediately susceptible, MIT and UT2; and 3. resistant, UT1. In addition, it was found that random-bred LVG hamsters were resistant to low doses of VSV. When graded doses of VSV were injected IP into LVG hamsters, only some of those receiving large numbers of VSV died (Table 2); the dose at which 50% of the animals died was determined to be 10^5 PFU. Table 2 also shows the survival of UT1 hamsters after IP injection of 10^2, 10^4, and 10^6 PFU of VSV. Because of the limited availability of UT1 animals, a wider range of doses could not be tested; it can be seen, however, that the UT1 strain is at least as resistant as, if not more so than, the LVG hamsters. Among the strains tested, there was no relationship between susceptibility to VSV and age (all hamsters were three months or older).

Table 1. Susceptibility of Inbred Syrian Hamsters to Lethal VSV In-
          fection

Strain	Mortality[1]	% Survival
MHA	13/18	28
LSH	17/19	11
CB	10/12	16
MIT	4/12	67
UT1	1/16	94
UT2	3/12	75

[1] Number of animals dead within 7 days/number of animals injected with
   VSV. Cumulative results after IP injection of 10 or 100 PFU.

     Since susceptibility/resistance to VSV is genetically determined,
LSH and UT1 hamsters were mated and the resulting F1 progeny were
tested for their susceptibility to lethal VSV infections. Six (UT1 X
LSH)F$_1$ hamsters (male and female) were injected IP with 100 PFU. All
six survived, suggesting that resistance is inherited as a dominant
autosomal trait. Whether one or more loci are involved in the expression of this trait cannot be determined until backcross progeny are
tested. We can conclude, however, that the controlling gene(s) is not
linked to the MHC since LSH, MHA, and UT1 all possess the same MHC
haplotype, Hm-1^a.

Table 2. Resistance of Random-Bred LVG and Inbred UT1 Hamsters to
          VSV

PFU of VSV injected[1]	Mortality in 10 days[2]	
	LVG	UT1
10^8	5/6	–
10^7	6/6	–
10^6	4/6	1/3
10^5	3/6	–
10^4	0/6	1/3
10^3	2/6	–
10^2	1/6	0/4

[1]Injection was IP.

[2]Number of animals that died/number of animals injected with VSV.

As stated above, susceptible hamsters usually die between 48 and 72 hours after IP injection of VSV; therefore, the mechanism of resistance in UT1 hamsters must be operative within 48 hours. Histologic studies were undertaken not only to determine whether the genetically resistant animals support replication of the virus and/or develop lesions, but also to define the VSV-induced disease. Of animals from the experiment described in Table 1, at least one hamster of each of the six inbred strains was necropsied at death; essentially the same pattern of disease was seen in all animals. Macroscopic lesions were distended, somewhat dark spleens and focal, mottled discoloration of the liver. Microscopically, lymphoid necrosis of the spleen was always present, with the affected areas varying from only the peripheral portion of the periarteriolar lymphoid sheath to complete destruction of all lymphoid tissue. Large amounts of necrotic detritus and fragmented nuclear structures were seen throughout the lymphoid tissue. The splenic red pulp was distended by blood and appeared less cellular than normal. In less severely affected animals, focal areas of necrosis in the red pulp also were evident and were thought to be the result of injury to reticular and sinusoidal lining cells. Characteristic lesions in the liver were dilated sinusoids and frank hemorrhage which dissected the hepatic plates. Kupffer cells were often necrotic, and frequently the lining of sinusoids was completely destroyed. In the more severely affected livers, there were multiple foci of hepatocellular necrosis with many clumps of chromatin from karyorrhectic nuclei. In general, animals with only moderate splenic necrosis had less severe hepatic lesions, while hamsters with more severe splenic lymphoid necrosis and distortion of the red pulp had hepatic lesions that included necrosis of hepatocytes. The distribution and changes in severity of the lesions suggest that the primary necrotic event occurs in the spleen, and is followed by hepatic lesions.

That the disease is first manifest in the spleen was verified in the following study. MHA and UT1 hamsters were injected IP with 100 PFU of VSV and animals were killed at 24, 32, 40 and 48 hours post-injection. Selected tissues (including the spleen and liver) were collected and examined by light microscopy. Necrotic lesions were first evident in the MHA hamsters at 32 hours and in the UT1 hamsters at 40 hours post-injection and were confined to the spleen in both strains; all other tissues examined appeared normal by this method of analysis. Titration of tissue homogenates from animals of both strains, however, revealed high titers of VSV in most tissues and serum, even as early as 24 hours post-injection (Table 3). The only exception was brain tissue, in which VSV was not detectable until 32 and 40 hours after injection in UT1 and MHA hamsters, respectively. Titers were consistently high in spleens, irrespective of whether they were from susceptible or resistant animals. These results indicate that the mechanism of resistance of UT1 hamsters to the lethal VSV disease is not an inability to replicate the virus or to disseminate it after replication.

   Alternatively, the differential susceptibility to VSV could be
due to the fact that the susceptible strains are unable to develop an
effective immune response to eliminate the virus once it has spread
throughout the body. This idea is invalidated by the following facts:
1. Susceptible hamsters that survived the initial IP injection of VSV
were able to survive a subsequent challenge of 10^4 PFU of VSV three
weeks later. Serum from rechallenged LSH hamsters was tested for its
ability to neutralize VSV in a plaque assay. Compared to a control in
which non-immune LSH serum was used at a dilution of 1:10, a PR_{50} of
5000 was obtained for the immune serum. Serum from resistant UT1 hamsters, rechallenged with 10^5 PFU of VSV, exhibited a PR_{50} of 8000 when
similarly tested. In addition, serum taken from a surviving LSH hamster one month after IP injection of 100 PFU of VSV had a PR_{50} of

Table 3. Amount[1] of Virus Detected in Various Tissues of Susceptible
          (MHA) and Resistant (UT1) Hamsters at Different Times after
          Intraperitoneal Injection of 100 PFU of VSV

| Tissue | Strain | Hours post-infection | | | |
		24	32	40	48
Spleen	MHA	4.0	5.8	–	6.6
	UT1	5.8	7.3	6.3	4.5
Liver	MHA	3.0	4.5	–	7.6
	UT1	4.7	6.1	7.3	3.7
Kidney	MHA	<2.0[2]	2.2	–	5.9
	UT1	3.1	4.6	4.2	4.3
Thymus	MHA	3.0	2.0	–	5.0
	UT1	2.9	5.7	3.3	4.1
Mesenteric	MHA	4.3	5.2	–	6.0
lymph node	UT1	<2.0	<2.0	4.7	6.3
Brain	MHA	<2.0	<2.0	–	3.2
	UT1	<2.0	3.1	3.6	2.0
Serum	MHA	2.8	4.0	–	6.6
	UT1	4.0	6.7	7.2	2.9

[1]Titers are expressed as $\log_{10}$ PFU/100 mg of tissue or $\log_{10}$ PFU/ml
of serum.

[2]<2.0, lower limit of detectability; no plaques were seen.

10,000. Thus, susceptible and resistant hamsters are capable of making a vigorous antibody response to VSV. In conjunction with the above, VSV-immune serum from LSH hamsters, transferred IV to susceptible LSH hamsters 24 hours prior to an IP injection of 100 PFU of VSV, protected the animals from the lethal effects of the virus. 2. Susceptible MHA hamsters showed 100% survival after subcutaneous injection of VSV in the footpads. This suggests that these animals are able to mount a localized immune response that effectively abrogates the fatal disease. 3. Susceptible MHA and LSH hamsters survived as many as 10^6 PFU of VSV injected IV; all of the control hamsters, injected IP with the same inoculum, died. Furthermore, when the survivors were rechallenged IP with 10^4 PFU, they did not succumb to the virus. The above suggests that neither antibody nor a localized immune response determines the resistant phenotype.

Since susceptible hamsters can survive an infection of VSV if the virus is administered IV, but not IP, it is evident that the route by which VSV is injected is important in the pathogenesis of the lethal disease. To test this possibility, six LSH hamsters were injected with 100 PFU of VSV directly into the pleural cavity. All six died; four within 72 hours, and the remaining two on days 5 and 6 post-injection. Necropsy revealed that death was not due to puncture of the lungs and, macroscopically, lesions similar to those observed in animals injected IP were seen. The fact that IP and intrapleural injections result in death in the susceptible strains, whereas IV injection does not, suggests that the major determinant of resistance to VSV may exist within the peritoneal and pleural cavities and, therefore, is not encountered if VSV is injected IV. This could be due to the presence of a specific cell type, e.g. macrophage, which differentially replicates the virus in the susceptible and resistant strains. This probably is not the case, however, in view of the comparable amount of virus found in the tissues of susceptible and resistant animals at various times after IP injection of VSV (Table 3). An alternative possibility could be that after IV injection, VSV is borne via the blood to the spleen where the virus is not amplified by replication, but, instead, elicits an immune reaction which effectively eliminates it. For reasons discussed below, we do not think that the failure of susceptible hamsters to succumb to large doses of VSV injected IV is because of the presence of a toxic factor in the serum which inactivates the virus.

Since the resistant phenotype does not appear to be due to either a humoral or cellular response, we have examined a completely unrelated mechanism through which resistance could be effected, i.e., the generation of DI particles. Our initial postulate was that the differential susceptibility of inbred hamsters could be due to an inherent ability of the resistant strain to generate and to amplify DI particles whereas the susceptible strains cannot. First it had to be demonstrated that DI particles could protect susceptible hamsters from the lethal effects of VSV.

Table 4. Effect of Simultaneous Injection of a Lethal Dose[1] of VSV
and Different Amounts of DI Particles on Susceptible
Hamsters

# DI Particles	Ratio DI:VSV	Mortality[2]	
		DI-2	DI-LT
10^{10}	10^6:1	1/6	0/8
10^9	10^5:1	2/6	0/8
10^8	10^4:1	6/6	3/8
10^7	10^3:1	6/6	4/8
10^6	10^2:1	6/6	nt[3]
—[4]	–	6/6	nt
10^{10}[5]	–	1/5	nt

[1]10^4 PFU, injected IP.

[2]Number of animals dead/number of animals injected.

[3]nt, not tested.

[4]Injected with 10^4 PFU of VSV only.

[5]Injected with DI particles only.

LSH hamsters were injected with a lethal dose of VSV (10^4 PFU
per animal) to which were added graded amounts of homologous DI particles. Two different DI particles were used, DI-2 and DI-LT. The
former contains RNA from the 5' end of the VSV genome and is approximately one-third the size of the standard virion, while the latter
contains RNA from the 3' end of the VSV genome and is one-half the
size of the standard virion. The number of DI particles used ranged
from 10^6 to 10^{10} so that ratios of DI to standard particles (10^4 PFU)
of 10^2:1 to 10^6:1 were generated. Table 4 shows that both DI-2 and
DI-LT, when co-injected with wild-type VSV, rendered susceptible (LSH
and MHA) hamsters resistant to the lethal effects of VSV. With DI-2,
50% of the animals survived at a DI:VSV ratio of approximately 10^5:1
whereas with DI-LT, a ratio of 10^3:1 resulted in 50% survival. The
greater survival of susceptible hamsters upon receiving fewer DI-LT
than DI-2 particles probably is a reflection of there being more functional DI's in the DI-LT stock than in the DI-2 stock. Alternatively,
it is possible that DI-LT persists longer, i.e., is more stable, in
vivo and may therefore be more active biologically than the smaller
DI-2.

Since the protective effect of DI particles can be seen only if
DI and standard virus particles infect the same cell, it was of inter-

est to see whether protection could be mediated when the DI particles were injected via a route different from that by which the standard virions were administered. If protection were observed, this would mean that both types of viral particles migrated or were transported to a common site, implying a cellular or tissue tropism for VSV. This was tested by injecting MHA hamsters with 10^{10} DI-2 particles IV and 10^4 PFU of VSV IP; all of the hamsters survived. Therefore, VSV does exhibit tropism in hamsters and, as suggested from the pathological studies, this tropism is probably for the spleen and/or lymphoreticular cells in the spleen. These results also indicate that there probably is nothing in the peripheral blood of susceptible hamsters that might inactivate VSV after IV injection; this is a possible explanation for the failure of susceptible hamsters to succumb to large doses of VSV administered by this route.

To determine the inherent ability of the six different strains to generate and/or to amplify DI particles, serial undiluted passages of VSV were made on primary lung fibroblasts of each of the strains. The amount of virus produced during each passage, in PFU/ml, gives an indication of the ability of each of the different fibroblasts to replicate the virus and/or to generate DI particles. A decrease in the titer of VSV produced during successive passages is indicative of the production of DI particles, a phenomenon usually accompanied by a decrease in the amount of wild-type virus. The magnitude of the decrease in PFU is a function not only of the multiplicity of infection of wild-type virions but also of the relative numbers of DI and standard particles present in the inoculum. Fig. 1 shows the results of one series of ten passages on cells from each of the hamster strains. Since the inoculum for the initial passage was virus from a single plaque, any variation in the number of PFU on the first passage could simply be a reflection of differing amounts of VSV in different plaques and, therefore, different multiplicities of infection. No general pattern is evident with respect to the number of PFU produced in fibroblasts from the susceptible or resistant strains upon serial undiluted passage. Fibroblasts of the UT1 strain are able to replicate VSV as efficiently as those from CB and LSH, and all ultimately show a decrease in the number of PFU with increasing numbers of passages. That the titer on HL-UT1 drops on the third passage may or may not be significant since no DI particles were detected upon analysis with sucrose-gradient banding (see below). A distinctly different pattern is seen with HL-UT2: five passages are required before the maximum titer is reached and the increase in PFU/ml with each successive passage is less than or equal to one $\log_{10}$, whereas the increases in PFU/ml on HL-MIT and HL-MHA during the second passages are greater. Analysis by sucrose-gradient banding of the virus produced during the second passage of VSV on HL-UT2 showed that DI particles were present.

Even though DI particles are produced during the second passage on HL-UT2, the titer continues to increase for three more successive

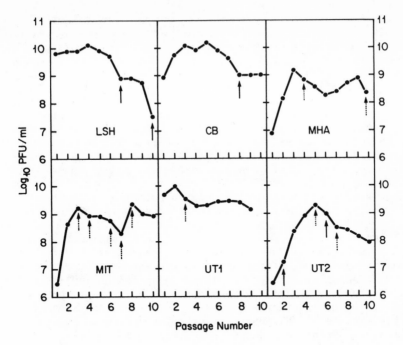

Fig. 1: Production of wild-type VSV during serial undiluted passages
on hamster lung fibroblasts from six inbred strains. Arrows
indicate those passages analyzed via sucrose-gradient banding
to determine the type(s) of viral progeny produced. Solid
arrows indicate DI particles were present; dashed arrows indicate only wild-type virus was present.

passages before it decreases on passage 6. From passage 6 through
passage 10 there is a total decrease in titer of approximately one
$\log_{10}$. This is in contrast to what usually is observed when employing established cell lines (L_2, R(B77), BHK21) where the generation and production of DI particles results in a decrease in titer of
three to four $\log_{10}$ after only two or three successive passages (30).
This could imply that the DI particles generated in the hamster fibroblasts do not have as great a capacity to interfere with standard
virus production as do those generated in the established cell lines;
however, the reason for the minimal decrease in titer with each successive passage seen also with HL-UT1, is not known.

DI particles also were seen when LSH passages 7 and 10 and CB
passage 8 were analyzed; we therefore conclude that fibroblasts from
susceptible strains are capable of generating DI particles. That no
DI particles are generated in early passages on these fibroblasts is
suggested by the fact that the PFU/ml do not change significantly

until those passages where DI's were observed. Passages of VSV on susceptible HL-MHA result in a decrease in titer on passage 4; no DI particles were detected, however, upon analysis by sucrose-gradient banding. This does not mean that they are not present, since the sensitivity of the assay is poor. It has been determined (25) that at least 10^{11} DI particles must be present to be detected by this method; therefore, another more sensitive assay will have to be devised before we can ascertain unequivocally whether there is a time differential in the generation of DI particles by resistant and susceptible strains. Whether the pattern of VSV replication observed in the lung fibroblasts is indicative of the ability of all cell types in the hamster strains to generate DI particles is unknown. If cells of a particular lineage can be shown to confer resistance to VSV, then these should be used in a comparable study in order to determine if DI particles actually play an important role in resistance to lethal VSV infection.

In summary, it has been demonstrated that resistance to IP or intrapleural injection of VSV is genetically determined and is inherited as a dominant autosomal trait not linked to the MHC. The lethal VSV-induced disease appears to be localized in splenic lymphoid tissue with some secondary hepatic lesions and does not appear to be due to an inability of the susceptible strains to develop an immune response. Comparable amounts of VSV neutralizing antibodies were present in serum from susceptible and resistant animals, and susceptible animals appeared capable of mounting a localized immune reaction since they were able to survive VSV infections after subcutaneous or IV injection of the virus. Susceptible hamsters can be protected from the lethal effects of VSV by exogenously supplied homologous DI particles; however, whether the ability of susceptible and resistant hamsters to generate DI particles in vivo is quantitatively and/or qualitatively different and, if so, whether it is utilized as a defense mechanism against VSV propagation is not known.

ACKNOWLEDGMENTS

We thank Diane Apgar for help in determining PR_{50} values for immune serum. This work was supported by NIH grant CA-09082.

REFERENCES

1.   Doyle, M.; Holland, J.J. Proc Natl Acad Sci USA 70 (1973) 2105.
2.   Zinkernagel, R.M. et al. Exp Cell Biol 46 (1978) 53.
3.   Zinkernagel, R.M. et al. J Immunol 121 (1978) 744.
4.   Goodman, G.T.; Koprowski, H. Proc Natl Acad Sci USA 48 (1962) 160.
5.   Goodman, G.T.; Koprowski, H. J Cell Comp Physiol 59 (1962) 333.
6.   Lindenmann, J. et al. J Immunol 90 (1962) 942.
7.   Bang, F.B.; Warwick, A. Proc Natl Acad Sci USA 46 (1960) 1065.
8.   Stohlman, S.A.; Frelinger, J.A. Immunogenetics 6 (1978) 277.

9.   Gallatin, W.M.; Longenecker, B.M. Nature 280 (1979) 587.
10. Mogensen, S.C. Infect Immun 17 (1977) 268.
11. Gee, S.R. et al. J Immunol 123 (1979) 2618.
12. Haller, O. et al. J Exp Med 149 (1979) 601.
13. Darnell, M.B.; Koprowski, H. J Infect Dis 129 (1974) 248.
14. Smith, A.L. et al. Intl Symposium Can Soc Immunol (1980)
     Abstract.
15. Faulkner, G. et al. Cell 17 (1979) 979.
16. Sekellick, M.J.; Marcus, P.I. Virology 85 (1978) 175.
17. Ramseur, J.M.; Friedman, R.M. Virology 85 (1978) 253.
18. Huang, A.S.; Wagner, R.R. Virology 30 (1966) 173.
19. Huang, A.S.; Baltimore, D. Nature 226 (1970) 325.
20. Von Magnus, P. Acta Pathol Microbiol Scand 29 (1951) 156.
21. Rabinowitz, S.G.; Huprikar, J. J Infect Dis 140 (1979) 305.
22. Spandidos, D.A.; Graham, A.F. J Virol 20 (1976) 234.
23. Welsh, R.M. et al. J Infect Dis 136 (1977) 391.
24. Popescu, M.; Lehmann-Grube, F. Virology 77 (1977) 78.
25. Holland, J.J.; Villareal, C.P. Virology 67 (1975) 438.
26. Streilein, J.W.; Duncan, W.R. Immunogenetics 9 (1979) 563.
27. Kang, C.Y.; Prevec, L. J Virol 3 (1969) 404.
28. Kang, C.Y.; Allen, R. J Virol 25 (1978) 202.
29. Lowry, O.H. et al. J Biol Chem 193 (1951) 265.
30. Kang, C.Y. et al. Virology 84 (1978) 142.

DEFECTIVE INTERFERING VIRUS PARTICLES AND THEIR BIOLOGICAL FUNCTIONS

C. Yong Kang

Department of Microbiology
University of Texas Health Science Center at Dallas
Dallas, TX   75235

Biologically active defective interfering (DI) virus particles
have been found in a large number of animal virus groups. These include picorna, toga, orthomyxo, paramyxo, rhabdo, arena, reo, retro,
papova, adeno, and herpes viruses (1). This list of animal viruses
suggests that DI particles are common in most, if not all, animal viruses. The properties, biological roles, and perspectives of DI particles have been reviewed previously (1,2,3). A brief summary of the
properties and the biological significance of DI particles in the outcome of natural viral infections will be presented here.

DI particles are forms of deletion mutants. They contain only
a part of the standard virus genome but contain all of the normal
structural proteins of the standard virions. Some DI particles reflect large deletions of viral nucleotide sequences but retain the
one critical region for a DI particle genome, the site for initiation
of nucleic acid replication. Some DI particles carry genetic information for functional products, whereas other DI particle genomes do
not code for any recognizable proteins. DI particles are unable to
replicate in the absence of standard virions. Propagation of DI particles requires co-infection of a cell with both types of virions.
Such an infection in some way decreases the yield of standard virus
production. This phenomenon is known as viral interference, and may
well be responsible for early protection against lethal viral infection.

Many defense mechanisms are known that protect hosts from viral
infections. These include production of anti-viral antibodies, generation of cytotoxic T lymphocytes, and production of interferon. Most
of these host defense mechanisms, however, require a rather long
period after the initial infection. Rapidly growing viruses may

cause viremia within a day, and all susceptible target cells in the host will be infected during or shortly after the viremic state. Thus, these defense mechanisms may not be able to protect the host from lethal infection unless there is some other protective mechanism available which functions during the initial infection.

The DI particles have been overlooked as a possible important determinant in the outcome of natural viral infections (1,2). If DI particles are generated to protect hosts, it seems reasonable to assume that host cells should play an important role in generating them. Some in vitro experiments showed that synthesis of DI particles is largely dependent upon the species of host cell (1). The most direct evidence that a host-cell function is required for the induction of DI particles comes from inhibitor studies. It has been shown that cells pretreated with actinomycin D are unable to generate DI particles when a DI particle-free stock of vesicular stomatitis virus (VSV) was used (4). Production of DI particles is a two-step process. The first step is the initial induction of a single DI particle from a standard virion; the second is the amplification of the DI particle at the expense of standard virus. Only the first step was inhibited by actinomycin D, while the second step was normal. These results suggest that host cells exert control over the induction of DI particles from standard virus genomes. Several models have been proposed to explain the molecular mechanism of DI particle induction on the basis of the structure of DI particle RNA (5-8). These include copy-back mechanisms, looping and copy-choice mechanisms, and splicing mechanisms (6).

DI particles seem to have two biological functions. The first is the establishment and maintenance of persistent viral infections. The second is the protective effects against viral disease. It is not clear whether these biological functions of DI particles are programmed biological processes. An increasing number of reports document a role for DI particles in persistent infections (9,10). These reports emphasize a major involvement of DI particles as inhibitors of standard virus replication in in vitro persistent infections caused by VSV, rabies virus, Sendai virus, Japanese encephalitis virus, canine distemper virus, measles virus, reovirus, and lymphocytic choriomeningitis virus (9,10). In these persistent infections mediated by DI particles, a large percentage of the cells contain viral antigens. Although inhibition of standard virus replication by DI particles is thought to be the major mechanism for the establishment of these persistent infections by diminishing the cytopathic effect of the primary infection, there is no explanation for the mechanism maintaining the expression of virus-specific macromolecules found inside persistently infected cells (9,10).

The protective effects of DI particles against viral disease seems to me a more attractive explanation for the existence of DI particles than the establishment and maintenance of persistent viral infection. Because of the problems of detecting DI particles in ani-

mals during the course of a disease, studies on DI particles in animals have focused on the inoculation of large amounts of DI particles
and observation of the subsequent effects of these particles on acute
lethal viral diseases. Earlier studies with unpurified preparations
of DI particles of influenza virus, polio virus and vesicular stomatitis virus strongly support the hypothesis that DI particles not only
can delay the onset of acute disease but also can prevent it alto-
gether (1,3). Studies with purified preparations of DI particles of
vesicular stomatitis virus clearly demonstrated that exogenous DI particles injected simultaneously with a lethal dose of vesicular stomatitis virus render susceptible hamsters resistant. Although the exact
mechanism of the protective effect produced by inoculating the animals with DI particles remains obscure, it does not correlate with in-
terferon-mediated resistance or heterologous interference by DI particles. It is extremely difficult to extend DI particle protection to
other virus groups because physical separation of DI particles and
standard virions is impossible. Thus, VSV and the inbred hamster
lines provide a unique model system to learn more about the protective
role of DI particles against lethal viral infection.

Understanding of the molecular mechanism of DI particle generation and homologous viral interference mediated by DI particles will
undoubtedly shed light on the control of viral diseases.

REFERENCES

1.   Huang, A.S.; Baltimore, D. In: Comprehensive Virology 10,
     ed. Fraenkel-Conrat and Wagner. Plenum Press, N.Y. (1977) 73.
2.   Huang, A.S.; Baltimore, D. Nature 226 (1970) 325.
3.   Huang, A.S. Annu Rev Microbiol 27 (1973) 101.
4.   Kang, C.Y.; Allen, R. J Virol 25 (1978) 202.
5.   Huang, A.S. Bacteriol Rev 41 (1977) 811.
6.   Kang, C.Y. In: Rhabdoviruses, 2, ed. Bishop. CRC Press (1980)
     in press.
7.   Leppert, M. et al. Cell 12 (1977) 539.
8.   Perrault, J.; Leavitt, R.W. J Gen Virol 38 (1977) 35.
9.   Holland, J.J. et al. In: Comprehensive Virology, ed. Fraenkel-
     Conrat and Wagner. Plenum Press, New York, in press.
10. Roux, L.; Holland, J.J. Virology 100 (1980) 53.

SECTION VII

INFECTIONS WITH UNCONVENTIONAL AGENTS

Chairpersons:

William R. Duncan

Richard F. Marsh

EFFECT OF VACCINIA-ACTIVATED MACROPHAGES ON SCRAPIE INFECTION IN

HAMSTERS

Richard F. Marsh

Department of Veterinary Science
University of Wisconsin
Madison, WI   53706

INTRODUCTION

The Syrian hamster has been shown to be the animal model of choice for studies on the physicochemical nature of the scrapie agent (1). The high titers of scrapie infectivity in brain tissue and the short incubation periods in this species have decreased the time required to obtain bioassay data necessary for the detection of this unusual neuropathic agent. Relatively little attention, however, has been given to the pathogenesis of scrapie infection in the hamster. The main purpose of this study was to investigate the role of the macrophage on early events in hamsters inoculated intraperitoneally (IP) with the hamster-adapted scrapie agent.

MATERIALS AND METHODS

Outbred (LVG) male hamsters purchased as weanlings from the Lakeview Hamster Colony, Newfield, N.J., were housed three to a cage on wood shavings with food and water ad libitum throughout the course of the experiment.

The origin of hamster-adapted scrapie has been described elsewhere (2). A 10% saline brain suspension representing the 25th consecutive hamster serial passage was the source of infection for these experiments. Vaccinia virus (WR strain) was grown in rabbit skin fibroblasts and titrated as described (3).

Hamsters 10 weeks old were inoculated IP (0.1 ml) with 10^7 PFU of vaccinia virus or with saline. After intervals of two hours, three days, five days and 10 days, animals were inoculated either intracerebrally (0.05 ml) or IP (0.5 ml) with scrapie.

On days 5 and 18 after IP scrapie inoculation, three hamsters each from the two hour and three day vaccinia groups and their saline controls were injected IP with 3 ml of sterile mineral oil. These animals were killed with chloroform two days later and their spleens and peritoneal exudate cells (PEC) collected for culture and bioassay.

The PEC were collected from each animal using three 5-ml washes of minimal essential medium (MEM) supplemented with 10% fetal calf serum, 100 units penicillin and 100 µg streptomycin/ml. The washes from each group of three animals were combined and dispensed in 10-ml aliquots in 75 cm^2 plastic tissue culture flasks. Cells were allowed to adhere for 60 minutes at 37°C before the supernatants were decanted and passed through a sterile nylon wool column. These columns were prepared by placing 300 mg of scrubbed nylon wool in 12-ml syringe barrels which were sealed and autoclaved. The columns were saturated with warm sterile PBS followed by warm MEM which was allowed to drain until the miniscus was just above the nylon wool. The supernatants (about 10 ml) from each of the flasks were added to a syringe, and after the void volumes were discarded, the cells were allowed to adhere at 37°C for 45 minutes. The nonadherent cells were recovered by adding 10 ml of warm MEM to the top of the column and collecting the effluent in a centrifuge tube. The cells were pelleted at 1200 rpm for 20 minutes, then resuspended to 10% (v/v) in MEM for bioassay.

The adherent cells were washed repeatedly with MEM, then scraped from the flask with a rubber policeman. Some flasks were not scraped but were incubated with MEM at 37°C for observation of a possible cytopathic effect and were later used for bioassay.

Ten percent (v/v) suspensions of cells and spleen tissues were bioassayed by intracerebral inoculation of 10-fold dilutions into weanling LVG hamsters. Endpoints were calculated 16 weeks after inoculation as described (4).

RESULTS

Hamsters injected IP with scrapie two hours after IP vaccinia inoculation had a 20% reduction in the length of incubation period when compared with animals that had not received vaccinia (Table 1). No reduction in incubation was seen in intracerebrally inoculated hamsters or in animals inoculated with scrapie five or 10 days after vaccinia injection.

Table 2 compares the infectivity of spleen tissue and of adherent and non-adherent cell populations from hamsters killed seven and 20 days after IP injection with scrapie. The adherent cells contained most of the infectivity after seven days, and the titers in these cells were higher in hamsters receiving a prior injection of vaccinia

Table 1. Incubation periods in hamsters inoculated either intracere-
          brally (IC) or intraperitoneally (IP) with scrapie at var-
          ious intervals after IP injection with 10^7 PFU of the WR
          strain of vaccinia virus

Post-vaccinia	Length of incubation (days)[1]	
	IC	IP
2 hours	60 (60–61)	80 (78–81)
3 days	60 (58–61)	92 (91–93)
5 days	60 (60)	98 (96–102)
10 days	60 (59–60)	99 (97–102)
Control[2]	60 (60–61)	98 (97–100)

[1]Mean length of incubation of six inoculated animals (range within
group in parentheses).

[2]Each vaccinia-injected group had its own saline control, but because
no significant differences were observed between any of the control
groups, the results are summarized for brevity.

Table 2. Infectivity of spleen and adherent and nonadherent PEC
          seven and 20 days after IP scrapie inoculation

Post-vaccinia	Post-scrapie (days)	Spleen	Adherent	Nonadherent
2 hours	7	3.5[1]	4	1.5
	20	4	<1	<1
Saline control	7	4	2.5	<1
	20	4	<1	<1
3 days	7	4.5	5	1
	20	4	<1	<1
Saline control	7	4.5	3	<1
	20	4	<1	<1

[1]Log_{10} LD_{50}/ml 10% (v/v) suspension.

as compared with saline. When tested at 20 days, however, the infectivity of the adherent cells had fallen off sharply. No significant differences were seen in the spleen titers.

Adherent cells from hamsters injected IP with scrapie three days after vaccinia inoculation [10^5 LD_{50}/ml 10% (v/v) suspension] and their saline control [10^3 LD_{50}/ml 10% (v/v) suspension] were grown in culture for 14 days, split 1:2 and grown for 10 additional days before harvesting for bioassay. No cytopathic effect was observed in any of the cultures during this time, and hamsters inoculated with 10% (v/v) cell suspensions remained unaffected for 20 weeks (< 10^1 LD_{50}/ml).

DISCUSSION

No attempt was made to characterize the adherent cell population in these experiments. Experiments by other investigators using identical methods have shown that 90% to 93% of these cells demonstrate active phagocytosis and have characteristic macrophage morphology (5). Therefore, for the purposes of interpreting the results of these present experiments, the adherent cells will be referred to as macrophages, in full awareness that they are not a homogeneous cell population.

It has been shown that vaccinia-activated macrophages (VAM) are cytotoxic when tested against vaccinia or herpes simplex virus-infected target cells (5). This cytotoxicity is not virus-specific and reaches a peak five days after immunization with 10^7 PFU of vaccinia virus. The results of these experiments on scrapie show no increase in the incubation period as might be expected if the VAM were having a cytotoxic effect on scrapie-infected target cells. On the contrary, hamsters inoculated IP with scrapie two hours after vaccinia injection have a shorter incubation period, and the VAM contain a higher titer of infectivity seven days after scrapie inoculation than do unstimulated macrophages. These results are similar to those of another report that hamsters had a shorter incubation time if inoculated IP with scrapie two hours after receiving an IP injection of methanol extraction residue of BCG (6).

These findings show that activation of macrophages by viral immunization does not alter the pathogenesis of scrapie infection in hamsters inoculated IP at a time when the VAM should have their maximum viral cytotoxic effect. The decrease in incubation time in animals inoculated two hours after vaccinia injection is similar to the response of hamsters injected with a non-viral macrophage stimulator (BCG), and suggests that the shortened incubation time is due to a transient, non-specific activation of macrophages which phagocytize the scrapie inoculum and mobilize it to the site of primary replication.

This is the first study to compare adherent and non-adherent PEC in scrapie-infected animals. The low titer of scrapie infectivity in the non-adherent cells is consistent with other studies on transmissible mink encephalopathy, which have shown that blood and concentrated preparations of peripheral lymphocytes are not infectious (7). But the most important finding of these studies is that the adherent PEC, either in vivo or in vitro, do not retain their scrapie infectivity beyond three weeks after infection.

ACKNOWLEDGMENTS

I would like to thank Wayne Tompkins and Stephen Chapes for valuable discussions and for supplying the vaccinia virus. This study was supported by NIH grant NS 18422 and by the College of Agricultural and Life Sciences of the University of Wisconsin--Madison.

REFERENCES

1. Marsh, R.F.; Hanson, R.P. Fed Proc 37 (1978) 2076.
2. Kimberlin, R.H.; Marsh, R.F. J Infect Dis 131 (1975) 97.
3. Blanden, R.V. et al. J Exp Med 124 (1969) 585.
4. Dougherty, R.M. In: Techniques in Experimental Virology, ed. Harris. Academic Press, New York (1964) 184.
5. Chapes, S.K.; Tompkins, W.A.F. J Immunol 123 (1979) 303.
6. Kimberlin, R.H. In: Slow Transmissible Diseases of the Nervous System, Volume 2, ed. Prusiner and Hadlow. Academic Press, New York (1979) 44.
7. Marsh, R.F. et al. Infect Immun 7 (1973) 352.

USE OF THE GOLDEN SYRIAN HAMSTER IN THE STUDY OF SCRAPIE VIRUS

Paul Brown, Robert G. Rohwer, Marie-Claude Moreau-Dubois,
Ernest M. Green, and D. Carleton Gajdusek

Laboratory of Central Nervous System Studies, National
Institute of Neurological and Communicative Disorders and
Stroke, National Institutes of Health, Bethesda, MD   20205

INTRODUCTION

Various considerations may guide the choice of an animal species
in which to study scrapie virus infection. The use of larger animals,
for example, may be required for ease of surgical manipulation, or
the examination of small organs or body fluids such as blood and ce-
rebrospinal fluid. Characteristics of immunologic development, or
biologic closeness to man, also may be important determinants in the
choice of animal. When such considerations are not relevant, however,
economy can be the major criterion, and of the many animal species now
known to be susceptible to experimental infection by scrapie virus,
the golden Syrian hamster offers the greatest economies of space,
time, and money. This is obviously true in comparison to studies in
primates, sheep and goats, mink, ferrets, cats, or guinea pigs. It is
less obvious that the hamster would show an overall economy greater
than is possible in the mouse.

In Table 1, we have outlined in parallel for the hamster and the
mouse the arithmetic which supports the choice of the hamster. It is
clear that experimental scrapie infection in the hamster enjoys two
major advantages over the mouse: a shorter incubation period and a
higher concentration of virus in the brain. The consequences of these
facts, from considering, in order, total brain infectivity per animal,
per cage, and per cage year, lead to a calculated infectivity yield
favoring the hamster over the mouse by a ratio of 240 to 1.

It should be pointed out that incubation periods in certain
inbred mouse-scrapie virus combinations are shorter than 180 days (1),
and that some investigators may prefer to house fewer than four ham-

365

Table 1. Relative Economics of the Hamster vs. Mouse Scrapie Systems

Infectivity yield	Hamster (263K)	Mouse (C506)
Minimum incubation time for high titer material	60 days	180 days
Average brain mass	1.0 grams	0.42 grams
LD_{50} per gram brain	1×10^{10}	2×10^8
Total LD_{50} per animal	1×10^{10}	8.4×10^7
Animals per cage	4	6
Total infectivity (LD_{50}) per cage	4×10^{10}	5×10^8
Maximum yield of infectivity (LD_{50}) per cage year	2.4×10^{11}	1×10^9
Ratio of infectivity yield	240 :	1
Titration efficiency		
Maximum incubation time for low titer material	270 days	540 days
Cages per dilution (6 mice or 4 hamsters per cage)	1	1
Ratio of efficiency (number of titrations per unit time and space)	2 :	1

sters per cage. Even assuming the shortest known incubation period in the mouse of 150 days, however, and housing only two hamsters per cage, the calculated infectivity yield still favors the hamster by a ratio of 100 to 1, because of the higher viral concentration in hamster brain tissue. This remains an important advantage when the goal is to obtain large amounts of infective material, for example, in biochemical or immunological studies where purification procedures may be necessary.

A second important, albeit routine, aspect of virtually all studies of scrapie virus involves infectivity titrations. Here again, the hamster has the advantage over the mouse, although the gain is not so impressive. In the lower part of Table 1, figures are presented that show that, because of the shorter incubation time of even low titer material in the hamster, twice as many titrations may be performed in hamsters as in mice for a given space over the same length of time. This advantage would disappear if only two hamsters were housed in a cage, but in our experience to date of several hundred

titration dilution points, four hamsters per cage is an entirely practical arrangement, as hamsters are fastidious in their housekeeping,
and if animals of one sex are caged together as weanlings, fighting
does not occur until an advanced clinical stage of disease is reached.

The body of this report describes the results of two recent experiments from our laboratory, in which scrapie infection was studied
in the golden Syrian hamster. In both experiments, randomly-bred
Syrian hamsters were obtained from Lakeview-Charles River Farms as 5-
to 7-week-old weanling animals, and accommodated to their new cages
for a week before use. The source of scrapie virus in both experiments was a single large pool of brain tissue from terminally ill animals infected with hamster scrapie strain 263K (2). Originally obtained from Dr. Richard Kimberlin at the Compton Laboratories in
Great Britain, the virus has since been passaged twice more in golden
Syrian hamsters in our laboratory and stored as a centrifuged 10% suspension in phosphate-buffered saline (PBS), pH 7.4, at -70°C.

RESULTS AND DISCUSSION

Evaluation of Sodium Hypochlorite and Chlorine Dioxide as Disinfect-
ants of Scrapie Virus

Hypochlorite has for years enjoyed wide use as a general disinfectant, and an early study (3), as well as a more recent unpublished
experiment in our own laboratory (C.J. Gibbs, Jr., et al, 1975), both
have documented a substantial effect of hypochlorite on mouse-adapted
scrapie virus. The obvious practical disadvantage of hypochlorite is
its corrosive nature, making it either inconvenient or even impossible
to use on metal instruments, cloth fabrics, or skin. Chlorine dioxide, also used as a disinfectant of bacteria and conventional viruses
(4, 5), is in contrast completely non-corrosive and non-irritating to
skin.

In the present experiment, household bleach was diluted 1 to 10
to give a final concentration of 0.5% (w/v) sodium hypochlorite. Chlorine dioxide was generated at a maximum concentration of 100 ppm (6)
from the spontaneous decomposition of chlorous acid in a reaction
mixture of 0.036M sodium chlorite and 0.26M lactic acid (Alcide^{R},
patent number 4,084,747, generously furnished by Mr. Howard Alliger,
Alcide Corporation, 38 East Mall, Plainview, NY 11803).

After an aliquot of 10% brain suspension was removed for titration as a virus control, equal volumes of brain suspension were mixed
with freshly prepared hypochlorite or chlorine dioxide solutions.
Under continuous stirring at room temperature, the mixture was sampled
at 15, 30, and 60 minutes, and again at 24 hours. The pH of the chlorine dioxide solution remained stable at its optimal value of 3.0
throughout the experiment, whereas the pH of the sodium hypochlorite

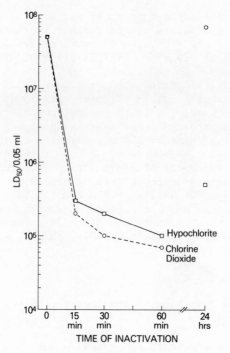

Fig. 1:   Comparison of inactivation curves of scrapie virus by sodium
           hypochlorite and chlorine dioxide.

solution decreased from an initial value of 11.2 to 7.9 after one
hour, and to 7.5 after 24 hours. This range of pH values per se has
been shown to have no effect on scrapie infectivity (7).

     Aliquots removed from the reaction mixtures were diluted imme-
diately in logarithmic series in PBS, and 0.05-ml volumes inoculated
by the intracerebral route into eight hamsters for each dilution
point. All but eight of 200 animals that contracted scrapie died
within five months of inoculation. Four animals died during the sixth
month, and another four died during the seventh month. The experiment was terminated after eight months, at which time coded sections
of the brains from all dead animals were examined histologically.
Only animals showing unequivocal spongiform pathology were considered
to have died from scrapie.

     The results are plotted in Fig. 1 as an inactivation curve, the
vertical axis showing virus infectivity titers in $\log_{10}$ units, and the
horizontal axis showing time of exposure of the virus to the tested
chemicals. The two curves are very similar, and demonstrate that
chlorine dioxide is as effective as sodium hypochlorite for inacti-

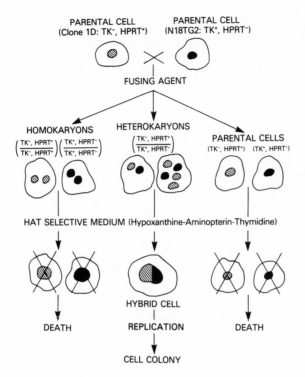

Fig. 2: Schematized method for the detection of in vitro cell-fusing
         activity. TK=thymidine kinase, HPRT=hypoxanthine-guanine
         phosphoribosyl transferase.

vating scrapie virus. Because of its non-corrosive, non-irritating
nature, we therefore propose chlorine dioxide as an alternative to
bleach in the chemical decontamination of scrapie-infected material.

    We would emphasize, however, that neither chemical fully inacti-
vated the virus. A loss of between 2½ and 3 logs (or more than 99 per
cent) of the starting infectivity is certainly a significant reduction,
but is much less reassuring when considered in light of the 5 to 6
logs of virus per gram of tissue that remain. Early work from other
laboratories (8, 9), and unpublished data from our own laboratory,
suggest that permanganate and phenolic solutions may be superior to
either bleach or chlorine dioxide, but for the moment we can only
repeat that reproducible sterilization of the scrapie virus still is
limited to autoclaving at 121°C and two atmospheres pressure for one
hour, and remains the method of choice.

Table 2.   In Vitro Cell-Fusing Activity of Brain Tissue During Evolution of Scrapie Infection in the Golden Syrian Hamster

Weeks after inoculation	Reciprocal $\log_{10}$ dilution of brain				
	1	2	3	4	5
Scrapie hamsters					
2	0	0.02	0	0.02	0
4	0.56	0.75	0.89	0	0
6	0.62	0.25	0.50	0.03	0.03
7	0.63	0.24	0	0	0
8	0.30	0.38	0.04	0	0
10	0.53	0.63	0.21	0.01	0.38
Control hamsters					
2	0	0	0	0	0
4	0.02	0	0.33	0	0
6	0.20	0.21	0	0	0
7	0	0	0	0.02	0
8	0.04	0	0	0	0
10	0	0	0	0	0

A more fundamental aspect of this experiment relates to the kinetics of inactivation. Most of the effect of both chemicals has already occurred within 15 minutes of contact with the scrapie virus, whereas by one hour, inactivation is progressing very slowly if at all. The shape of this curve is thus similar to the more rapid inactivation curves of conventional viruses, with a large sensitive population, and a small residual resistant population of infective particles. The higher titer 24-hour exposure values were unexpected, and if they are verified in further experiments, we shall have to contend with possibilities like changing chemical equilibria of chlorine and chlorine oxides among functionally active scrapie particles and uninfective tissue components, or aggregation-disaggregation phenomena in the reappearance of scrapie infectivity.

Fusinogenic Activity of Brain Tissue During the Evolution of Scrapie Infection in the Hamster

We have reported studies of in vitro cell-fusing activity present in brain suspensions of scrapie-infected mice (9), and we have

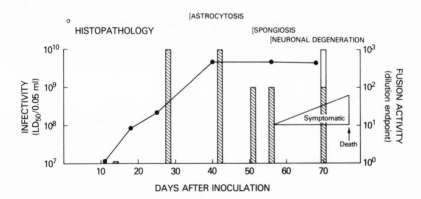

Fig. 3:   Time sequence of brain infectivity, cell-fusing activity,
           histopathology, and clinical course of experimental scrapie
           virus infection in the golden Syrian hamster (data for in-
           fectivity and histopathology from Malone et al., ref. no.
           12). Line represents infectivity titers, and bars represent
           fusion activity levels (open section of 70-day bar indicates
           borderline fusing activity at 10^{-3} dilution).

since confirmed a similar activity in terminally ill scrapie-infected
hamsters. The present experiment was undertaken to determine at what
point cell-fusing activity appears during the evolution of scrapie infection in the hamster.

Groups of four to six animals inoculated intracerebrally with
scrapie-infected brain suspensions were killed at weekly intervals
throughout the course of infection until death from disease terminated the experiment at about 9 to 10 weeks after inoculation. Animals were anesthetized with CO_2 vapor, and their brains removed aseptically. A portion of each brain was snap-frozen for fluorescent antibody microscopy, and the remainders pooled and frozen at $-70^{\circ}C$ for titration of infectivity and cell-fusing activity. A parallel series of
animals inoculated with normal hamster brain suspensions served as a
control, and all results were obtained from randomly-coded specimens.

Details of the method used to detect cell-fusing activity have
been described elsewhere (10, 11). Briefly, dilutions of sonicated,
centrifuged brain tissue were incubated with a mixture of two diploid
mouse cell lines, each deficient in a different enzyme necessary for
nucleic acid replication (Fig. 2). When grown in a selective culture
medium, the cells are unable to divide, and die within three to five
days. If, however, heterozygotic cell fusion occurs, each parental
cell complements the other's defect, and normal replication and cell
growth result. Visible colonies appear after about three weeks, and
the number of colonies in test specimens is compared to a standard

Sendai-virus treated control, expressed as a ratio of cell fusion. Specimens having a ratio of 0.2 or more are considered to be positive.

The results are presented in Table 2. Fusing activity was absent in the brain tissue of hamsters two weeks after inoculation, but appeared abruptly at four weeks and thereafter was consistently detectable for the duration of the infection. It was present in highest concentration (through 10^{-3} dilutions of brain) in the four- and six-week specimens, and then appears to have decreased slightly in later specimens.

The positive value in the 10^{-5} dilution of the 10-week scrapie hamster, as well as the three positive values scattered among the control hamster dilution series, are probably non-specific in nature, and not due to any fusing factor present in the brain tissue per se. We know from long experience with this test that unpredictable, non-specific fusion can occur occasionally, and have never considered an isolated positive value as significant without verification on repeat testing. What is clearly significant in this experiment is the pattern and consistency of fusion in the scrapie hamster group. We are presently examining the alternate-week specimens for fusing activity, and all specimens for neuropathology and titration of infectivity, which will not be completed for another seven to eight months. Until these results are known, we regard as preliminary the data presented here. Nevertheless, in order to appreciate the probable temporal sequence of these measures of scrapie infection in the hamster, we have made use of another report (12) for information about the evolution of neuropathologic changes, and for data from which we have calculated the progression of infectivity levels in the brain.

Fig. 3 presents a composite of these various data. It is evident that the appearance of fusion activity corresponds temporally with the rising segment of the infectivity curve, well before any sign of clinical disease, and at the threshold of, or possibly before, the earliest detectable histologic abnormalities. We have suggested elsewhere (13) that cell fusing activity found in association with the spongiform virus encephalopathies might be due to secondary physico-chemical changes in brain membranes, particularly the disrupted membrane structures seen in humans and animals in the advanced stages of illness. It now appears possible to entertain the idea that scrapie and related viruses may instead be directly responsible for cell fusion, which would encourage a shift in focus to the early phase of infection in further biochemical study of these diseases.

REFERENCES

1. Dickinson, A.G.; Fraser, H. In: Slow Transmissible Diseases of the Nervous System. Academic Press, New York (1979) 367.
2. Kimberlin, R. H.; Walker, C.A. J Gen Virol 34 (1977) 295.

3. Hartley, E.G. Nature 213 (1967) 1135.
4. Benarde, M.A. et al. Appl Microbiol 15 (1967) 257.
5. Cronier, S. et al. Abstract N 58 In: Abstracts of the Annual
    Meeting of the American Society of Microbiology (1977).
6. Alliger, H. Personal communication (1980).
7. Mould, D.L. et al. Res Vet Sci 6 (1965) 151.
8. Hunter, G.D. et al. J Comp Pathol 79 (1969) 101.
9. Adams, D.H. Res Vet Sci 13 (1972) 198.
10. Kidson, C. et al. Proc Natl Acad Sci USA 75 (1978) 2969.
11. Coon, H.G.; Weiss, M.C. Proc Natl Acad Sci USA 62 (1969) 852.
12. Malone, T.G. et al. J Virol 25 (1978) 933.
13. Moreau-Dubois, M-C. et al. Proc Natl Acad Sci USA 76 (1979) 5365.

HAMSTER SCRAPIE: EVIDENCE FOR ALTERATIONS IN SEROTONIN METABOLISM

Robert G. Rohwer, Jaap Goudsmit, Leonard M. Neckers, and
D. Carleton Gajdusek

National Institute of Neurological and Communicative Dis-
orders and Stroke, Laboratory of Central Nervous System
Studies, National Institutes of Health, Bethesda, MD 20205
and National Institute of Mental Health, Laboratory of
Clinical Pharmacology, National Institutes of Health, St.
Elizabeths Hospital, Washington, D.C. 20032

INTRODUCTION

The subacute spongiform virus encephalopathies--scrapie, transmissible mink encephalopathy, kuru and Creutzfeldt-Jakob Disease--
are central nervous system disorders characterized histopathologically
by neuronal loss, vacuolation of neuron processes, and glial hypertrophy (1). Clinical disease appears only after the production of
high titers of virus in the brain itself (2). Significant reductions
in brain choline acetyltransferase activities have been reported during
the late stages of clinical disease caused by several strains of mouse
scrapie (3), thus suggesting a disturbance in the cholinergic nervous
system. We have investigated the involvement of serotonergic neurons
by comparing the effects of a serotonin precursor and an agonist on
the behavior of scrapie-infected and control hamsters and by measurement of brain serotonin (L-5-hydroxytryptamine) concentrations in both
groups. We have also compared blood serotonin concentrations in infected and control animals.

MATERIALS AND METHODS

Weanling female outbred golden Syrian hamsters were obtained from
the Lakeview Hamster Colony. All animals were inoculated intracerebrally in the left hemisphere with 0.05 ml of 10% brain homogenate in
phosphate buffered physiological saline, pH 7.4. Infected hamsters
received 10^8 infectious doses of hamster scrapie strain 263K (a gift

of R. H. Kimberlin passaged twice in this laboratory [4]). Control
hamsters were inoculated with normal hamster brain.

Behavioral Tests

Two drugs were tested for their ability to alleviate scrapie symptoms in hamsters: quipazine maleate, a serotonin agonist (5,6) was obtained from Miles Laboratories Inc., and L-5-hydroxytryptophan methyl
ester (5-HTP), a serotonin precursor (7,8), from Calbiochem-Behring
Corp. The toxicity of both drugs also was compared in scrapie and
normal hamsters. Both drugs were dissolved in deionized water and injected intraperitoneally (IP) in a concentration such that the volume
administered was 0.2 to 0.3 ml per 100 g body weight. The drugs were
administered 60 to 70 days after inoculation when the scrapie-infected
hamsters showed ataxia, diminished rearing, action jerks of the head
and body, and were also very irritable and aggressive compared to the
control hamsters. The infected animals did not show resting tremor
or any other clinical sign that could interfere with assessment of
the serotonin toxicity syndrome (see below). No behavioral abnormalities were seen in the control animals. The mean weight of the
scrapie-infected hamsters was not significantly different from that
of the control hamsters. Each animal was used only once to test the
effect of a single dose of one of the two drugs. None of the animals
used in the drug tests were used for the biochemical analyses.

Both drugs were tested for their therapeutic effects on scrapie
hamster locomotor symptoms. Hamsters were examined for 30 minutes
before, and between 30 and 60 minutes after, the administration of
one of the two drugs for the presence of action jerks and ataxia
scored as follows:

> Jerks: 1. mild jerking of the head only
> 2. severe jerking of the head only
> 3. jerking of both head and body
> 4. severe jerking of both head and body

> Ataxia: 1. slight unstable gait
> 2. wobbling gait
> 3. wobbling gait plus spontaneous backrolls with the
>   ability to stand up within 15 seconds
> 4. wobbling gait plus spontaneous backrolls with ina-
>   bility to stand up within 15 seconds

At high doses, both drugs became toxic, eliciting a syndrome
that is specific for the activation of central serotonergic neurons
(7,9,10, and see below). For this purpose, hamsters were examined
for the following signs: resting tremor, rigidity (evaluated by
grasping the hamster around the torso and then extending and flexing
the hindlimbs), hindlimb abduction (a splaying-out of the hindlimbs),
Straub tail (erect and rigid tail stump) and reciprocal forepaw

treading (rhythmic dorsoventral movements of the forelimbs) (8,10).
No attempt was made to assess the intensity of these signs; hamsters
were scored solely on the basis of signs present, from zero to five.
Because some of these behavioral signs are not specific to stimulation
of serotonin receptors, the animal was considered to have displayed
the serotonin syndrome only when at least three of the five signs were
present.

All of the behavioral tests were conducted with coded inocula and
scored by two independent observers with an intra-pair observer agreement score of 0.98 (11).

Biochemical Tests

Animals were killed for the biochemical studies by two methods.
One group of infected and control hamsters was first lightly anesthetized with methoxyflurane (Metafane, Pitman-Moore, Inc.). Two to three
milliliters of blood were then collected by retroorbital bleeding into
a glass pasteur pipet freshly rinsed with 10,000 units/ml of beef lung
heparin solution (The Upjohn Co.). Immediately after collection, two
or three 0.3-ml aliquots were transferred to separate tubes and frozen
in powdered dry ice. The animals were then killed by cervical fracture and the brains immediately dissected and placed in tared tubes.
The tubes were then reweighed and frozen in powdered dry ice. A
second group of hamsters was killed by cervical fracture only and the
brains immediately dissected and frozen.

Serotonin was extracted from brains by adding sufficient ice-cold
4% perchloric acid to each frozen brain to make a 10% suspension. The
brains were then homogenized in a teflon-glass homogenizer and the resulting suspension centrifuged for 30 minutes at 5000 rpm at 4°C in a
Sorval HS4 rotor. The clear supernatants were transferred to fresh
tubes and stored at -70°C until assay.

Serotonin was extracted from blood by adding 3.0 ml of acid n-
butanol (0.85 ml of concentrated HCl to 1 liter of n-butanol [12]) to
each 0.3-ml aliquot of frozen blood followed by homogenization for 15
minutes at full speed at room temperature in a Buchler Vortex Mixer.
The blood/n-butanol mixture was then centrifuged at 2000 rpm for 2
minutes at 4°C in a Sorval HS4 rotor. Two and one-half milliliters
of the clarified supernatant was transferred to a fresh tube containing 0.4 ml of 0.1N HCl and 5 ml of n-heptane. This mixture was homogenized for 10 minutes at full speed in the Buchler Vortex Mixer and
then centrifuged as above. The aqueous phase was transferred to a
small tube and stored at -70°C until assay (13).

The concentrations of serotonin in the brain and blood extracts
were determined by high pressure liquid chromatography (14). Without
further purification, 0.05-ml aliquots were injected onto a 250-mm x

4-mm Bio-Sil ODS-10 reverse phase chromatography column (Biorad Laboratories) and eluted as described (15). Serotonin fluorescence was measured at 350 nm in a Shoeffel FS970 fluorometer with an excitation wavelength of 295 nm.

Serotonin concentrations were corrected for extraction efficiencies estimated from the recovery of exogenous ^{14}C-labeled serotonin (New England Nuclear) added to 0.3-ml aliquots of blood immediately before freezing or to 10% brain homogenates immediately before the addition of perchloric acid. Fractional recoveries were 0.79 for brain and 0.51 for blood.

Differences in the mean values of both the biochemical and the behavioral tests were analyzed for significance (probability of t, $p(t)$, greater than 0.05) using Student's t test for two tails. The ED_{50} values for producing the serotonin toxicity syndrome were estimated by probit analysis (16). Simple correlations, r, were computed for some of the biochemical data.

RESULTS

Two easily scored signs of scrapie disease in hamsters are ataxia and action jerks of the head and body. When the serotonin precursor, L-5-hydroxytryptophan methyl ester (5-HTP), or the serotonin agonist, quipazine maleate, are administered to scrapie-infected hamsters displaying these symptoms, one observes small, but statistically significant ($p(t) < 0.05$), reductions in the severity of their ataxia and the frequency of action jerks (Fig. 1). These improvements occur at relatively low drug dosage levels (5 mg/kg for 5-HTP and 1 to 2.5 mg/kg for quipazine). These dosages have no noticeable effect upon the behavior of normal hamsters. Dosages one-half as great or twice that of the effective dose do not result in significant improvements. Even higher doses were impossible to score accurately because of drug toxicity.

Doses four to eight times greater than those which effect small reductions in the symptoms of ataxia and action jerks produce a toxic response in the scrapie-infected animals but still have no effect upon control hamsters (Fig. 2). Control animals do show the toxic response, however, after doses five to eight times greater than those causing toxicity in the infected group. This is 30 to 40 times greater than the doses showing therapeutic benefits.

Serotonin toxicity of this sort is a well-characterized syndrome in the rat (7,9) and is associated with a less well-characterized but similar syndrome in the hamster (10). In the rat the main features are tremor, body rigidity, reciprocal forepaw treading, Straub tail, hindlimb abduction, and lateral head weaving (8). The less well characterized hamster syndrome does not include lateral head weaving but does include, in addition, a hunched posture and prominent sniffling (10).

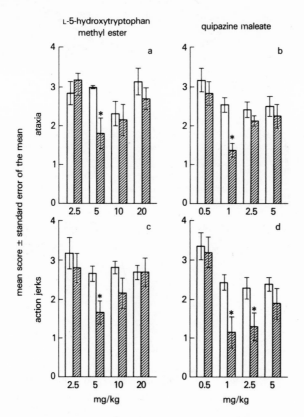

Fig. 1:   The effects of 5-HTP and quipazine on ataxia and action jerks
          in scrapie-infected hamsters. Six to eight animals at each
          dose were scored for locomotor signs as described in the text
          for 30 minutes before treatment (open bar) and between 30 and
          60 minutes after drug administration (hatched bar). Aster-
          isks indicate differences with p(t) < 0.05.

        The behavioral responses of both scrapie and control hamsters
to high doses of both quipazine maleate and 5-HTP were nearly identical, both fitting the pattern of the serotonin toxicity syndrome. The
exception was that quipazine in doses of 10 to 15 mg/kg in scrapie-
infected hamsters and 40 to 70 mg/kg in control hamsters often caused
seizures, while 5-HTP did not. The order of appearance of the behavioral signs was fairly constant in both control and scrapie-infected
hamsters: body rigidity, Straub tail, hindlimb abduction, resting
tremor, and reciprocal forepaw treading. Both drugs elicited a maximum manifestation of the serotonin syndrome between 30 and 60 minutes
after IP injection. The time between injection and onset of the syn-

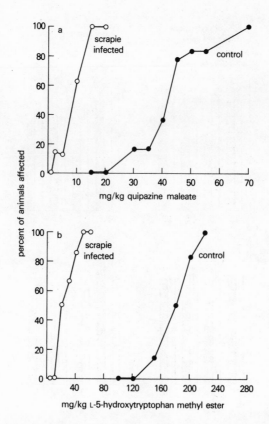

Fig. 2: Dose response to quipazine maleate (a), and 5-HTP (b), of
         scrapie-infected (open symbols) and normal (closed symbols)
         hamsters for production of the serotonin toxicity syndrome.
         Each point is the percentage of six to eight animals at that
         dose that displayed the syndrome.

drome varied from 10 to 30 minutes, independent of the dose or the
drug and without marked differences between scrapie-infected and control hamsters.

Scrapie-infected hamsters displayed a distinct hypersensitivity
to quipazine (Fig. 2a). The estimated value of the ED_{50} for scrapie-
infected hamsters, 8.13 mg/kg, was 20% of the ED_{50} for the control
hamsters, 40.74 mg/kg (p(t) <0.000). An even greater difference in
sensitivity was seen with 5-HTP (Fig. 2b). The estimated value of the
ED_{50} for scrapie-infected hamsters, 20.89 mg/kg, was 12% of the ED_{50}
for the control hamsters, 169.82 mg/kg, (p(t) <0.000).

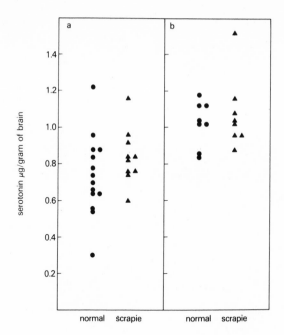

Fig. 3:   Serotonin concentrations in whole brains of scrapie-infected
          (triangles), and normal (circles) hamsters killed after metho-
          xyflurane anesthesia (a), or without anesthesia (b).

        This toxicity syndrome is considered to be a specific reflection
of central serotonin receptor activation in rats (7,9) and provides a
valuable method for assessing changes in sensitivity of the serotonergic system (8).   Presuming that the syndrome has a similar origin in
hamsters, the hypersensitivity of scrapie-infected hamsters to 5-HTP
and quipazine, both activators of central serotonin receptors, indicates a derangement of the central serotonin pathway in these animals.

        As a first step in identifying the nature of this disturbance,
we have looked for gross changes in serotonin metabolism by direct
biochemical measurement of brain serotonin levels in infected and control hamsters.   At the same time we have also measured blood serotonin
levels in the same animals on the remote chance that a defect in serotonin metabolism might affect the serotonin pathways in blood as well
as brain even though there is little to suggest any interaction between these systems.   A blood defect could provide a noninvasive biochemical indicator of scrapie disease.

        In brain (Fig. 3a, 3b, Table 1), the sample means of the seroto-
nin concentrations in hamsters killed either with or without anesthe-

Table 1.   Brain and Blood Concentrations of Serotonin in Scrapie-
Infected and Normal Hamsters

| | Serotonin concentration | | | |
| | Brain | | Blood | |
	Mean μg/g	Standard error μg/g	Mean μg/ml	Standard error μg/ml
Normal hamsters				
Methoxyflurane anesthesia	0.74	0.06	1.11	0.07
Cervical fracture alone	1.03	0.04		
Scrapie-infected hamsters				
Methoxyflurane anesthesia	0.84	0.05	0.44	0.05
Cervical fracture alone	1.08	0.07		

tization by methoxyflurane do not vary significantly ($p(t) > 0.10$ for both groups) between infected animals and controls. We did note a 25% decrement ($p(t) < 0.0000$), however, in the brain serotonin levels of methoxyflurane-treated animals, whether scrapie-infected or not, and animals killed directly by cervical fracture. Within each group of infected animals, individuals were scored for the extent of disease on a scale of zero to five. For both groups, individual serotonin concentrations were not correlated with the disease state of the animal ($r < 0.4$ for both groups).

In blood (Fig. 4, Table 1) there is a highly significant 2½-fold decrease in serotonin levels in scrapie versus normal animals ($p(t) < 0.0000$). We saw no correlations of individual blood serotonin levels with either the score for disease state or the brain serotonin concentration in the same animals.

DISCUSSION

The hypersensitivity of scrapie-infected hamsters to the serotonin precursor, L-5-hydroxytryptophan methyl ester (5-HTP), and the serotonin agonist, quipazine maleate, indicates a major derangement in the serotonin pathways of the central nervous system. In the rat, a similar hypersensitivity to serotonin and its precursors and agonists follows pharmacological destruction of serotonin nerve terminals with 5,7-dihydroxytryptamine (8). The hamster displays a behavioral reaction to toxic concentrations of serotonin nearly identical

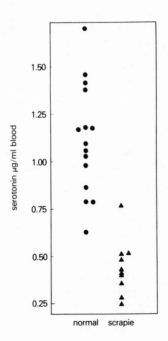

Fig. 4:   Serotonin concentrations in whole blood of scrapie-infected
          (triangles), and normal (circles) hamsters.

to the serotonin toxicity syndrome seen in the rat (10). Thus the hypersensitivity of infected hamsters to 5-HTP and quipazine is, depending upon the strength of analogy to the rat system, consistent with
the destruction of nerve terminals in the central serotonin pathways.

This pharmacological evidence for destruction of serotonin nerve
terminals was not corroborated by a concomitant reduction in the whole
brain serotonin concentrations in infected hamsters. In the rat, however, the serotonin syndrome originates mainly in the cells of the
median raphe nuclei of the brain stem (17). Thus our inability to
detect a reduction in scrapie hamster brain serotonin levels may be a
superficial consequence of having assayed whole brain as opposed to
some more restricted locus. We have detected a highly significant 20%
reduction in brain serotonin levels during the late clinical phase of
scrapie in mice (p(t) <0.0005) (18). We also observed a 20% reduction
in whole brain serotonin in both normal and scrapie-infected hamsters
after anesthesia with methoxyflurane.

In our tests of the therapeutic efficacy of 5-HTP and quipazine,
the small reductions in scrapie-induced ataxia and action jerks noted

after administration of low doses of either drug were both subjec-
tively and objectively (statistically) apparent, although by no means
dramatic. Nevertheless, the fact that these drugs do effect some improvements, even if minimal, does support the idea of a serotonergic
defect resulting from the scrapie infection.

The $2\frac{1}{2}$-fold decrement in blood serotonin concentrations in
scrapie-infected hamsters is the first major change in blood chemis-
try noted in the subacute spongiform virus encephalopathies. Since
blood serotonin is concentrated almost entirely within the platelets
(19), this reduction in whole blood serotonin levels may be a secondary consequence of a change in platelet, spleen or megakaryocyte function.

REFERENCES

1. Lampert, P.W. et al. Am J Pathol 68 (1972) 626.
2. Eklund, C.M. et al. J Infect Dis 117 (1967) 15.
3. McDermott, F.R. et al. Lancet ii (1978) 318.
4. Kimberlin, R.H.; Walker, C.A. J Gen Virol 37 (1977) 295.
5. Hong, E. et al. Eur J Pharmacol 6 (1969) 274.
6. Kuhn, D.M.; Appel, J.B. Neurosci Abstr 1 (1975) 293.
7. Sloviter, R.S. et al. J Pharmacol Exp Ther 206 (1978) 339.
8. Trulson, M.E. et al. J Pharmacol Exp Ther 198 (1976) 23.
9. Grahame-Smith, D.G. J Neurochem 18 (1971) 1053.
10. Jacobs, B.L. Life Sci 19 (1976) 777.
11. Johnson, S.M.; Bolstad, O.D. In: Behavior Change--Methodology,
    Concepts and Practice, ed. Hamerlynck, Handy, and Mash. Re-
    search Press, Champaign, Ill. (1973) 7.
12. Chang, C.C. Int J Neuropharmacol 3 (1964) 643.
13. Maickel, R.P. et al. Int J Neuropharmacol 7 (1968) 275.
14. Neckers, L.M.; Meek, J.L. Life Sci 19 (1976) 1579.
15. DeLisi, L.E. et al. Arch Psychiatr (1980) in press.
16. Colquhoun, D. Lectures on Biostatics. Oxford University Press,
    Oxford (1971) 344.
17. Jacobs, B.L.; Klemfuss, H. Brain Res 100 (1975) 450.
18. Neckers, L.M. et al. The Pharmacologist 21 (1979) abstract 266.
19. Undenfriend, S.; Weissbach, H. Fed Proc 13 (1954) 412.

DETERMINATION OF SCRAPIE AGENT TITER FROM INCUBATION PERIOD

MEASUREMENTS IN HAMSTERS

Stanley B. Prusiner, S. Patricia Cochran, Deborah E.Downey
and Darlene F. Groth

Howard Hughes Medical Institute Laboratory, Departments of
Neurology, and Biochemistry and Biophysics, University of
California, San Francisco, CA 94143

INTRODUCTION

One of the most distinctive and remarkable features of slow virus
infections is the prolonged incubation period during which the host
is free of disease (1). These long incubation periods terminate with
the onset of clinical disease which progresses to death in a relatively short time. Considerable interest has surrounded the mechanisms
regulating the length of the incubation periods of the spongiform encephalopathies: scrapie of sheep and goats, transmissible encephalopathy of mink, and kuru and Creutzfeldt-Jakob disease (CJD) of humans
(2,3). Factors controlling the length of the incubation period in
scrapie include: the dose of agent, the genetic background of the host,
the strain and passage history of the agent, the lymphoid system of
the host, and the metabolic and endocrinological state of the host (4,
5). The shortest incubation periods are found in scrapie, where hamsters develop clinical disease in two months, while the longest incubation periods approach three decades in kuru and probably CJD (6-8).

Although the length of the incubation period was carefully recorded in early studies on scrapie in sheep and goats, its relationship to the dilution of the inoculum was unclear. Data relating the
length of the incubation period in goats to the dilution of the sample
(9) are plotted in Fig. 1. Other data (10) show a clear relationship
between the length of the incubation period in mice and the dilution
of the inoculum (Fig. 2). This plot also relates the interval from
inoculation to death to the dilution of the inoculum. The regular increases in incubation periods and times from inoculation to death with
increasing dilution prompted these workers (10) to suggest that this
relationship might be used as an assay. Other investigators have docu-

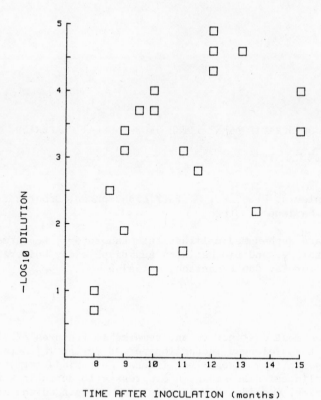

TIME AFTER INOCULATION (months)

Fig. 1: Incubation periods for scrapie in goats inoculated intra-
        cerebrally with various dilutions of the agent. (Data from
        Pattison and Millson, 1961.)

mented this relationship in both mice and hamsters (11-13). In fact,
it has been used (14) to estimate titers in murine tissues in order to
document kinetics of agent replication.

Our use of the incubation period to determine titers of the scrapie agent has evolved because studies on the isolation of the scrapie
agent demand maximum speed and economy. Until recently, all quantitative studies on the purification of the scrapie agent have used quantal endpoint titrations. We have found that over a considerable range
of dosages, the length of the incubation period varies inversely with
the logarithm of the inoculated dose. The time for assay of the agent
in both mice and hamsters is diminished considerably with this new
assay procedure, especially with samples containing high titers. Just
as important, the number of animals required for assay of a single
sample is decreased by a factor of 10 to 15. In fact, we believe the

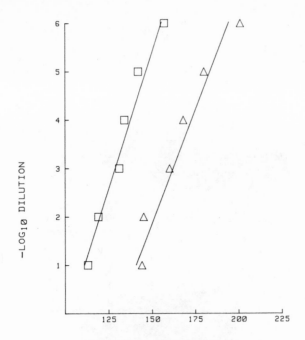

TIME AFTER INOCULATION (days)

Fig. 2:   Incubation periods for scrapie in mice inoculated intrace-
          rebrally with various dilutions of the agent. Time from inocu-
          lation to onset of clinical illness (☐-☐) and to death
          (Δ-Δ). (Data from Eklund et al., 1963.)

incubation period assay is of equal or increased accuracy compared to
the quantal endpoint titration procedure. While this assay represents
a considerable advance over the previous endpoint titration procedure,
the ultimate isolation of the scrapie agent continues to be compli-
cated by the lack of a cell culture system for replication of the
agent to high titers and by the hydrophobic nature of the agent (15).

MATERIALS AND METHODS

     Hamster-adapted scrapie agent was obtained from Dr. Richard
Marsh. The agent was in its sixth passage in an LHC/LAK inbred hamster. The brain was homogenized in 320mM sucrose and the homogenate
clarified by centrifugation at 1,000 x g for 10 minutes. Random-bred
LVG/LAK female weanling hamsters obtained from Charles River Laboratories were inoculated intracerebrally with 50 μl of 10^{-1} dilution.
After approximately 60 days, the hamsters were killed when they developed signs of clinical scrapie. Homogenates of the agent were pre-

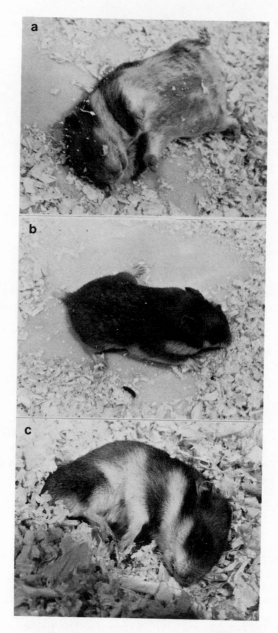

Fig. 3:   Clinical scrapie in the hamster: a) difficulty righting her-
          self from supine position; b) ataxia with broad-based gait
          especially the hind legs as shown; c) lying quietly on her
          side during the terminal stage of scrapie.

pared from these animals and the agent passaged again prior to use in
the studies described here. The titer of the final inoculum (8th hamster passage) was 10^{10} ID_{50} units/gram of brain tissue as determined
by endpoint titration using the method of Spearman and Kärber (16).

Quantal endpoint titrations of the scrapie agent were performed
by the inoculation of four weanling female hamsters at each 10-fold
dilution. The animals were inoculated intracerebrally with 50 µl of
a given sample at a specified dilution using a 27-gauge needle. The
inoculations all were made in the left parietal region of the cranium
and the needle inserted to a depth of approximately 3 mm. The diluent
used was phosphate buffered saline containing 0.5 units penicillin/ml,
0.5 µg streptomycin/ml and 2.5 µg amphotericin/ml, and 50 mg of re-
crystalized fraction V bovine serum albumin (BSA)/ml.

The animals were housed in polyurethane cages 20 cm high, 20 cm
wide and 42 cm deep and covered with a wire screen. Eight animals
were housed per cage and groups of four distinguished by notching the
right ear of one group. Water was provided by an automatic watering
system and Purina rat chow was provided ad libitum. A generous supply
of pine wood shavings was placed on the bottom of each cage. The cages
were changed two times a week. All personnel entering the room were
required to wear masks, gowns, rubber boots and rubber gloves, as well
as head covers.

None of the hamsters showed any signs of neurological dysfunction
for more than six weeks after inoculation (17). The onset of clinical
scrapie was diagnosed by the presence of at least two of the following
signs: generalized tremor, ataxia of gait, difficulty in rising from
a supine position (Fig. 3a), and head bobbing. The bobbing movements
of the head increased progressively and may have resulted from visual
difficulties due to degenerative changes in the retina (N. Hogan, personal communication). Between 1% and 10% of the hamsters had generalized convulsions at this early stage of the illness. With further
progression, the ataxia became so pronounced that balance was maintained with considerable difficulty (Fig. 3b). Kyphotic posture,
bradykinesia and weight loss appeared 7 to 15 days after the onset of
illness. Over the next week the hamsters became unable to maintain an
erect posture, lay quietly on their sides, and exhibited frantic movements of the extremities when disturbed (Fig. 3c). Death followed in
three to five days.

In order to organize and process the large number of data obtained from these studies, computer programs in Basic language were
written for an HP 9845 microcomputer. These programs allowed us to
record the time of onset of illness for each animal as well as the
time of death. These measurements were used as described below for
the development of equations relating the titer of the inoculum to
the length of the incubation period. The programs are available upon
request on either cassette tape or flexible disk.

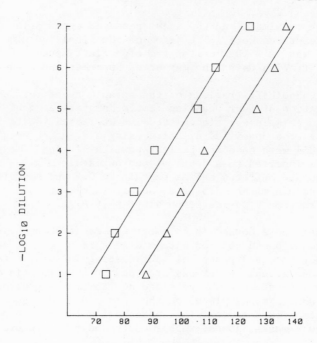

TIME AFTER INOCULATION (days)

Fig. 4:   Onset of clinical illness and time of death as a function of
          the dilution of the sample. Onset of illness (□-□) and
          time of death (Δ-Δ). Each symbol is the average of eight
          animals.

RESULTS

     While several reports have demonstrated that the length of the
incubation period is a linear function of the logarithm of the inoculated dose of the scrapie agent, this relationship has not been generally exploited as an assay (10,11,14). Our initial intention was to
use the length of the incubation period as a guide to determine the
range over which endpoint titrations needed to be performed. As described in this communication, however, incubation period measurements
provide at least as great accuracy as do endpoint titrations.

     To construct calibration curves for the incubation period assay,
samples with different titers were subjected to endpoint titration.
Four hamsters were inoculated intracerebrally (IC) with a given sample
at a specified dilution. After six weeks, the hamsters were examined
twice each week for clinical signs of scrapie. From the number of
animals positive at each dilution, the titer was calculated by the
method of Spearman and Kärber (16). The injected dose was then cal-

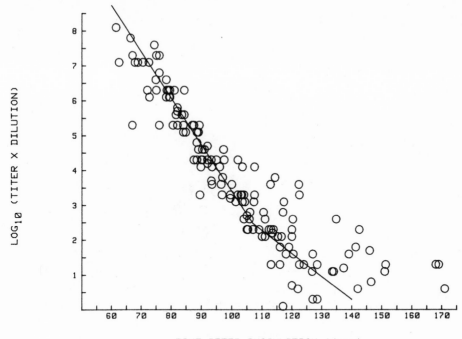

TIME AFTER INOCULATION (days)

Fig. 5: Relationship between the onset of illness and the inoculated
         dose (titer x dilution) of the scrapie agent. Each circular
         symbol is the mean of four animals.

culated by multiplying the titer of the sample times the dilution.
The average length of the incubation period as measured by the onset
of clinical illness as well as the time until death were also recorded. It is noteworthy that the ID_{50} and LD_{50} values for a given
sample are identical, since scrapie is uniformly fatal.

     In Fig. 4, both the onset of clinical illness and the time until
death are plotted as a function of the dilution of the sample. As
shown in Fig. 2, the time intervals from inoculation to the onset of
clinical illness as well as to death are a linear function of the logarithm of the dilution of the inoculum.

     Curves relating the injected dose to the length of the incubation
period are shown in Fig. 5 and 6. The titers of the samples used to
construct these curves varied over a range from 10^3 to $10^{8.5}$ ID_{50}
units/ml as determined by endpoint titration. When data from samples
are combined with different titers, a simple exponential relationship

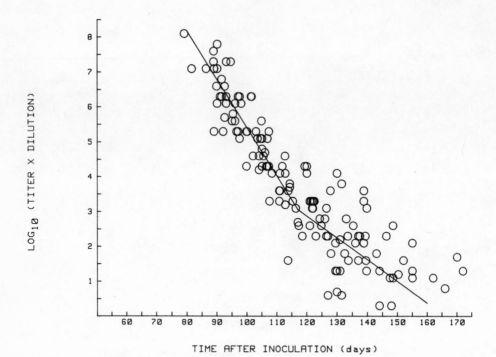

Fig. 6:   Relationship between the time of death and the inoculated
          dose (titer x dilution) of the scrapie agent. Each circular
          symbol is the mean of four animals.

does not hold over the entire range of values examined. As illustrated
in Fig. 5, the length of the incubation period is a complex function
of the inoculated dose and must be expressed as the sum of at least
two exponentials. Since the scatter of points precludes the advantageous use of curve fitting techniques, we have chosen to approximate
the relationship with two straight lines.

    While the onset of illness requires clinical judgment with re-
spect to the diagnosis of scrapie, the time of death is a completely
objective measurement. Thus, a similar analysis was performed for
the incubation period of the scrapie agent as measured from the time
of inoculation until death. As shown in Fig. 6, the interval from inoculation to death is also a complex function of the injected dose of
the agent. Again, this function can be expressed as the sum of at
least two exponentials. Like the data for onset of illness, the scatter of points precludes the advantageous use of curve fitting techniques, and thus we have chosen to approximate the relationship again
with two straight lines.

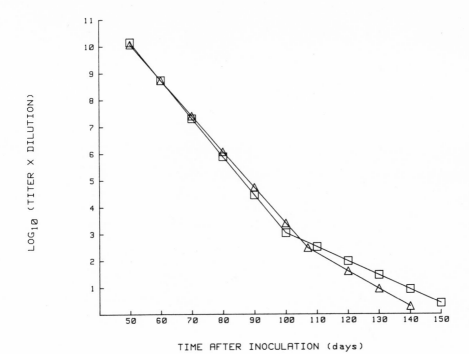

Fig. 7: Comparison of two curves relating the onset of illness and
         the inoculated dose of the scrapie agent. Curve developed
         1½ years ago (□-□) and curve from Fig. 5 (Δ-Δ).

     Fig. 7 compares the curve in Fig. 5 with one constructed nearly
1½ years ago which was used for calculation of titers in our initial
studies on the scrapie agent from hamster brain (18). As shown, the
curves are virtually superimposable, especially with respect to their
steep portions, which are most critical. The equation given below
represents the average of the two experimentally determined curves:

$$\text{Log } T = \begin{cases} 17.0 - \log D - 0.138 \ (\bar{x}) & \text{for } x < 104 \\ 8.9 - \log D - 0.059 \ (\bar{x}) & \text{for } x \geq 104 \end{cases} \quad (I)$$

where T is the titer expressed in ID_{50} units/ml, D is the dilution of
the sample expressed as the fractional concentration and $\bar{x}$ is the mean
interval from inoculation to the onset of clinical illness in days.

     In an attempt to improve the precision of the titer determina-
tions, the interval between the onset of clinical illness and death
was examined. Fig. 8 compares the curves shown in Fig. 5 and 6, while
Fig. 9 gives the difference interval between onset of illness and
death as a function of incubation period. As shown, this interval is

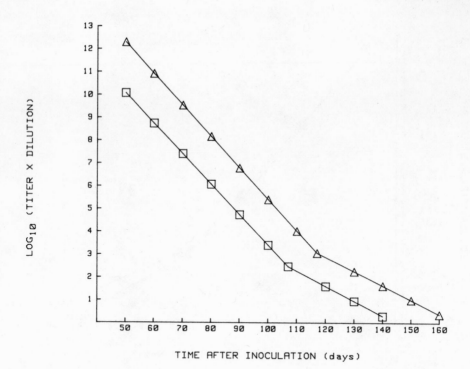

Fig. 8: Comparison of the onset of illness and time of death curves.
The curves depict the two straight lines used to describe the
data in Fig. 5 and 6. Onset of illness (□-□) and time of
death (△-△).

virtually constant for the steep and gradual portions of the curves.
The average interval between onset of illness and death for the steep
portions of the curves (i.e., < 100 days) is 16 days while the average
interval for the more gradual portions of the curves (i.e., > 120) is
21 days. We have used the constancy of these intervals to convert the
times until death to the corresponding times for onset of illness.
From the data in Fig. 9, equation II was derived where z is the interval in days from inoculation to death.

$$x = \begin{cases} z - 16.0 & \text{for } z \leq 100 \\ z - 18.5 & \text{for } z > 100, < 120 \\ z - 21.0 & \text{for } z \geq 120 \end{cases} \quad \text{(II)}$$

Subtracting 18.5 days for the period from 100 to 120 days represents
a compromise value to take into account the transitions between the
steep and gradual portions of the curves in Fig. 8.

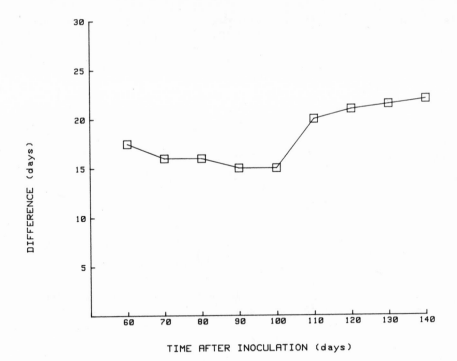

TIME AFTER INOCULATION (days)

Fig. 9:   The difference interval between onset of illness and time of
death.

After conversion of all z-values into onset of illness values
(x), all eight of these x-values can be used to compute the titer. It
has been our experience that the variability among all eight values
is relatively low.   Studies are in progress to determine whether eight
values increase the precision of our assay sufficiently to warrant the
continued use of four animals or whether it may be possible to reduce
the number of animals to three or even two for each assay.

In Table 1, a comparison of titers calculated by endpoint titration as well as by the new incubation period method at dilutions of
10^{-1}, 10^{-3} and 10^{-4} is given.   As shown, the incubation period measurements of titer in the inoculum do not generally vary more than $\pm$ 0.5
log ID_{50} units from those determined by quantal endpoint titrations
according to the method of Spearman and Kärber (16).   The average deviation of the 18 values determined by incubation period measurements
from the six corresponding endpoint titration values was 0.32 log ID_{50}
units/ml (Table 1).   Estimates of the standard error for the incubation period method based only on the onset of illness times gave an
average standard error of 0.22 log ID_{50} units/ml (4).   The standard

Table 1.   Comparison of Titers Determined by Endpoint Titration and
           Incubation Period Measurements

Endpoint titration		Incubation period measurements (Dilution)		
		10^{-1}	10^{-3}	10^{-4}
(log ID_{50} units/ml $\pm$ S.E.)		(log ID_{50} units/ml)		
1.	8.3 $\pm$ .35	8.3	8.7	9.0
2.	8.3 $\pm$ .35	7.7	8.4	8.2
3.	8.1 $\pm$ .25	8.1	8.0	7.9
4.	8.3 $\pm$ .35	8.1	7.7	7.3
5.	8.1 $\pm$ .25	8.2	7.8	8.2
6.	8.0 $\pm$ .44	8.2	8.5	8.6

errors for endpoint titrations are generally slightly higher, ranging
between 0.3 and 0.5 log ID_{50} units/ml.

DISCUSSION

     The validity of the incubation period method for determining
scrapie titers as described by equation I is supported by several
lines of evidence. First, the titers of the hamster agent obtained by
the incubation period method agree, in general, within $\pm$ 0.5 log ID_{50}
units/ml with those found by endpoint titration. Second, the incubation period gives the same data whether the onset of illness is used
as a criterion for determining the incubation period or the time of
death after inoculation is used. Third, the onset of illness is so
distinct and readily determined that the calibration curve developed
1½ years ago is virtually superimposable on the one reported in this
communication. Fourth, no differences between the molecular properties of the agents from hamster and murine sources have been detected,
with primarily the incubation period method used with the former and
endpoint titration used with the latter (19). Sedimentation profiles,
detergent stability studies and gel electrophoresis experiments yield
the same data whether assays are performed by the incubation period
method or endpoint titration.

     In the hamster, the onset of clinical scrapie and the progression
of the disease is so stereotyped with hamster-adapted strains of the
agent, that pathological confirmation of all cases is not necessary.
Routine histological confirmations of random animals is advisable,
however. In addition, it may be necessary to reassess continuously
the validity in the calibration curves as purification of the agent

progresses. Some properties of the scrapie agent appear to change
during purification, such as the ability of the agent to aggregate
with cellular elements when heated (15,18,20). Indeed, the incubation
period method may prove to be superior to endpoint titration with respect to aggregation of the agent. If aggregation occurs in the titration assay and the agent is not disaggregated during serial dilution, the actual titer will appear falsely low. Measurements of the
incubation period may possibly obviate this problem, assuming that
disaggregation will occur within the animal.

The advantages of the incubation period assay over the endpoint
titration assay are numerous. First, the number of animals required
for determination of a particular sample is decreased by a factor of
10 to 15. Second, the imprecision that arises during pipetting the
serial dilutions of samples is obviated by the incubation period
method. Third, determination of the titer in samples with high titers
is considerably faster using the incubation period method. As illustrated above, there is an inverse relationship between the length of
the incubation period and the titer of the inoculum. To establish the
endpoint of a titration for the scrapie agent, it is necessary to wait
until all the animals become sick at the highest positive dilution.
Fourth, the incubation period assay will always give a quantitative
estimate of the amount of scrapie in a given sample, unlike the endpoint titration assay. Attempts to economize with endpoint titrations
will, at times, result in a series of dilutions that do not span the
endpoint of the sample. In such cases, considerable time will have already elapsed and it will be necessary to begin a second titration.

While data on the onset of illness are subjective and require
clinical assessment of neurological dysfunction in animals, we have
shown that the phenomena are highly reproducible and correlate with
the objective observations on death times. It would seem important to
emphasize that the calibration curves described in this communication
should not be applied directly by others to their experimental protocols. Other investigators should develop their own calibration curves
based on their own criteria for the reliable and reproducible diagnosis of scrapie.

Over a wide range of injected doses, the incubation period is a
linear function of the logarithm of the injected dose of the scrapie
agent. This appears to be the result of exponential agent multiplica-
tion. In general, it is assumed that the titers in the brains of the
inoculated animals must reach a threshold level before clinical signs
of disease are manifest. Thus, a high dose or large initial inoculum
will result in more rapid attainment of this threshold level. A small
dose of the scrapie agent, conversely, will require a longer time for
this threshold level to be reached. To our knowledge, experimental
studies confirming this assumption have not been reported.

Even though the incubation period assay does not provide an extremely rapid method for determining the amount of scrapie agent in a given sample in a one or two-day period, it does substantially reduce the time and resources necessary for measurement of the agent. While most of our initial work on the biochemical and biophysical properties of the scrapie agent was performed with the endpoint titration in mice, more recent studies have used the incubation period method in hamsters. We estimate that our ability to gain information about the scrapie agent with an equal number of animals has increased by a factor of 60 to 75.

SUMMARY

Progress in studies on the scrapie agent has been hampered by the slow and tedious endpoint titration assays in rodents. A new assay based on incubation period measurements has been developed. The incubation period is defined as the time interval from inoculation to the onset of clinically detectable neurological illness or as the interval from inoculation to death. Both of these intervals or incubation periods are inversely proportional to the size of the dose injected intracerebrally into random bred weanling syrian hamsters. The incubation period was found to be a linear function of the logarithm of the inoculum size over a wide range of dosages (10^2 - 10^8 ID_{50} units). From these studies an equation relating the titer of the inoculum to the dilution of the sample and the length of the incubation period has been developed facilitating the use of a computerized record system. Validation of the assay was provided by comparing samples where the agent was measured both by endpoint titration and incubation period methods. Agreement between the 2 methods was generally within $\pm$ 0.5 $\log_{10}$ ID_{50} units. In addition, no differences between the molecular properties of the agents from hamster and murine sources have been detected using primarily the incubation period method with the former and endpoint tiration with the latter. The advantages of the incubation period assay are considerable with respect to time and economy.

ACKNOWLEDGMENTS

Dr. Prusiner is an investigator at the Howard Hughes Medical Institute. This work was supported in part by research grants from the National Institutes of Health NS14069 and the National Science Foundation PCM7724076. The authors wish to thank Dr. Louis Sokoloff for helpful discussions and Mrs. Sandra Prusiner for developing the computer programs. Manuscript preparation by Mss. C. Boghosian and L. Gallagher is acknowledged. The continuing interest and help of Dr. M. Redfearn and Mr. R. Bevis is also gratefully acknowledged.

REFERENCES

1. Sigurdsson, B.   Br Vet J 110 (1954) 341.
2. Gajdusek, D.C.   Science 197 (1977) 943.
3. Prusiner, S.B.; Hadlow, W., ed.   Slow Transmissible Diseases of
    the Nervous System, Vol. 1 and 2. Academic Press, New York (1979).
4. Prusiner, S.B. et al.   In: Aging of the Brain and Dementia, ed.
    Amaducci,Davison, and Antuono.   Raven Press, New York, (1980) 205.
5. Outram, G.W.   In: Slow Transmissible Diseases of Animals and Man,
    ed. Kimberlin. American Elsevier, New York (1976) 325.
6. Alpers, M.P.   In: Slow Transmissible Diseases of the Nervous
    System, ed. Prusiner and Hadlow, Vol. 1. Academic Press, New
    York (1979) 67.
7. Masters, C.L. et al.   In: Slow Transmissible Diseases of the Ner-
    vous System, ed. Prusiner and Hadlow, Vol. 1. Academic Press,
    New York (1979) 143.
8. Masters, C.L. et al.   Ann Neurol 5 (1979) 177.
9. Pattison, I.H.; Millson, G.C.   J Comp Pathol Ther 71 (1961) 350.
10. Eklund, C.M. et al.   Proc Soc Exp Biol Med 112 (1963) 974.
11. Dickinson, A.G. et al.   J Comp Pathol 79 (1979) 15.
12. Kimberlin, R.H.; Walker, C.A.   J Gen Virol 34 (1977) 295.
13. Marsh, R.F.; Hanson, R.P.   Fed Proc 37 (1977) 2076.
14. Kimberlin, R.H.; Walker, C.A.   J Comp Pathol 89 (1979) 551.
15. Prusiner, S.B. et al.   In: Slow Transmissible Diseases of the
    Nervous System, ed. Prusiner and Hadlow, Vol. 2. Academic Press,
    New York (1979) 425.
16. Dougherty, R.   In: Techniques in Experimental Virology, ed.
    Harris.   Academic Press, New York (1964) 169.
17. Marsh, R.F.; Kimberlin, R.H.   J Inf Dis 131 (1975) 104.
18. Prusiner, S.B. et al.   Proc Natl Acad Sci USA 77 (1980) 2984.
19. Prusiner, S.B. et al.   In: Neurochemistry and Clinical Neurology,
    ed. Battistin, Hashim and Lajtha. A. Liss, Inc., New York (1980)
    73.
20. Prusiner, S.B. et al.   J Neurochem, 35 (1980) 574.

TOWARD DEVELOPMENT OF ASSAYS FOR SCRAPIE-SPECIFIC ANTIBODIES

Kenneth C. Kasper, Karen Bowman, Daniel P. Stites, and
Stanley B. Prusiner

Howard Hughes Medical Institute Laboratory, Departments of
Neurology, Biochemistry and Biophysics, Laboratory Medicine
and Medicine, University of California, School of Medicine,
San Francisco, CA 94143

INTRODUCTION

At least 40 attempts have been made to detect antibodies directed
against the scrapie agent (Table 1). All have failed. More than 10
were by neutralization (1-6), seven by precipitation in gel or tubes
(3,7-9), eight by complement fixation (3,5,7), and six by direct or
indirect immunofluorescence procedures (3,6,8). Passive hemagglutination, passive hemolysis, passive anaphylaxis, immunoconglutinin (7),
and anti-nuclear (10) and anti-cardiolipin (7) antibody tests were
also employed. Antisera from goats, sheep, mice, rabbits, roosters,
monkeys and humans have been tested.

The reasons for the lack of success are not clear. We can only
surmise that the scrapie agent is a poor immunogen (11), which may be
due in part to its hydrophobic character (12). For most if not all
of the previous assays for anti-scrapie antibody, two common features
may explain the lack of success (13). First, only crude antigen preparations have been employed, and these have consisted primarily of
tissue suspensions or crude extracts. Second, the concentrations of
the scrapie agent in unpurified fractions were generally low.

The possibility that the scrapie agent may evade both primary
and secondary immune defense systems through as yet undescribed mechanisms must also be considered. Of interest is the lack of an inflammatory response to devastation of the central nervous system by scrapie infection (11). Even during the clinical phase of the illness,
when drastic changes in brain structure are evident, no inflammatory
response can be detected.

Table 1. Attempts to Demonstrate Anti-Scrapie Antibodies

Serological technique	Source of scrapie agent	Antigen preparation	Source of antibody	Reference
Neutralization	Goat	Brain suspension	Goat "scrapie-recovered" sheep	1
	Chandler strain mouse	"	Mouse Goat "scrapie-recovered" sheep	2
	"	"	Sheep Mouse Rabbit Rooster Monkey Human	3,4
	"	"	Guinea pig Rat Human	5
	"	Freon-clarified brain	Mouse	6
Precipitation	Goat	Brain cerebrospinal fluid	Goat	7
	Goat	Cerebrospinal fluid	Rabbit	8
	Sheep	Spleen homogenate	Rabbit	9
	Chandler strain mouse	Brain suspension	Sheep Mouse Rabbit Rooster	3

Assay	Scrapie source	Antigen	Antibody source	Ref.
Complement fixation	Sheep	Spleen extract	Sheep	7
	Sheep	Brain extract	Sheep	7
	Chandler strain mouse	Brain suspension	Sheep, Mouse, Rabbit, Rooster	3
	"	"	Guinea pig, Rat	5
Immunofluorescence	Goat	Brain section	Rabbit anti-CSF	8
	Chandler strain mouse	Brain suspension	Sheep, Mouse, Rabbit, Rooster	3
	"	Monolayer from brain explant cultures	Mouse	6
Anti-nuclear antibody	Sheep	DNA (_E. coli_)	Sheep	10
	Chandler strain mouse	RNA (virus)	Mouse	
Passive hemmagglutination	Goat	Cerebrospinal fluid	Goat	7
Passive hemolysis	Sheep	Brain extract	Sheep	7
	Sheep	Brain extract	Goat, Sheep	
Passive anaphylaxis	Goat	Cerebrospinal fluid	Goat	7
Immunoconglutinin	Sheep	Brain or spleen extracts	Sheep, Goat	7
Anti-cardiolipin	None	Cardiolipin	Sheep	7

Earlier attempts in our laboratory to develop an immunoassay for the scrapie agent focused on a search for changes in lymphocyte immunoreactivity (14,15). Since changes in immunoreactivity to mitogens were of insufficient magnitude to be used as an assay for the agent, we focused our attention on the development of a quantitative immunoassay which would use antibodies directed specifically toward the agent. These studies have been facilitated by the development of a new bioassay for the agent (16) and novel purification schemes yielding highly enriched preparations (17).

The indirect, solid phase enzyme-linked immunosorbent assay (ELISA) is particularly well suited for measurement of antibody to a specific antigen in impure preparations. A minimal number of reagents are needed, partially-purified antigens can be adsorbed nonspecifically to a solid-phase support, and the method is both sensitive and quantitative (18-22). We have investigated ELISA using two purified model antigens, bovine serum albumin (BSA) and vesicular stomatitis virus (VSV). Our studies have defined the limits of detection for antibodies when antigens are present in low concentration. Addition of impurities, similar to those present in preparations of the scrapie agent, to a purified model antigen (BSA) diminished ELISA sensitivity. Thus, both the concentration of the specific antigen and the surrounding impurities affect the sensitivity of the ELISA.

Initial studies on detection of antibodies to the scrapie agent show that ELISA is ineffective with a deoxycholate-extracted fraction, designated P_3, from hamster brain as the antigen. Whether the concentration of the agent in these preparations is insufficient, or specific antibodies have not been produced by our immunization procedures, or both, remains to be established.

MATERIALS AND METHODS

Rabbit anti-bovine serum albumin (anti-BSA) and the heterologous IgG fraction of goat anti-rabbit IgG (GaRIgG) were obtained as lyophilized materials from Miles Laboratories, and rabbit anti-vesicular stomatitis virus (anti-VSV) was generously provided by Dr. Ludvik Prevec, McMaster University, Ontario. Other chemical reagents were of the highest purities commercially available.

The antigens, bovine serum albumin (BSA), fraction V (Sigma) and purified vesicular stomatitis virus (VSV, Indiana serotype) were used at various concentrations to coat Cooke polystyrene, round bottom, 96-well microtiter plates (Cat. No. 1-223-24, Dynatech Laboratories). Vesicular stomatitis virus was purified from chicken embryo fibroblast culture supernatant by sucrose density centrifugation and dialyzed against phosphate-buffered saline (PBS). Purified virus was kindly supplied by Dr. Douglas W. Ehresmann. Detergent extracted hamster brain antigens were prepared according to a differential centrifuga-

tion scheme (17). Briefly, cell debris, nuclei and mitochondria were
removed from a 10% (w/v) brain homogenate and the resultant supernatant fraction was treated with 0.5% (w/v) sodium deoxycholate and centrifuged at 228,000 x g for two hours at 4°C. The pellet was resuspended in 20mM Tris acetate (pH 8.3), stored frozen at -20°C, and diluted in carbonate-bicarbonate coating buffer for mixtures with BSA.

The enzymes, alkaline phosphatase from calf intestine (Sigma Type
VII, 1025 units/mg protein) and beta-D-galactosidase from Escherichia
coli, E.C. No. 3.2.1.23 (Sigma Grade IV, 385 units/mg protein), were
used to prepare conjugates with GaRIgG in the colorimetric and fluorimetric ELISA procedures, respectively. Enzymes and GaRIgG were mixed,
dialyzed and conjugated in a one-step glutaraldehyde cross-linking procedure (20). Goat antibody-enzyme conjugates were dialyzed against
several changes of PBS and finally 0.05M Tris-HCl (pH 8.0). Conjugates
were stored at 4°C in buffer containing 0.02% sodium azide and ovalbumin (10 mg/ml) or an equal volume of glycerol to stabilize protein.

Disodium p-nitrophenyl phosphate in 10% diethanolamine buffer
(pH 9.8) and 4-methylumbelliferyl-beta-D-galactopyranoside in 0.1M
Tris-citrate (pH 7.0) containing 0.5 mg BSA/ml and 1mM $MgCl_2$ (Tris-
BSA-Mg buffer) were used as enzyme substrates in the colorimetric and
fluorimetric ELISA procedures, respectively. These ELISA procedures
followed a five-step, indirect method for assay of antibody (20) and
are described in Fig. 1.

The ability of anti-VSV to neutralize VSV was determined by a
microtiter neutralization assay. Serial 10-fold dilutions of stock
VSV from infected culture supernatant were made in minimal essential
medium containing 100 units penicillin/ml and 100 µg streptomycin/ml.
Normal rabbit serum or anti-VSV was added at a final dilution of 10^{-3}.
Aliquots (0.1 ml) were distributed into eight wells and incubated for
one hour in 5% CO_2 at 37°C. Then 0.1 ml-aliquots of vero monkey kidney
cells in medium were added to all wells. After 48 more hours of incubation, the number of wells, in eight, showing positive cytopathic
effect (CPE) was recorded. Virus titers were computed by the Reed-
Muench method and expressed as $TCID_{50}$/ml.

RESULTS AND DISCUSSION

Antibody Detection by ELISA

The limits of sensitivity of ELISA for antibody can be defined
by two extreme conditions: 1. limiting antigen with excess antibody
and 2. saturating antigen with limiting antibody. The minimum concentration of BSA necessary for adsorption to the solid phase that permitted detection of anti-BSA is shown in Fig. 2 and 3. Both colorimetric and fluorimetric ELISA were employed in these studies. A minimal concentration of 10 ng/ml was required in both assays, while 100

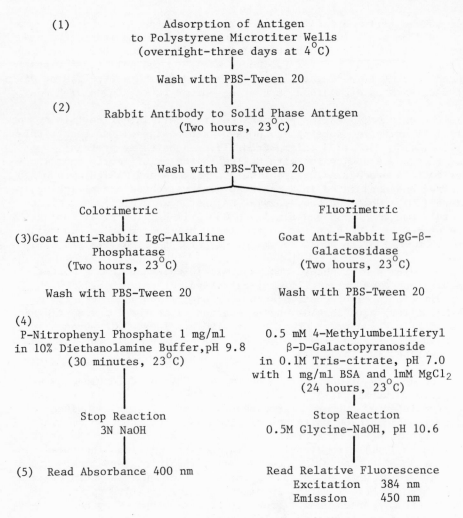

(1)   Adsorption of Antigen
                          to Polystyrene Microtiter Wells
                          (overnight-three days at 4°C)
                                        |
                           Wash with PBS-Tween 20
                                        |
(2)   Rabbit Antibody to Solid Phase Antigen
                            (Two hours, 23°C)
                                        |
                           Wash with PBS-Tween 20

          Colorimetric   Fluorimetric
              | |
(3)Goat Anti-Rabbit IgG-Alkaline   Goat Anti-Rabbit IgG-β-
        Phosphatase   Galactosidase
     (Two hours, 23°C)   (Two hours, 23°C)
              | |
   Wash with PBS-Tween 20   Wash with PBS-Tween 20
              | |
(4)
P-Nitrophenyl Phosphate 1 mg/ml   0.5 mM 4-Methylumbelliferyl
in 10% Diethanolamine Buffer,pH 9.8   β-D-Galactopyranoside
     (30 minutes, 23°C)   in 0.1M Tris-citrate, pH 7.0
              | with 1 mg/ml BSA and 1mM MgCl$_2$
              | (24 hours, 23°C)
              | |
         Stop Reaction   Stop Reaction
           3N NaOH   0.5M Glycine-NaOH, pH 10.6
              | |
(5)   Read Absorbance 400 nm   Read Relative Fluorescence
                                              Excitation   384 nm
                                              Emission   450 nm

Fig. 1:   Scheme for colorimetric and fluorimetric ELISA procedures.

μg of BSA/ml gave maximal signals. The sensitivities of these two
ELISA procedures are indistinguishable when limiting concentrations
of antigen are used for adsorption to the solid phase. Thus, fluorimetric ELISA would not be advantageous for detection of putative anti-
scrapie antibody, under conditions where scrapie agent concentrations
were limiting. In contrast, fluorimetric ELISA has greater sensitivity than colorimetric ELISA when saturating concentrations of antigen
are adsorbed (18,19,22,23).

    The effect of adsorbed BSA concentration on antiserum titration
is shown in Fig. 4. Various concentrations of BSA were adsorbed to

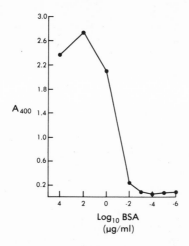

Fig. 2:   Detection of anti-BSA by colorimetric ELISA. Various concen-
          trations of BSA were coated for three days at 4°C. BSA-
          coated plates were incubated with 10^{-2} anti-BSA (2.5 mg/ml).
          The color reactions of the enzyme catalyzed hydrolysates were
          read at 400 nm.

wells at 4°C for three days. Ten-fold dilutions of anti-BSA were reacted in the colorimetric procedure. Adsorption of BSA to the microtiter well at 1 µg/ml or more permitted titration of anti-serum. At
such concentrations of antigen, antisera could be diluted 1000-fold
and still give measurable activities. Dilution of antisera 10,000-
fold gave only marginal activities. When antigen concentrations of
10 ng/ml were used for adsorption to microtiter wells as noted above,
antibodies to BSA could be detected but antiserum titration could not
be performed.

We have performed a similar study on VSV in order to compare requirements for detection of antibodies to an infectious virus particle
with those for anti-BSA (Fig. 5a). The effect of the VSV concentrations used for adsorption to the microtiter well on anti-VSV ELISA
activity is shown. The minimum concentration of VSV required for adsorption in order to detect anti-VSV activity was 10^9 $TCID_{50}$/ml. Since
the particle-to-infectivity ratio of VSV is approximately 10^3, a concentration of 10^{12} virus particles/ml will be required for detection
of VSV antibodies. This corresponds to a molar concentration of 1.5nM,
which is 10 times higher than found for BSA.

The anti-viral activity of this same antiserum against VSV was
tested in a virus neutralization assay. Serial 10-fold dilutions of
VSV from infected cell culture supernatant were cultured with normal

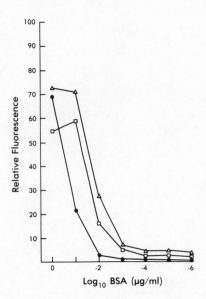

Fig. 3:   Detection of anti-BSA by fluorimetric ELISA. BSA was coated
           for two days at 4°C. The fluorimetric ELISA procedure used
           10^{-2} anti-BSA (2.5 mg/ml) and 1/200 GaRIgG-BG; substrate was
           incubated for one hour at 23°C (●). BSA was also coated for
           three hours at 37°C followed by 4°C overnight. Substrate in-
           cubation times of 24 hrs (□) and 48 hrs (△) were employed.
           The relative fluorescence of enzyme catalyzed hydrolysates
           was measured at the optimal wavelengths of excitation (384
           nm) and emission (450 nm) for 4-MU.

rabbit serum or anti-VSV, both diluted 1000-fold (Fig. 5b). The titer
of VSV in the presence of normal rabbit serum was 10^9 $TCID_{50}$/ml, and
in the presence of anti-VSV the titer was 10^3 $TCID_{50}$/ml. Thus, anti-
VSV at 10^{-3} dilution neutralized more than 99.999% of the virus.

Detection of Antibodies to Antigens in Impure Preparations

       To assess the influence that impurities might have on detection
of antibodies to scrapie-specific antigens, BSA was mixed with deter-
gent-extracted fractions prepared from hamster brain (Fig. 6). The
addition of these hamster brain impurities had two effects. First,
nonspecific binding of the GaRIgG-AP was substantially increased.
Second, as the ratio of impurities to BSA increased, there was a progressive decrease in our ability to detect anti-BSA activity. When
BSA comprised 1% of the total protein adsorbed to the solid phase,
anti-BSA was readily detected. When BSA comprised 0.1% of the total
protein, however, antiserum activity was not detectable.

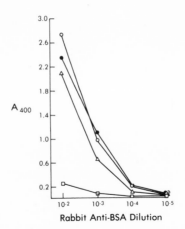

Fig. 4: Concentrations of BSA required for titration of anti-BSA in
         colorimetric ELISA. Four concentrations of BSA were coated
         in polystyrene microtiter plates for three days at 4°C: 10
         10 mg/ml (●), 100 µg/ml (O), 1 µg/ml (Δ), and 10 ng/ml (□).
         Ten-fold dilutions of anti-BSA (2.5 mg/ml) and 1:500 GaRIgG-
         AP were incubated as described in the colorimetric procedure.
         The color reactions of the enzyme catalyzed hydrolysates were
         read at 400 nm.

Detection of Antibody to the Scrapie Agent

The data obtained with BSA and VSV as model antigens (summarized
in Table 2) indicated that concentrations of 0.15 to 1.5nM antigen are
necessary for ELISA detection of specific antibodies. Antigen concentrations 10- to 100-fold higher are needed for adsorption to the solid
phase when antiserum is to be titrated. Since the hamster brain provides the highest titers of the scrapie agent (10^{10} ID_{50} units per
gram of tissue) (24), it appears to be the best available source of
scrapie antigen for detection of anti-scrapie antibody.

Although the particle-to-infectivity ratio and the macromolecular
composition of the scrapie agent are unknown, some estimates of the
amount of agent in a hamster brain can be made (25) (Table 3). Assuming a particle-to-infectivity ratio of one, 10^{10} ID_{50} units of
scrapie agent in one hamster brain corresponds to 16.7 attomoles of
agent. Assuming further that each particle contains a single copy of
a nucleic acid genome with a molecular weight of 150,000 (26), one
brain will contain approximately 2.5 ng of the putative genome. Each
hamster brain weighs approximately 1 g and contains 3 mg of nucleic
acid. Thus, the purification of the putative scrapie genome will require a 10^6-fold enrichment to achieve homogeneity. A genome of this
size could code for a protein of 15,000 MW. Considerable evidence

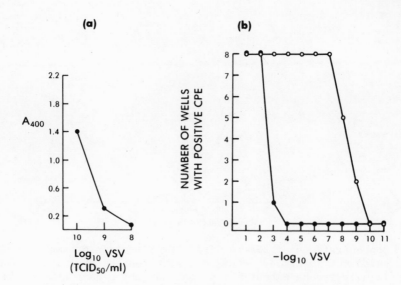

Fig. 5: Quantitative requirement for VSV coating in ELISA and neu-
         tralization of VSV. a. ten-fold dilutions of purified VSV
         were adsorbed to polystyrene microtiter wells for three days
         at 4°C. Then, 10^{-3} anti-VSV was tested in colorimetric ELISA.
         The color reactions of enzyme catalyzed hydrolysates were
         read at 400 nm. b. Serial ten-fold dilutions of VSV from
         infected cell culture supernatant were added with 10^{-3} normal
         rabbit serum (0) or 10^{-3} anti-VSV (●) to vero cells and cul-
         tured for 48 hours at 37°C with 5% CO_2. The number of wells,
         in eight, showing positive CPE was recorded.

suggests that the scrapie agent does contain a hydrophobic protein
which is required for maintenance of infectivity (12,17). With one
copy of this protein per agent as a minimal estimate, there would be
0.25 ng in each hamster brain. Since one brain contains 100 mg of
total protein, a 10^8-fold enrichment would be required for purification of this scrapie protein to homogeneity.

    These estimates are important with respect to the degree of
scrapie agent purification and concentration required for ELISA. Experiments with BSA and brain fraction mixtures indicate that antibody
could be detected if a given antigen represents more than 0.1% of the
total protein (Fig. 6). If the putative scrapie protein is the antigen, the particle-to-infectivity ratio is one, only one copy of protein exists per particle, and the yield of scrapie agent is 10%, then

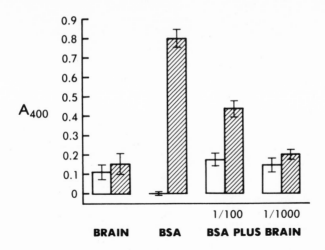

Fig. 6:   Detection of antibodies to impure antigens by ELISA. PBS-
          Tween 20 buffer (open bars) or a 1:500 dilution of anti-BSA
          (shaded bars) was incubated with the following antigens, ad-
          sorbed to polystyrene wells: detergent-extracted, normal
          hamster brain antigens (100 μg/ml); BSA (0.1 μg/ml); BSA
          mixed 1:100 with the brain antigens (1 μg BSA plus 100 μg
          brain protein/ml); BSA mixed 1:1000 with the brain antigens
          (0.1 μg BSA plus 100 μg brain protein/ml). Then all wells
          were incubated with a 1:500 dilution of GaRIgG-AP. The color
          reaction of enzyme catalyzed hydrolysates was read at 400 nm.

at least a 10^6-fold purification of antigen will be needed for detection of anti-scrapie antibody. The assumptions for the particle-to-infectivity ratio, the genomic size, and the copies of putative protein
per particle are the most conservative estimates that can be made. If
any one of these is greater than the minimal estimates, then the purification factor will be reduced accordingly. For example, many animal
viruses have particle-to-infectivity ratios of 1000 (27). If this is
the case for the scrapie agent, then the degree of antigen purification

Table 2. Quantitative Antigen Requirements in ELISA

	BSA	VSV
Concentration of antigen for detection of antibody	10 ng/ml 0.15nM	10^9 TCID$_{50}$/ml
Concentration of antigen for titration of antibody	1 μg/ml 15.0nM	10^{10} TCID$_{50}$/ml —

Table 3.   Estimates of Putative Scrapie Antigens for Antibody De-
           tection by ELISA

	Particle-to-infectivity ratios		
	10^0	10^2	10^4
	ng of antigen/brain[2]		
Nucleic acid (150,000 MW)[1]	2.5	250	25,000
Protein (15,000 MW)[1]	0.25	25	2,500
	Degree of antigen purification[3]		
Detection of antibody by ELISA	10^6	10^4	10^2

[1]Assuming a genome MW of 150,000 which codes for a 15,000 MW protein.

[2]Each hamster brain weighs approximately 1 g. Homogenates are typi-
cally 10% (w/v).

[3]Assuming a 10% recovery of the agent during purification, the scrapie
antigen is the putative protein, and one copy of the protein is present per agent particle.

needed for antibody detection by ELISA will be reduced from 10^6- to
10^3-fold.

     Preliminary ELISA studies with the scrapie agent have been con-
ducted with deoxycholate-extracted fractions ("P_3") of infected and
uninfected hamster brains as antigen. These antigens were reacted
with rabbit antisera which were absorbed with glutaraldehyde cross-
linked normal hamster brain homogenate. In several experiments, anti-
scrapie sera have yielded greater reactions with scrapie antigen than
with control antigen. These results, however, have not been reproduced
consistently. An equal number of experiments have given opposite results. The differences appear to be related to the background reactivity of GaRIgG-AP with scrapie-infected and uninfected brain antigens, which fluctuates with each batch of antigen. Thus we are faced
with two possible explanations: 1. anti-scrapie antibodies were not
produced; or 2. antigen concentrations were below the critical limit
required for antibody detection. While the "P_3" fraction represents
approximately a 10-fold purification of the scrapie agent, more recent
preparations are enriched 100- to 1000-fold with respect to protein
and DNA. As purification procedures improve, detection of scrapie-
specific antibodies will become more likely.

ACKNOWLEDGMENTS

     This work was supported in part by research grants from the Na-
tional Science Foundation (PCM 7724076) and the National Institutes

of Health (NS 14069 and HD 03939). K.C. Kasper was supported by a Public Health Service training grant on aging (AG 00047). The authors thank Mss. C. Boghosian and L. Gallagher for preparation of the manuscript.

REFERENCES

1.   Pattison, I.H. et al. Res Vet Sci 5 (1964) 116.
2.   Clarke, M.C.; Haig, D.A. Vet Rec 78 (1966) 647.
3.   Gibbs, C.J., Jr. et al. NINDB Monograph No. 2, Slow, Latent, and Temperate Virus Infections. (1965) 195.
4.   Gibbs, C.J., Jr. Curr Top Microbiol Immunol 40 (1967) 44.
5.   Gardash'yan, A.M. et al. Bull Exp Biol Med 6 (1971) 67.
6.   Porter, D.D. et al. J Immunol 111 (1973) 1407.
7.   Chandler, R.L. Vet Rec 71 (1959) 58.
8.   Moulton, J.E.; Palmer, A.C. Cornell Vet 49 (1959) 349.
9.   Gardiner, A.C. Res Vet Sci 7 (1965) 190.
10. Cunnington, P.G. et al. IRCS Medical Science; Biochemistry; Cell and Membrane Biology; Immunology and Allergy; Microbiology, Parasitology and Infectious Diseases 4 (1976) 250.
11. Stites, D.P. et al. In: Slow Transmissible Diseases of the Nervous System, ed. Prusiner and Hadlow, Vol. 2. Academic Press, New York (1979) 211.
12. Prusiner, S.B. et al. Biochemistry 17 (1978) 4993.
13. Gajdusek, C. Curr Top Microbiol Immunol 40 (1967) 59.
14. Garfin, D.E. et al. J Immunol 120 (1978) 1986.
15. Garfin, D.E. et al. J Inf Dis 138 (1978) 396.
16. Prusiner, S.B. et al. This volume.
17. Prusiner, S.B. et al. Proc Natl Acad Sci USA 77 (1980) 2984.
18. Engvall, E. Med Biol 55 (1977) 193.
19. Schuurs, A.H.W.M.; Van Weeman, B.K. Clin Chim Acta 81 (1977) 1.
20. Voller, A. et al. Bull WHO 53 (1976) 55.
21. Widsom, G.B. Clin Chem 22 (1976) 1243.
22. O'Sullivan, M.J. et al. Ann Clin Biochem 16 (1979) 221.
23. Kato, K. et al. Lancet i (1977) 40.
24. Kimberlin, R.; Walker, C. J Gen Virol 34 (1977) 295.
25. Masiraz, F.R. et al. In: Search for the Cause of Multiple Sclerosis and Other Chronic Diseases of the Central Nervous System. First International Symposium of the Hertie Foundation, ed. Boese. Verlag Chemie, Weinheim, Frankfurt (1980) 321.
26. Latarjet, R. In: Slow Transmissible Diseases of the Nervous System, ed. Prusiner and Hadlow, Vol. 2. Academic Press, New York (1979) 387.
27. Wildy, P.; Watson, D.H. Cold Spring Harbor Symp Quant Biol 27 (1962) 25.

SECTION VIII

VIRAL ONCOGENESIS AND IMMUNE RESPONSES

Chairperson:

William R. Duncan

AN IMMUNE- AND HORMONE-DEPENDENT PHASE DURING THE LATENCY PERIOD OF

SV40 ONCOGENESIS IN SYRIAN HAMSTERS

Sachi Ohtaki

Department of Pathology, National Institute of Health,
Japan, Gakuen 4-7-1, Musashi-Murayama, Tokyo, 190-12,
Japan

INTRODUCTION

SV40 oncogenesis in hamsters requires a latency period ranging
from three to more than 12 months. Hamsters neonatally inoculated with
SV40 do not develop tumors until much later, as adults, but then the
incidence of tumor-bearing hamsters is very high (1). During this latency period, the hamsters appear to be immunologically neutral to
SV40 or SV40-TSTA; they are neither tolerant nor resistant, and tumor
induction can be prevented by specific immunization with the virus or
the tumor cells up until a few weeks before the tumor becomes palpable
(2,3).

Since the hamsters become immunocompetent long before the manifestation of palpable tumors, i.e., during the latency period, the
question arises as to whether tumor cells exist during this period.
There are two possible answers. It is possible that the cells with
the SV40 genome integrated have not yet completed their neoplastic conversion; or that potentially neoplastic cells, if present, cannot proliferate under certain circumstances. Several efforts have been made
to elucidate the conditions under which TSTA-bearing SV40 tumor cells
can survive and then grow in the host (4-11). Explanations based on
in vitro experiments with tumor cells, however, are restricted to the
last stage of tumorigenesis. In vivo experiments on SV40 oncogenesis,
on the other hand, facilitate study of the primary or true oncogenic
process during the lengthy latency period, as events other than the
cell transformation observed in vitro may be involved.

MATERIALS AND METHODS

Strain VA-777 of the SV40 virus was grown in primary green monkey kidney cell cultures and had a titer of 2.4 x 10^8 PFU/ml.

Random-bred Syrian golden hamsters were used. Pregnant females
in the terminal week of gestation were received from a closed colony
whenever they were needed, and their offspring of both sexes were
used. Every experimental group was composed of littermate hamsters.

Each animal was inoculated with 4.8 x 10^7 PFU of the virus in
0.2 ml of PBS in the subcutis of the right flank within three days
after birth. Adult animals were inoculated in the same manner with
4.8 x 10^8 PFU of the virus in 2 ml of PBS. Animals were observed
weekly for tumor development for more than one year. Mean latency
period and S.D. were calculated on each group. Significance of deviation from the control was estimated by means of Student's t test.

Viable SV40 tumor cells obtained from tumor-bearing hamsters were
inoculated SC into the backs of hamsters. In each experiment, tumor
growth was observed daily until any one of the animals became moribund
from overgrowth of the tumor mass, and all animals in the experiment
were killed at that time. Mean tumor weight and S.D. in each group
were calculated, and significance of deviation from the control was
estimated by Student's t test.

Thymectomy or gonadectomy was carried out under sodium pento-
barbital anesthesia. A few animals with incomplete thymectomy, determined at autopsy by histology, were discarded.

Anti-thymocyte and anti-spleen cell sera were prepared from rabbits. About 15 x 10^8 thymus or spleen cells from young hamsters were
injected SC into three rabbits with incomplete Freund's adjuvant.
After nine and 24 days, the rabbits received IV about 2 x 10^8 thymus
or spleen cells per animal per day without the adjuvant. One week
later, rabbits were bled. The globulin fraction was obtained by ammonium sulfate precipitation and diluted to the original serum volume.
Agglutinating capacity against respective target cells was about
1:1024. Weanling hamsters were given three SC doses of either globulin (0.5, 0.25, and 0.25 ml per animal) every other day. For adults,
these doses were doubled to 1.0, 0.5 and 0.5 ml, respectively.

Cyclophosphamide (CY) as an immunosuppressant was administered
in an IP dose of 125 mg/kg body weight. A 0.85% NaCl solution of cortisone acetate was given in a SC dose of 125 mg/kg for hamsters of
single-dose groups and in a SC dose of 2.5 mg per animal (about 25
mg/kg) for those of weekly dosage groups.

Testosterone propionate and estrone were dissolved in warmed
sesame oil for SC injection. The dose was 0.2 or 0.3 mg per animal
in 0.1 ml to newborn hamsters and 0.5 mg per animal to adults.

RESULTS AND DISCUSSION

Immunosuppression During the Latency Period

Only tumor cells which can evade the host's immunological surveillance system are believed to be able to proliferate. Most attempts
in which immunosuppression was induced during viral oncogenesis in
order to enhance tumor induction in animals naturally resistant to the
respective viruses have been successful (12-20). Immunosuppression
resulted in a high incidence or progressive growth of tumors which,
without immunosuppression, were either rare or regressed.

The present system, in which hamsters of both sexes were neonatally inoculated with SV40, manifested a high incidence of vigorous
tumor growth in the absence of host immunosuppression. The present

Table 1. Effects of Immunosuppression at the Different Phases of
          SV40 Oncogenesis

Treatment	Host animals Sex / Age	Effects on		
		SV 40-induced tumorigenesis treated at 0.2.4.6[2]	12-15	Growth of SV40 tumors[1] grafted to animals at 25-30[3] weeks old
Thymectomy	Male	↓	↓	↑*
	Female	↓*	↓**	↑
ATG	Male	↓·	↓·	N.T.
	Female	↓**	↓**	N.T.
ASPG	Male	↓*	↓	N.T.
	Female	↓	↓**	N.T.
Cyclophos-phamide	Male	↓	↓	N.T.
	Female	↓	↓**	N.T.
Cortisone	Male	↓	↓**·	↑
	Female	↓**	↓**	↑↑↑

[1]Same sex donor-recipient system.

[2]Up to 4 weeks of age, hamsters may be immature sexually.

[3]At this age, the virus-induced tumors developed most frequently.

[4] —, no effect; ↑, accelerated; ↓, suppressed; **, P < 0.02;
   *, P < 0.05; ·, prominent decrease of tumor incidence; NT, not
   tested.

experiments were carried out to determine whether immunosuppression of hamsters shortens the latency period of SV40 tumor induction and to gain some information on the characteristics of the cells during the latency period. These hamsters therefore were thymectomized, or treated with anti-lymphocyte sera, cyclophosphamide, or cortisone acetate during the latency period.

We obtained unexpected results; in all immunosuppressant-treated hamsters, the development of SV40 tumors was delayed and their incidence was decreased (Table 1). This is a new, remarkable finding; since the SV40 tumor is a fibrosarcoma, neither lymphoma nor leukemia, the oncogenic process during the latency stage should be immunodependent. Circumstantial evidence for this view is provided if the suppressive effect is not random but rather manifests some features or patterns characteristic for different experimental procedures.

We found that thymectomy of the host animals, irrespective of their sex, resulted in a similar delay and decrease of SV40 tumorigenesis, especially when thymectomy was performed in older animals (Fig. 1a,b). Administration of anti-thymocyte globulin (ATG), which affects thymus-derived peripheral lymphocytes the most, exhibited different suppressive effects depending on the sex of the animals. In males, ATG treatment reduced the tumor incidence (Fig. 2a), while in females it only delayed tumor development markedly (Fig. 2b). Thymectomy and ATG administration may abrogate T cells specifically and sometimes resulted in a somewhat decreased tumor incidence. On the other hand, the administration of anti-spleen cell globulin (ASPG), which affects various lymphocyte subpopulations, manifested an effect different from ATG and similar to that of cyclophosphamide (CY). ASPG and CY treatment did not decrease the tumor incidence and prolonged the latency period similarly. For example, in hamsters treated with ASPG or CY in the fifth week, the delay of tumorigenesis seemed to be about the same in both sexes; however, when the animals were treated after having reached adulthood, the delay was less pronounced in males and more pronounced in females as compared to the groups treated at 5 weeks of age (Fig. 3a,b; 4a,b). The similarity in the effects of ASPG and CY is explicable if they both affect common target cells, i.e., B lymphocytes, and suggests that the oncogenic process was only temporarily inhibited by their actions. Cortisone acetate, which drastically affects many lymphocyte subpopulations, suppressed SV40 tumorigenesis most markedly. There were two groups which were almost tumor-free; one consisted of male hamsters treated with a single dose at adult age, the other, of females treated with weekly doses starting at the age of 3 weeks (Fig. 5a,b,; 6a,b). Although these observations suggest that one of the important factors in tumor induction may be cortisone sensitivity, cortisone-treated hamsters exhibited the wasting syndrome and the mortality rate was so high as to preclude firm conclusions regarding the effect of cortisone acetate.

A common feature of the effects of immunosuppression was that the intensity of suppression was affected by the sex of the host and age

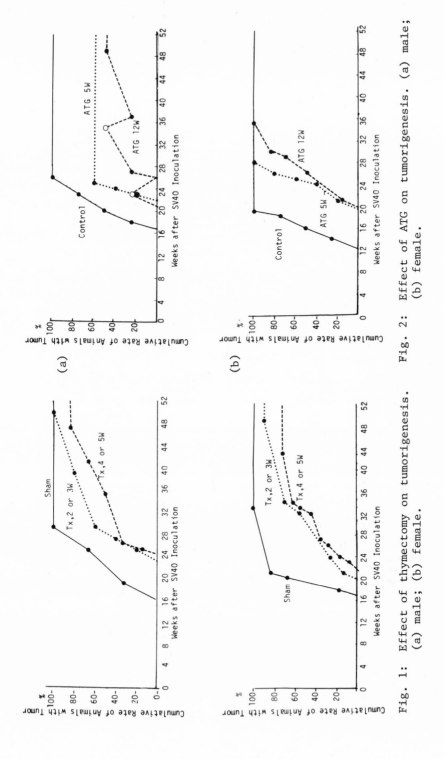

Fig. 1: Effect of thymectomy on tumorigenesis. (a) male; (b) female.

Fig. 2: Effect of ATG on tumorigenesis. (a) male; (b) female.

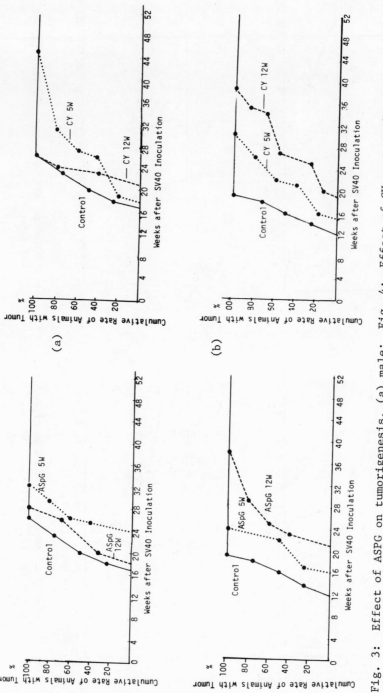

Fig. 3: Effect of ASPG on tumorigenesis. (a) male;
(b) female.

Fig. 4: Effect of CY on tumorigenesis. (a) male;
(b) female.

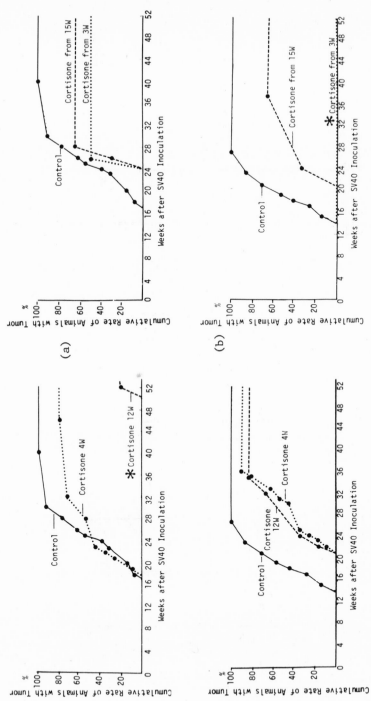

Fig. 6: Effect of cortisone acetate on tumorigenesis; weekly doses starting at 3
weeks. (a) male; (b) female.

Fig. 5: Effect of cortisone acetate on
tumorigenesis, single dose.
(a) male; (b) female.

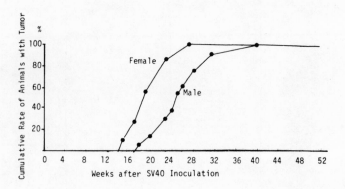

Fig. 7:   Comparison of SV40 induced tumor appearance in male and female hamsters.

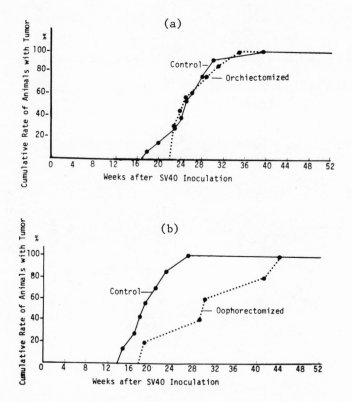

Fig. 8:   Effect of gonadectomy on tumorigenesis. (a) male; (b) female.

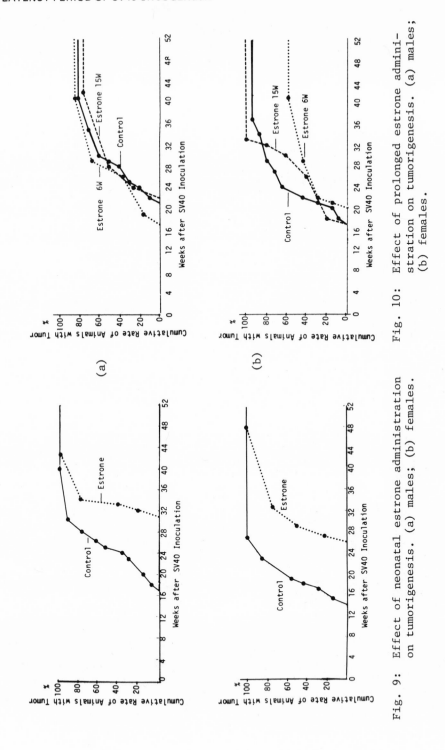

Fig. 10: Effect of prolonged estrone administration on tumorigenesis. (a) males; (b) females.

Fig. 9: Effect of neonatal estrone administration on tumorigenesis. (a) males; (b) females.

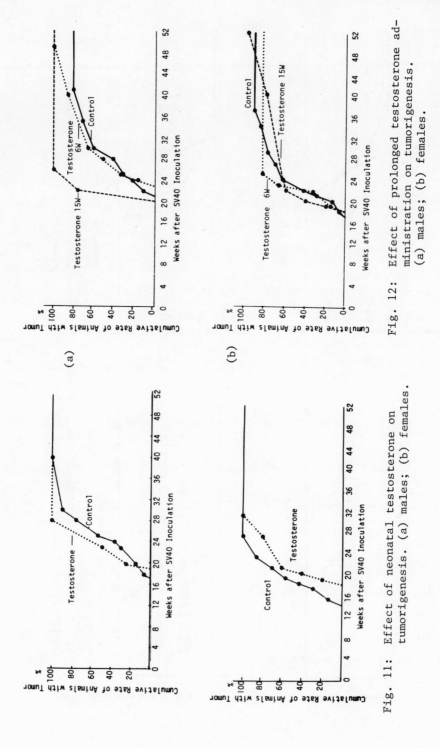

Fig. 11: Effect of neonatal testosterone on tumorigenesis. (a) males; (b) females.

Fig. 12: Effect of prolonged testosterone administration on tumorigenesis. (a) males; (b) females.

at treatment. In female hamsters, tumorigenesis was more sensitive to, to, and more readily delayed by, these treatments. These observations suggest a hormonal regulation of tumorigenesis.

Hormonal Modification Induced During the Latency Period

Our study revealed that under identical experimental conditions, SV40 tumors always developed earlier in female than in male hamsters (Fig. 7), suggesting the participation of a sex factor in the tumor-induction mechanism(s). This sex difference could be changed by altering the hormonal milieu of the host animals. Sexually-matured hamsters that had been neonatally inoculated with SV40 were gonadectomized; while orchiectomy had little effect on tumor development (Fig. 8a), oophorectomy markedly delayed development (Fig. 8b), resulting in a reversed sex difference. This evidence indicates the involvement of female gonads in oncogenesis.

To obtain more direct proof for this hypothesis, estrone and testosterone were administered during the latency period. The neonatal administration of estrone resulted in a marked prolongation of the latency period in hamsters of both sexes (Fig. 9a,b). Furthermore, the latency period was prolonged in females that were estrone-treated at a later stage (Fig. 10a,b). Although testosterone, administered neonatally, somewhat prolonged the latency period in female and shortened it in male hamsters (Fig. 11a,b), its administration to adult animals accelerated tumor development only in males (Fig. 12a,b). These findings indicated that the effect of these sex hormones was in

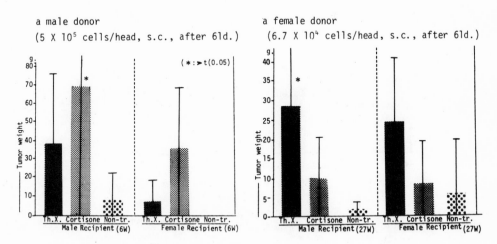

Fig. 13:   Effect of thymectomy or cortisone acetate on rate of SV40 tumor growth.

Table 2. Effects of Hormonal Modifications at the Different Phases
of SV40 Oncogenesis

	Host animals	SV40-induced tumor-	Growth of SV40 tumors[1]
		igenesis treated at	grafted to animals at
Treatment	Sex / Age	0.2.4.6[2].....12-15	.........25-30[3] weeks old
Gonadectomy	Male	— —	↑
	Female	↓** ↓**	↑*
Estrone	Male	↓** — —	↑
	Female	↓** ↓* ↓	(↑)
Testosterone	Male	↑ ↑ ↑(*)	↓
	Female	↓ — —	↓

[1]The same sex donor-recipient system.

[2]Up to 4 weeks of age, host animals may be immature sexually.

[3]At this age, the virus-induced tumors developed most frequently.

[4] ——, no effect; ↑, accelerated; ↓, suppressed; **, P < 0.02;
*, P < 0.05; ( ), speculative effect.

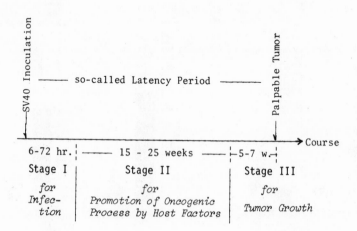

Fig. 14: Proposed stages of oncogenesis.

the reverse direction and was dependent, respectively, on the sex and age of the treated animals. These results are explicable if each of these hormones exerts a specific action; the time required for tumor induction may depend on the hormonal milieu of the hosts. Female sex hormone(s) appear to play a greater role in regulating this milieu, since our data indicate that estrone exerted a far greater effect than testosterone.

The suppressive effect of cortisone acetate, a steroid hormone similar to sex hormones, on SV40 tumor induction may be antagonistic to testosterone and synergistic with estrone, as suggested by our data regarding the host age and sex dependence of the effects of estrone, testosterone, and cortisone acetate. For a precise evaluation of the role of hormonal regulation in oncogenesis, however, further studies are required. As for an underlying physiological condition, we had reported conspicuous sex difference in zona regicularis of the adrenal cortex of hamsters used in this study (21).

Three Proposed Stages in SV40-Induced Oncogenesis

The interesting results we presented so far were on neonatally SV40-inoculated hamsters that had been treated as described in the early or middle, but not in the late stages of latency. Identical immunosuppression or hormonal modification, however, produced effects opposite from those already described, when induced during the course of grafted SV40 tumor cell growth, which may represent the final stage of SV40 oncogenesis. In immunosuppression experiments, for example, thymectomy or weekly administration of cortisone acetate to tumor cell-graft recipients resulted in enhanced tumor growth, irrespective of the sex of the cell donor or recipient hamsters (Fig. 13). These results coincide with previous reports (22-25) and with what is generally known about SV40 tumor immunity (26-31). Furthermore, the effects of the hormonal modifications were different with respect to SV40 tumor induction and tumor growth. Gonadectomy of the graft recipients, irrespective of their sex, enhanced tumor growth. The administration of estrone or testosterone had only slight effects, if any, on tumor growth in graft recipients; the former sex hormone stimulated, while the latter inhibited, tumor growth somewhat (Table 2).

These different, almost opposite effects of identical experimental treatments in two oncogenic phases, i.e., during neoplastic conversion and tumor cell growth, may be indicative of the operation of two mechanisms which may become distinct in the absence of any mature neoplastic cells during the latency period. Some weeks, however, are required for the nodule, which derived from one neoplastically converted cell, to become palpable, and this time span must be subtracted from the latency period (Fig. 14). After infection with SV40, therefore, tumorigenesis can be construed to occur in two different phases. We propose that the greatest proportion of the latency period of SV40

Table 3. SV40 Oncogenesis in Adult Hamsters Immunosuppressed at the
          Time of Virus Inoculation

Treated with	Sex of animals	Mortality	Incidence of tumors	Latent period (weeks) (mean ± S.D.)
—	Male	2/5	0/3	
ATG	"	3/5	2/2	34 ± 7.07 (n.s.)
ASPG	"	2/5	0/3	
ATG	"	0/10	1/10	31 ± 0 (")
ASPG	"	1/10	0/9	
CY	"	0/10	0/10	

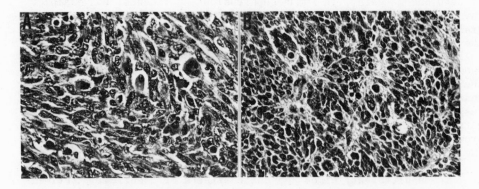

Fig. 15. Microscopic morphology of hamster subcutaneous tumors in-
          duced by SV40 (A; more matured fibrosarcoma) and those in-
          duced by adenovirus-12 (B; rather embryonic undifferen-
          tiated sarcoma) (HxE, same magnification)

oncogenesis is comprised of a specialized stage during which neoplastic conversion is promoted and that this promotion is aided by biological activities taking place in the host animal, e.g., immune and hormonal functions.

The virus infection stage, as well as the tumor growth stage, may not require, but rather elude, these biological activities, especially the function of the lymphoid organs. The reduced immunocompetence of newborn hamsters may contribute significantly to their susceptibility to SV40 virus infection and may be due primarily to insufficient T-cell function. This suggestion is supported by our observation that a few doses of ATG, but not ASPG or CY, administered at the same time as virus inoculation resulted in a high incidence of tumors in adult hamsters (Table 3).

Between the infection and the tumor growth stages, both of which take place in opposition to the host defense, an immune- and hormone-dependent stage intervenes in the prolonged latency period of SV40 oncogenesis. We may be the first workers to characterize this second stage as a phase with a specialized role in SV40 oncogenesis (1).

On the other hand, in hamsters, the oncogenesis of another primate DNA tumor virus, adenovirus 12, may have a negligible second stage. The time required for tumor induction with adenovirus 12 is comparable to the lag time between the grafting of a few of these cells and the manifestation of a palpable nodule. Furthermore, a marked enhancement of tumorigenesis has been reported in hamsters thymectomized at the age of 3 weeks or treated weekly with cortisone acetate (19,20). The neoplastic cell conversion induced by this virus may be completed immediately after virus inoculation so that subsequent immunosuppression may enhance the proliferation of already transformed tumor cells, as is the case in tumor grafts.

When considering tumor etiology, especially in humans, one must take into account several possibilities with respect to the oncogenic process, even if the tumors are induced by certain viruses. The hamster-SV40 system may involve physiologic functions in which the host acts as a tumor promoter. This system may represent an excellent animal model for human cancer of the adult type, because in contrast to the rather infantile morphology of adenovirus 12-induced tumors, the morphology of SV40 tumors is of a more mature type (Fig. 15).

REFERENCES

1.   Ohtaki, S. Cancer Res 38 (1978) 4698.
2.   Deichman, G.I.; Kluchareva, T.E. Virology 24 (1964) 131.
3.   Deichman, G.I. Adv Cancer Res 12 (1969) 101.
4.   Lausch, R.N. et al. J Immunol 115 (1975) 682.
5.   Prather, S.O.; Lausch, R.N. Int J Cancer 17 (1976) 380.

6.   Prather, S.O.; Lausch, R.N.   J Immunol 118 (1977) 203.
7.   Glaser, M.   J Exp Med 149 (1979) 774.
8.   Gooding, L.R.   J Immunol 122 (1979) 2328.
9.   Heimer, R.; de Vaux St. Cyr, C.   Cancer Res 39 (1979) 2919.
10.   Volpe, E.A.   Neoplasma 23 (1976) 345.
11.   Volpe, E.A.   Experimentia 34 (1978) 113.
12.   Allison, A.C. et al.   Nature 215 (1967) 185.
13.   Allison, A.C.; Law, L.W.   Proc Soc Exp Biol Med 127 (1968) 207.
14.   Allison, A.C.; Taylor, R.B.   Cancer Res 27 (1967) 703.
15.   Larson, V.M. et al.   Proc Soc Exp Biol Med 136 (1971) 1304.
16.   Law, L.W.   Cancer Res 26 (1966) 551.
17.   Law, L.W.   Fed Proc 29 (1970) 171.
18.   Miller, J.F.A.P. et al.   Proc Soc Exp Biol Med 116 (1964) 323.
19.   Yohn, D.S. et al.   J Natl Cancer Inst 35 (1965) 617.
20.   Yohn, D.S. et al.   J Immunol 100 (1967) 771.
21.   Ohtaki, S.   Lab Anim Sci 29 (1979) 765.
22.   Ting, R.C.   Nature 211 (1966) 1000.
23.   Girardi, A.J.; Roosa, R.A.   J Immunol 99 (1967) 1217.
24.   Tevethia, S.S. et al.   J Immunol 101 (1968) 1105.
25.   Wright, P.W. et al.   J Natl Cancer Inst 51 (1973) 951.
26.   Tevethia, S.S. et al.   J Immunol 113 (1974) 1417.
27.   Blasecki, J.W.; Tevethia, S.S.   J Immunol 114 (1975) 244.
28.   Gooding, L.R.   J Immunol 118 (1977) 920.
29.   Trinchieri, G. et al.   Nature 261 (1976) 312.
30.   Knowles, B.B. et al.   J Immunol 122 (1979) 1798.
31.   Coggin, J.H.   Cancer Res 39 (1979) 2952.

THE IMPLICATIONS OF THE DIFFERENT TUMOR-INDUCING CAPACITIES OF ADENO-VIRUS 2 AND SV40 TRANSFORMED HAMSTER CELLS

Andrew M. Lewis, Jr., James L. Cook, C.H. Kirkpatrick and A.S. Rabson

National Institute of Allergy and Infectious Diseases, and the National Cancer Institute, National Institutes of Health, Bethesda, MD   20205

INTRODUCTION

Many reports have documented the lack of association between cell transformation in vitro and tumor induction in vivo by tumor viruses. It has also been established that cells transformed in tissue culture by many viruses are not oncogenic when inoculated into syngeneic hosts. The reasons for this lack of association are poorly understood. By comparing the tumor-inducing properties of adenovirus type 2 (Ad2) and SV40 transformed cells, we have developed data that offer a possible explanation for the discrepancy between in vivo and in vitro oncogenicity of tumor viruses and the cells they transform in tissue culture.

Based on studies in Syrian hamsters, Ad2 has been classified as nononcogenic. In spite of its lack of oncogenicity in vivo, Ad2 can transform cells from hamsters and rats in tissue culture (1). Rat cells transformed by Ad2 do not produce tumors in immunocompetent rats (2). During a preliminary study of the tumor-inducing capacity of Ad2 transformed inbred hamster embryo cells, we noted that most cell lines would produce tumors when inoculated into newborn syngeneic hamsters but were not oncogenic when inoculated into adults. Ad2 transformed cell-induced tumors (Ad2 transformed-cell tumors) carried by serial passage in newborn syngeneic hamsters produced small tumors that usually regressed when transplanted to adults. SV40, in contrast to Ad2, is known to be highly oncogenic for hamsters, and SV40 transformed inbred hamster embryo cell lines established from our transformation assays produced tumors in both newborn and adult hamsters. SV40 transformed-cell tumors carried by serial passage in syngeneic newborn hamsters consistently produced fatal neoplasms when transplanted to adults. Studies in thymectomized hamsters and hamsters at various

433

stages of maturation indicated that the regression of Ad2 transformed-cell tumors in adults was related to the maturation of the cellular immune response.

The purpose of this report is to summarize the findings that imply that the rejection of Ad2 transformed hamster embryo cells and transformed-cell tumors is a thymus-dependent cellular immune response, and to demonstrate that SV40 transformed LSH embryo cells and transformed-cell tumors (but not Ad2 transformed cells or transformed-cell tumors) are resistant to cellular immune rejection when transplanted to allogeneic CB hamsters.

MATERIALS AND METHODS

The laboratory and field strains of Ad2 used in these studies were propagated in human embryonic kidney cells (3). SV40 strains 776 and 777 were grown by low multiplicity infections in BSC-1 cells (3,4). Primary or secondary cultures of LSH hamster embryo cells (prepared from whole embryos after 14 days of gestation) were transformed with UV light-inactivated Ad2 and SV40 strain 777 under agar overlayers. Transformation assays using SV40 strain 776 were performed in bottle cultures using infectious inocula and liquid media (4). Well-separated foci developing under agar overlayers or in separate bottle cultures were gathered with Pasteur pipettes 8 to 12 weeks after infection and established as lines of transformed cells. All of the transformed lines contained serologically detectable, virus-specific T antigens. Each line was tested extensively for contaminating agents and none were found (3). A study of five lines transformed by Ad2 indicated that each line was produced by a different transformation event (5).

The LSH and CB strains of inbred Syrian hamsters were obtained from the Charles River-Lakeview colonies. These strains have been inbred for more than 50 brother-sister matings and differ by at least one strong histocompatibility locus as indicated by skin graft rejection, graft-versus-host reaction and mixed lymphocyte culture (6,7). Animals were classified as newborns during the first 96 hours of life and as adults after 4 weeks old. To study the tumor-inducing properties of cells transformed in vitro, 0.2 ml of suspensions, containing different cell concentrations (ranging from 10^8 to 10^2 cells/ml), were inoculated subcutaneously (SC) between the scapulae. Standard tumor suspensions were prepared by sieving whole tumors through 60-mesh wire screens and resuspending packed tumor cells in twice their volume. For serial passages, 0.2-ml aliquots of the tumor suspensions were inoculated SC between the scapulae. To determine the tumor-inducing efficiency of standard tumor suspensions, each suspension was serially diluted and 0.2 ml of each dilution was injected SC into one or two litters of newborn or four to five adult hamsters. Inoculated hamsters

were observed for 10 to 12 weeks for tumor development. The 50% endpoints of tumor production (TPD_{50}) were calculated by the Kärber
method (8).

Adult LSH hamsters thymectomized within 24 hours of birth were
obtained from the Lakeview colony.

The techniques for stimulating blood or spleen lymphocytes with
concanavalin A (Con A) either alone or mixed with adherent or non-
adherent populations of adult hamster peritoneal exudate cells have
been described in detail elsewhere (9,10).

RESULTS AND DISCUSSION

To study the tumor-inducing properties of Ad2 and SV40 transformed inbred hamster cells, 15 clonal lines of Ad2 transformed LSH
embryo cells and six lines of SV40 transformed LSH embryo cells were
derived from transformed foci. Each hamster embryo (HE) line was designated by the transforming virus preceding a consecutive numerical
designation (i.e., Ad2HE1 or SV40HE1). The tumor-inducing capacity
of each line was assayed at one or more tissue culture passage levels
by SC injection of 10^8 or 10^7 cells in newborn and adult LSH hamsters.
Thirteen of 15 Ad2 transformed cell lines induced tumors in 8% to 100%
of newborns, while none of six lines tested between tissue culture passages 5 and 71 produced tumors in adults (Table 1). At a cell concentration of 10^7, all of the SV40 lines tested produced tumors in 100%
of the inoculated animals.

Ad2 transformed-cell tumors were transplanted successfully to
100% of newborn LSH hamsters; these same newborn tumors, however,
transplanted to only 11% of adult LSH hamsters (Table 2). SV40 transformed-cell tumors transplanted to 100% of both newborn and adult LSH
animals.

Table 1. Tumor Development in LSH Hamsters Inoculated with LSH Ham-
          ster Embryo Cells Transformed In Vitro by Ad2 and SV40

Cells transformed by	No. oncogenic lines/no. lines tested in (range of tumor incidence)	
	Newborns	Adults
Ad2	13/15 (8%-100%)	0/6 (0%)
SV40	4/4 (100%)	6/6 (100%)

Other studies showed that the number of TPD_{50}'s in suspensions of four Ad2 newborn tumors ($10^{3.1}$ to $10^{4.7}$ $TPD_{50}/0.2$ ml) was similar to the number of TPD_{50}'s in suspensions of two SV40 tumors ($10^{3.9}$ and $10^{4.8}$ $TPD_{50}/0.2$ml). Thus adult LSH hamsters receiving comparable doses of Ad2 and SV40 tumor suspensions could reject Ad2 tumor cells but could not reject SV40 tumor cells.

During evaluation of the tumor-inducing capacity of the Ad2 transformed-cell tumors, we observed three distinct transplantation patterns. Some newborn tumor lines caused a low incidence of tumors in adults after only a few in vivo passages, while multiple newborn passages were required before other lines were adapted to grow in adults. The Ad2HTL6 (hamster tumor line 6--induced by Ad2HE6) remained unable to produce tumors in syngeneic adult hamsters after more than 60 newborn passages. The availability of adult-adapted, Ad2 transformed-cell tumor lines and newborn tumor lines which could not be transplanted to adult hamsters provided a phenotypic diversity that could be used to evaluate the hamster's ability to reject Ad2 transformed cells and transformed-cell tumors.

Initial studies indicated that Ad2 transformed-cell newborn tumors which regressed in normal adult hamsters could be transplanted successfully to adults that had been thymectomized during the first day of life. The tumor incidence (range 28% to 76%) in thymectomized animals, however, suggested that many hamsters were not completely thymectomized. We were unable to obtain a satisfactory correlation between the presence or absence of thymic remnants by histological examination with the regression or progression of Ad2 tumors in thymectomized animals (9). As another test of the immunocompetence of adult hamsters that had been thymectomized during the first 24 hours of life, we examined the response of their blood lymphocytes to the T-cell mitogen Con A. To allow any partially thymectomized hamster time to recover its thymic function, the animals were held for more

Table 2. Transplantability of Tumors Induced by 13 Lines of Ad2
          Transformed LSH Hamster Embryo Cells and Two Lines of SV40
          Transformed LSH Hamster Embryo Cells to Syngeneic Hamsters

Transformed-cell tumor	Tumor lines established in		Transplantation results No. with tumors/no. surviving (percent) in	
	Newborns	Adults	Newborns	Adults
Ad2	+		397/397 (100%)	27/257 (11%)
SV40	+		130/130 (100%)	10/10 (100%)
SV40		+		100/100 (100%)

than 80 days. Heparinized whole blood taken from these hamsters was cultured in the presence of 10 μg of Con A/ml. One week later, the animals were challenged with Ad2 transformed-cell newborn tumors that were rejected by normal adults (Table 3). The results of experiments using two different Ad2 transformed-cell newborn tumor lines indicated that blood lymphocytes from tumor-susceptible adult LSH hamsters had significantly lower stimulation indices (S.I., p = <0.001) than did tumor-resistant thymectomized or normal animals. Each of the suspensions of tumor cells used in these experiments produced tumors in 100% of newborn hamsters, while only one of 34 normal or partially thymectomized (defined as a blood lymphocyte S.I. of $\geq$ 60) inoculated with these suspensions developed a tumor. We concluded from these results that the degree of the response to Con A of blood lymphocytes from thymectomized hamsters was a good indicator of their relative T-cell deficiency following thymectomy and their susceptibility to fatal tumor development when challenged with Ad2 transformed-cell tumor lines that were rejected by normal adults. These results also demonstrated that the age-related ability of hamsters to reject Ad2 transformed cells and transformed-cell tumors was thymus dependent.

The inverse correlation between the response of the hamster's blood lymphocytes to Con A and their susceptibility to Ad2 transformed-cell neoplasms prompted us to compare tumor susceptibility with the mitogenic response of various populations of lymphocytes in hamsters of different ages (Fig. 1). Tumor transplantation experiments indicated that LSH hamsters were susceptible to challenge with Ad2 transformed-cell tumor lines during the first six days of life, but became resistant rapidly thereafter. Thymocytes from 2-day-old hamsters were as responsive to Con A as thymocytes from adults (2-day-old mean S.I. = 443.1 $\pm$ 55.5; adult mean S.I. = 326.5 $\pm$ 28.8). The hamster blood lymphocytes did not begin to respond to Con A until the animals were 4 weeks old. Lymphocytes from LSH hamster spleens began to respond to Con A after five days of life, responded to about 50% of adult levels by age 10 days, and attained adult responses between 12 and 20 days.

In preliminary experiments (10), splenic lymphocytes from 3-day-old hamsters that were unresponsive to Con A (S.I. ranging from 1.7 to 2.1) were capable of reacting with this mitogen (S.I. ranging from 31.3 to 35.9) when mixed with nylon wool-adherent fractions of X-irradiated (2500 R) adult peritoneal exudate cells (Fig. 2). Thus splenic T cells from hamsters less than 2 weeks old seem to require a population of functional accessory cells for an in vitro proliferative response to Con A.

We conclude from these studies that newborn hamsters are relatively T-cell deficient and are unable to reject Ad2 transformed cells and transformed-cell newborn tumors. As the thymus-dependent cellular immune system begins to mature during the first two weeks of life, the

Table 3. Tumor Development in Newborn, Adult and Neonatally Thymectomized Adult Hamsters that Were Rendered Either Partially or Completely T-Cell Deficient as Determined by Blood Lymphocyte Response to Con A[1]

| Transplanted newborn tumor line | Tumor incidence | | | Blood lymphocyte response to Con A (mean S.I.) | | |
| | | | | Thymectomized | | |
	Newborns	Normal or partially thymec-tomized adults	Thymec-tomized adults	Normal	Tumor resistant	Tumor susceptible
Ad2HTL3	6/6	1/13	5/18	3335[2]	701[3]	6.9[4]
Ad2HTL6	20/20	0/6	4/23			
"	17/17	0/10	10/13			
"	13/13	0/21	4/25	1907[2]	1211[3]	6.3[4]

[1]A partially thymectomized hamster was defined as a tumor-resistant adult that was thymectomized during the first 24 hours of life whose blood lymphocytes gave an S.I. of 60 or more when tested at age 84 to 103 days. One of 34 animals in this group (whose S.I. was 965 prior to challenge) developed and carried a slowly enlarging tumor for > 180 days before being killed for autopsy.

[2]Range 685–4235.

[3]Range 60–3956.

[4]Range 1.4–14.3.

neonatal animal becomes progressively resistant to challenge with
these tumor cells and is completely resistant by age 14 to 21 days.
In view of this sequence of events, we speculated that serial passage
of certain Ad2 transformed-cell tumors in newborns selected Ad2 tumor
cells that were somehow capable of resisting rejection by the cellular
immune response of the immunologically mature syngeneic hamster.

Since Ad2 transformed-cell tumors acquired resistance to rejection by the cellular immune response of adult hamsters during serial
newborn passage, it seemed logical to assume that SV40 transformed LSH
embryo cells, which would produce tumors in hamsters of any age, possessed an inherent resistance to rejection by immunocompetent hamsters.
This resistance to rejection could possibly be hamster-specific since
SV40 transformed cells from other species were usually nononcogenic
for autologous or isologous hosts. To attempt to document the extent
of the resistance of SV40 transformed LSH hamster cells to rejection
by the cellular immune system, the tumor-inducing efficiency of SV40
transformed cells and transformed-cell tumors and Ad2 transformed cells
and transformed-cell tumors was compared in syngeneic LSH and allogeneic CB hamsters (Tables 4 and 5). The results of these experiments

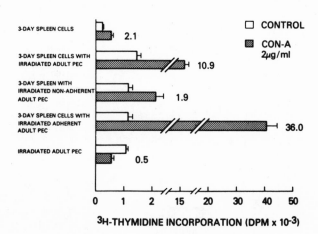

Fig. 1: Tumor susceptibility and lymphocyte responses of hamsters of
         different ages. Hamsters were observed for 10 to 12 weeks
         following SC inoculation of 0.2 ml of a standard tumor sus-
         pension of Ad2HTL6. Each Δ represents an average of 13 ani-
         mals (range 8 to 35). Lymphocyte responses (S.I.) = ratio
         of the Con A-stimulated cultures to the corresponding con-
         trols. Each ● represents the response of splenic T cells
         from five different hamsters; each o represents the response
         of lymphocytes from peripheral blood taken from five to 10
         hamsters.

indicated that SV40 transformed LSH embryo cells induced tumors with
equal efficiency in both syngeneic LSH and allogeneic CB hamsters.
For LSH hamsters, 3000 to 30,000 cells were required to produce tumors
in 50% of the animals. In CB hamsters, the number of cells per TPD_{50}
varied between 3000 and 300,000. The differences between the TPD_{50}
LSH and TPD_{50} CB for the SV40 transformed cells were not significant
(p = 0.15). In contrast, Ad2 transformed LSH cells were not oncogenic
for either LSH or CB adults. The differences between the oncogenicity
of the SV40 lines and Ad2 lines for both inbred strains were highly
significant (p = <0.01). Similarly, the tumor-inducing capacity of
suspensions of SV40 transformed-cell LSH tumors in LSH and CB adults
varied only 1- to 10-fold, differences that are not significant (p =
0.12). Adult-adapted, Ad2 transformed-cell tumors transplanted 100-
to 10,000-fold more efficiently in syngeneic LSH hamsters than in allogeneic CB hamsters; these differences were highly significant (p =
<0.01). Thus Ad2 transformed-cell tumors were recognized and rejected
as foreign grafts by allogeneic hamsters, while grafts of SV40 transformed-cell LSH tumors were accepted with almost equal efficiency by
syngeneic and allogeneic animals.

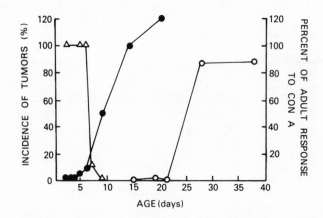

Fig. 2:   Effect of syngeneic adult peritoneal exudate cells on re-
          sponses of newborn spleen cells to Con A. Spleen cells (1
          x 10^6) from 3-day-old hamsters were cultured in 2.0 ml of
          RPMI 1640 medium (containing penicillin [250 µg/ml], 2mM
          glutamine and 5% fetal calf serum) either alone or with 2.5
          x 10^5 X-irradiated, syngeneic adult PEC's from one of three
          fractions. Control and Con A-stimulated triplicate cultures
          were incubated for 120 hours at 37°C in 5% CO_2, labeled for
          the final four hours with 2 µCi ^{3}H-thymidine and harvested
          (10).

Table 4. Tumor Induction by SV40 and Ad2 Transformed LSH Hamster
Embryo-Cells in Syngeneic LSH and Allogeneic CB Hamsters

	Tumor incidence in newborn hamsters[2]	No. cells/TPD_{50} (log_{10}) in adult hamsters	
Cell lines[1]	No with tumors/ no. surviving	LSH	CB
SV40HE1	11/20	4.2	5.0
SV40HE2	15/17	3.6	5.5
SV40HE3	20/20	3.5	3.5
SV40HE5		4.5	5.5
AD2HE1	35/54	>8.3	>8.5
AD2HE3	10/22	>8.5	>8.5
AD2HE6	19/19	>8.5	>8.5

[1]Tissue culture passages = 6 to 71.

[2]Inoculum = 10^7 cells/hamster.

The tumor-inducing capacity of SV40 appears to be restricted to
a few species (11-15). This virus, however, can transform cells from
a variety of species in tissue culture. These transformed cells are
usually not oncogenic for autologous or isologous hosts, but will form
tumors when injected into immunocompromised hosts such as nude mice
(16-25). To explain the behavior of this tumor virus, it is generally
assumed that tumor-susceptible hosts (such as hamsters) may be relatively immunoincompetent compared to tumor-resistant hosts or that
the presence of increased concentrations of virus-specific transplantation antigens on nononcogenic cells transformed by SV40 in vitro
allows them to be rejected efficiently by theoretically susceptible
syngeneic recipients. Another possible explanation of the species-
specific oncogenicity of SV40 and SV40 transformed cells is that SV40
induces, in cells of susceptible species, a unique change during transformation that renders the resulting neoplastic cells resistant to
host rejection. The studies of Duncan and Streilein (6,7) indicate
that the immunological responsiveness of hamsters is not significantly
different from other species. Furthermore, we are not aware of data
suggesting that nononcogenic SV40 transformed cells have increased
concentrations of SV40 transplantation antigens on their surfaces. In
these studies we have shown that SV40, in contrast to Ad2, conveys
what appears to be a species-specific resistance to allograft rejection to Syrian hamster cells transformed in tissue culture. From
these results we conclude that, in addition to transformation, the induction of some type of resistance to rejection by the cell-mediated
responses of the host is essential to the process by which SV40 (and
possibly other tumor viruses) convert normal cells to tumor cells.

Table 5. Transplantability of SV40 and Ad2 Transformed LSH Cell-
          Induced Tumor Lines to Adult Syngeneic LSH and Allogeneic
          CB Hamsters

Tumor line (passage tested)[1]		TPD_{50} $(\log_{10})/0.2$ ml of tumor suspension in		$\log_{10}$ $(TPD_{50}LSH/$ $TPD_{50}CB)$
		LSH	CB	
SV40HTL1	(2)	3.3	2.7	0.6
	(22)	3.7	3.3	0.4
SV40HTL2	(2)	2.7	2.8	(-)0.1
	(17)	4.5	4.5	0.0
	(4)*	4.5	4.5	0.0
Ad2HTL1	(3)	4.1	0.5	3.6
	(6)	>3.5	0.0	>3.5
Ad2HTL3	(11)	4.9	1.9	3.0
	(14)	>3.5	0.2	>3.3

[1]The (*) designated SV40HTL2 line was passaged in newborn hamsters;
the other tumor lines were carried in adult animals.

REFERENCES

1.   Philipson, L. et al. Virol Monogr 14 (1975) 45, 53.
2.   Harwood, L. M.; Gallimore, P.H. Int J Cancer 16 (1975) 498.
3.   Cook, J.L.; Lewis, A.M., Jr. Cancer Res 39 (1979) 1455.
4.   Lewis, A.M., Jr.; Cook, J.L. Proc Natl Acad Sci USA, 77 (1980)
     2886.
5.   Johansson, K. et al. J Virol 27 (1978) 628.
6.   Duncan, W.R.; Streilein, J.W. Transplantation 25 (1978) 12.
7.   Duncan, W.R.; Streilein, J.W. Transplantation 25 (1978) 17.
8.   Karber, G. Arch Exp Pathol Pharmakol 162 (1931) 480.
9.   Cook, J.L. et al. Cancer Res 39 (1979) 3335.
10. Cook, J.L. et al. Cancer Res 39 (1979) 4949.
11. Eddy, B.E. et al. Virology 17 (1962) 65.
12. Rabson, A.S. et al. J Natl Cancer Inst 29 (1962) 765.
13. Tooze, J. In: The Molecular Biology of Tumor Viruses. Cold
     Spring Harbor Laboratory, Cold Spring Harbor, N.Y. (1973) 350.
14. Butel, J.S. et al. Adv Cancer Res 15 (1972) 1.
15. Hargis, B.J.; Malkiel, S. J Natl Cancer Inst 63 (1979) 965.
16. Eddy, B.E. Prog Exp Tumor Res 4 (1964) 1.
17. Lewis, A.M., Jr. In: Biohazards in Biological Research, ed.
     Hellman, Oxman, and Pollock. Cold Spring Harbor Laboratory,
     Cold Spring Harbor, N.Y. (1973) 96.
18. Shah, K.; Nathanson, N. Am J Epidemiol 103 (1976) 1.
19. Black, P.H.; Rowe, W.P. Proc Soc Exp Biol Med 114 (1963) 721.
20. Diderholm, H. et al. Int J Cancer 1 (1966) 139.

21. Takemoto, K.K. et al. J Natl Cancer Inst 41 (1968) 1401.
22. Kit, S. et al. Int J Cancer 4 (1969) 384.
23. Wesslin, T. Acta Pathol Microbiol Scand [B] 78 (1970) 479.
24. Tevethia, S.S.; McMillan, V.L. Intervirology 3 (1974) 269.
25. Shin, S.I. et al. Proc Natl Acad Sci USA 72 (1975) 4435.

MODIFICATIONS OF THE LYMPHOID B AND T CELL POPULATIONS IN SPLEEN AND THYMUS OF TUMOR-BEARING HAMSTERS

H. Haddada, Ch. de Vaux Saint Cyr, F. Loisillier and
J. Zuinghedau

Institut de Recherches Scientifiques sur le Cancer
B.P. n° 8, 94800 Villejuif, France

INTRODUCTION

The golden Syrian hamster has proved to be a useful host for studying cell-oncogenic virus interaction, as many viruses induce neoplasms in this species. The first polyoma-induced tumors in Syrian hamsters were described in 1958 (1). Shortly thereafter, other authors (2) also noted that hamster cells could be transformed by this agent in vitro. After the discovery of the tumor-inducing potency of the polyoma virus, simian vacuolating virus or SV40 also was shown (3,4) to induce tumors when injected into newborn hamsters and to transform hamster fibroblasts in vitro.

Tumors induced by virus-transformed cells invariably contain cells that express antigens specifically associated with the transforming virus. Two- to five-month-old hamsters inoculated subcutaneously or intramuscularly with SV40 transformed cells ($ZDCl_{25}$) developed a poorly-differentiated fibrosarcoma that appeared at the site of inoculation 20 to 30 days later, in 90% to 100% of the animals (5, 6). The tumor cells were extremely basophilic, cell density was considerable and there were few if any fibers between the tumor cells. Frequent mitoses were noted, and abnormal, bizarre nuclei and multinucleated cells varied in number from tumor to tumor and even from one site to another in the same tumor. Even the smallest tumors showed necrosis. Over the past four years we have tried to characterize some aspects of the immunologic responsiveness of hamsters during the growth of tumors induced by injection of two kinds of neoplastic cells; SV40-transformed cells ($ZDCl_{25}$) and spontaneously transformed cells (EHB). We have studied the evolution of the immune response over the course of tumor development and examined the modifications of the lymphoid cells populating the peritumoral area, the spleen and the thymus. The amount of IgG_1 and IgG_2 was evaluated in sera of tumor-bearing hamsters. It is interesting to note that the results obtained with highly antigenic tumor cells (SV40-transformed $ZDCl_{25}$) are very similar to those obtained with non-antigenic spontaneously transformed EHB cells.

MATERIALS AND METHODS

Syngeneic 5- to 6-month-old Syrian hamsters from the animal farm of our Institut were used in these studies. Tumors were induced by SV40-transformed and strongly antigenic cells ($ZDCl_{25}$) (7) or by spontaneously transformed and non-antigenic cells (EHB). $ZDCl_{25}$ arose from a tumor appearing in a syngeneic hamster injected at birth with 10^5 PFU of SV40 virus: this cell line was maintained in culture after cloning and contained all the specific SV40-induced antigens (Big T, small t, TSTA and TATA). When 2×10^4 $ZDCl_{25}$ or EHB cells were injected into the right flank, tumors appeared in 100% of 5-month-old hamsters. Hamsters were killed at various intervals and their organs and the tumors weighed.

Animals were killed by cervical dislocation. The spleen and the thymus were removed aseptically: one half was fixed in absolute alcohol and embedded in paraffin, and 1.5-μm sections were cut on a Jung Autocut microtome. Sections were stained for standard histological examination; parallel sections were handled according to the technique of Sainte-Marie (8) and used for immunofluorescence studies. The other half of thymuses and spleens were used to prepare cell suspensions by aseptically mincing and pressing the organs through 60-mesh wire sieves. Following two cycles of washing in ice-cold RPMI 1640, 50-μl aliquots of suspensions of thymus or spleen cells were placed in 5-ml plastic tubes and 100 μl of either RaHIgG (1:250) or RaHThy (1:200) antiserum was added. After 20 minutes incubation at $0^{\circ}C$, 100 ml of absorbed guinea pig complement diluted 1:6 was added. Following a further 40 minutes incubation at $37^{\circ}C$, the cells were stained with trypan blue and counted, and the percentage of T and B cells was evaluated from the spleens of tumor-bearing hamsters throughout the growth of the tumor. The following antisera were used: rabbit antiserum against hamster IgG_1 and IgG_2 (RaHIgG) was decomplemented by heating at $56^{\circ}C$ for 30 minutes and used at a dilution of 1:200 with fresh guinea pig serum (dilution 1:6) as source of complement. This antiserum was cytotoxic for 32% spleen cells with negligible cytotoxicity against thymocytes. Rabbit anti-thymocyte serum (RaHThy) was decomplemented in the same way. At 1:100 dilution, in the presence of fresh guinea complement, it was cytotoxic for hamster thymocytes (95%), bone marrow cells (0.5%), and spleen cells (40%).

The amount of hamster immunoglobulins present in the sera of tumor-bearing hamsters was evaluated using the Laurell technique (9) with the same RaHIgG reacting with hamster IgG_1 and IgG_2 at 1:200 dilution in agarose C (Pharmacia, France).

RESULTS

Both types of tumors (ZDCl$_{25}$ and EHB) elicited similar responses
in the spleen and the thymus, and a relationship between the tumor
weight and the reactions in the peritumoral area, the spleen and the
thymus was seen in both cases. The period of tumor growth can be divided into three phases.

First phase (tumors up to 5 g): a peritumoral granulomatous zone
can be distinguished with numerous blood vessels, histiocytes, small
mononuclear cells and a large number of plasma cells. The lymphoid
and histiocytic cells often infiltrate the tumor mass.

The immunocompetent cells, which make up the peritumoral reactions
observed early in the tumor growth, were studied with RaHIgG and
RaHThy. An intense cytoplasmic fluorescence caused by the presence
of IgG, as revealed by RaHIgG, was seen in the peritumoral plasma
cells and large young lymphocytic cells. The NRS control was uniformly
negative. Very few cells stained with RaHThy. These cells had the
morphology of small lymphocytes (Fig. 1,2).

In the thymus, an initial increase in mass was noted with a progressive infiltration of cortical cells into the medullary region.

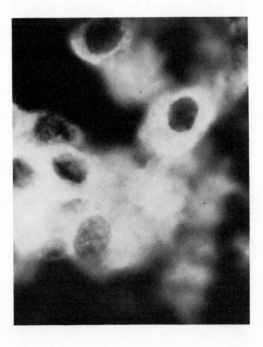

Fig. 1: Peritumoral area taken from a 500-mg tumor treated with
         RaHIgG, 1.5-μm section. 400 X. (Reduced 14% for reproduction.)

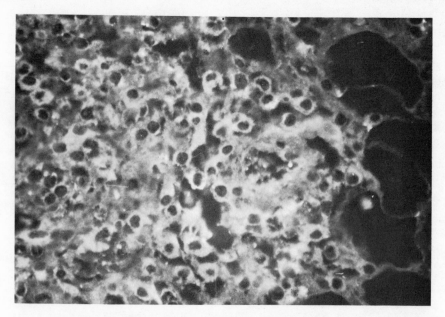

Fig. 2:   Peritumoral area taken from the same tumor treated with
          RaHThy, 1.5-μm section. 400 X. (Reduced 14% for reproduction.)

Sections treated with RaHIgG showed a few stained plasma cells. More
than 95% of the cells stained brilliantly with RaHThy.

     The reaction was modest in the spleen at the beginning of the
tumor growth, and hyperplasia of lymphoid follicles and of the T
spaces was noted thereafter. In the reticulum, scattered clusters of
10 to 15 cells were seen; they resembled plasma cells because of their
eccentric nuclei and the abundant cytoplasm which stained with RaHIgG.

     Second phase (tumor from 5 to 12 g): this phase is characterized
by disappearance of the peritumoral plasmatic reaction and by the loss
of normal cytoarchitecture of the spleen and the thymus.

     Thymic mass remained relatively constant but thymic lymphocytes
and blood-borne cells had colonized the medulla, and medullary epithelium had been largely replaced by proliferating lymphoid cells. In
immunofluorescence studies, the number of cells stained by RaHIgG increases as a function of tumor growth.

     In this phase the spleen is characterized by a reduction of the
number of lymphoid follicles, a loss of T lymphocytes in periarteriolar areas (Fig. 3) and the appearance in the reticulum of young lymphocytic cells which invade the T-dependent areas (Fig. 4).

Terminal phase (tumors over 13 g): this phase is characterized by a major remodelling of the cell populations of the spleen and the thymus.

The volume of the thymus was decreased and the epithelial cells had disappeared. The lymphoid cells were larger than in earlier phases, suggesting that a new population had invaded this organ. Studies of intracytoplasmic fluorescence showed that more than 30% of the cells stained by the RaHIgG were young lymphocytic cells containing IgG in their cytoplasm (Fig. 5).

The spleen increases as a function of tumor growth, and three new types of cells were seen in the splenic reticulum: scattered tumor cells which at this stage of tumor growth are detected very easily; hematopoietic cells that come to represent approximately 10% of the total population as the spleen enlarges; and young lymphoid cells grouped in masses; as tumor growth increased, so did the number of lymphoblasts in the reticulum. By the time the tumor had exceeded 20 g, they had replaced most of the lymphoid follicles, and the spleen presented a pseudo-leukemic aspect. These lymphocytes appear to be younger than in the earlier phases, with notched nuclei, little chromatin, and cytoplasm uniformly distributed around the nucleus. Sec-

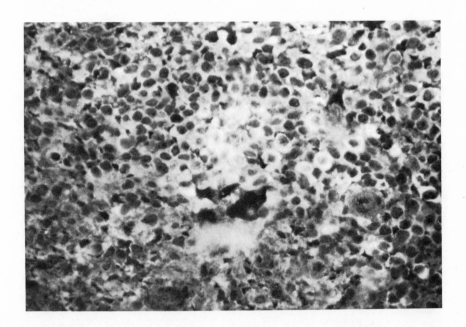

Fig. 3:   Spleen section treated with RaHThy. Few cells are positive in the T-dependent area. 400 X. (Reduced 14% for reproduction.)

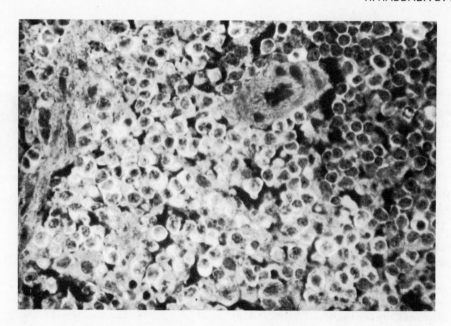

Fig. 4:   Section of the same spleen treated with RaHIgG. Young lym-
          phocytes are invading the periarteriolar area. 400 X.
          (Reduced 14% for reproduction.)

tions of spleens at this stage of tumor growth were treated with
RaHThy, and very few if any cells were fluorescent when stained by
RaHIgG. The majority of the young lymphoid cells were fluorescent,
demonstrating the presence of IgG in their cytoplasm.

     The variations in the T and B lymphocytes from the spleens of
tumor-bearing hosts are shown in Table 1 for the two tumoral systems.
It is striking that the percentage of B cells lysed by RaHIgG + C'
is fairly constant and increases very little only when tumors exceeded
10 g. This contrasts with results obtained on spleen sections treated
with the same antiserum. For the same tumor weight the percentage of
cells containing intracytoplasmic IgG is about 80%, as can be seen on
frozen sections. The easiest explanation of this discrepancy is that
a fairly important number of young lymphoid cells do not bear surface
IgG and are not lysed by RaHIgG. The percentage of T lymphocytes decreases regularly in the spleen as a function of tumor weight. After
a mild hyperplasia when tumors are small (0.1 to 0.9 g), the decrease
of T lymphocytes in the spleen began when the tumors reached 5 to 7 g.
At the same time, the disappearance of the peritumoral plasmatic reaction and modifications in the normal architecture of the spleen were
observed.

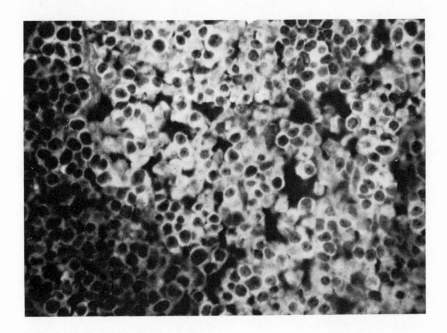

Fig. 5: Thymus section (tumor = 15 g) treated with RaHIgG. The same young lymphocytes with intracytoplasmic IgG are invading the thymus.

Table 1. Evolution of the Percentage of T and B Splenic Lymphocytes as a function of Tumor Weight

Tumor weight (g)	%T ZDCl$_{25}$	EHB	%B ZDCl$_{25}$	EHB
Control	42, 39, 38, 29		38, 33, 30, 24	
0.1 - 0.9	42, 44	40, 38	32, 31	31, 34
1 - 3	32, 34, 25	34, 30, 32	38, 37, 34	39, 40, 37
5 - 7	26, 21	20, 21	39, 36	38, 41
7 - 9	18, 20	18, 14	39, 40	39, 42
10 - 12	18.5, 17	16, 13	44, 44	41, 45
12 - 15	13.5, 11.8	9, 11	43, 45, 46	44, 43

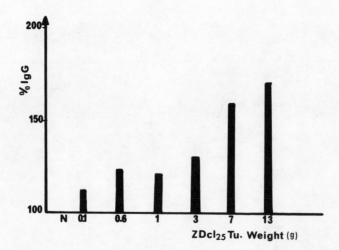

Fig. 6: Amount of IgG present in the sera of hamsters bearing a
ZDCl$_{25}$-induced tumor as a function of tumor growth.

The amount of IgG in the sera of tumor-bearers was calculated as
a percentage of the amount of IgG in normal serum, taken as 100%. Fig.
6 shows that the amount of hamster IgG increases during the growth of
the tumor (ZDCl$_{25}$); this agrees with our previous results (6), indicating a similar augmentation of antibody titer in the sera of tumor-
bearing animals. The same increase in circulating IgG was observed
in EHB tumor-bearing hamsters, but until now no antibody activity
against tumor cells could be demonstrated in those sera.

DISCUSSION

The histological and immunological studies of the spleen and
thymus of the golden Syrian hamster during the growth of two tumors
induced by injection of different transformed cells raise some questions:

The first point of interest is the similarity of the results obtained in hamsters bearing a tumor induced by SV40-transformed cells.
These cells are highly antigenic, and the sera of tumor-bearing hosts
contained antibodies directed against the multiple SV40-induced antigens. Antibodies directed against Forsmann-like antigens and against
embryonic antigens also can be demonstrated in the sera of ZDCl$_{25}$
tumor-bearers. With a few exceptions, circulating antibodies could
be measured only after tumors had exceeded 4 g in weight; thereafter,
the titer increases as a function of weight. The total amount of
IgG$_1$ and IgG$_2$ increases as well (Fig. 6). The EHB cells, on the con-

trary, seem to be devoid of demonstrable antigens; there is no difference in the immunofluorescence study using living or acetone-fixed
cells between the fixation of normal hamster serum and of sera of
tumor-bearing animals. But in sera of EHB tumor-bearing animals, the
amount of immunoglobulins decreases to below the normal level as the
tumor weight increases, even if the total number of lymphoid cells
with IgG-positive cytoplasm increases in the spleen during the same
period of time, suggesting that IgG is not excreted in the sera.

The evolution of the lymphoid populations of the thymus and the
spleen as a function of the growth of these two tumors are comparable
in many aspects. The changes observed in the lymphoid organs depend
on the weight of the tumor and not on time elapsed from the cell injection until the appearance of the tumor and the speed of enlargement.
The existence of a critical weight, between 5 and 10 g depending on
animals, can be shown for both tumors. It causes profound changes in
the thymus and spleen, as well as the disappearance of the peritumoral
plasma cell reaction. Two successive waves of immune response occur
which differ in cell type involved. The presence of T lymphocytes and
plasma cells in the peritumoral reaction seen early in the tumor
growth coincides with hyperplasia of the thymus and of the T-dependent
areas in the spleen. At the same time, clusters of plasma cells are
seen in the splenic reticulum. We believe that this response is thymus
dependent. Thereafter, the thymus begins to involute and the spleen
presents a picture of immune depression with depletion of T cells.
Simultaneously, the peritumoral plasma cell reaction stops abruptly.
The second wave is characterized by the appearance in the splenic reticulum and in the thymic medulla of groups of immature cells which
progressively colonize both organs. These cells, negative with RaHThy,
showed a bright cytoplasmic fluorescence when treated with RaHIgG,
demonstrating the presence of IgG in their cytoplasm. In a previous
work (6) we were able to prove that a fairly high proportion of these
cells (in the case of $ZDCl_{25}$ tumor) were synthesizing antibodies directed against specific SV40-induced antigens. The level of serum IgG
and circulating antibodies correlates with the increasing tumor mass
and with progressive proliferation of lymphoblastoid cells in the
thymus and spleen. The results obtained in evaluating the percentage
of T and B cells killed by the specific antisera during tumor development agree with our previous findings showing the depletion of T cells
in the spleen and repopulation by young IgG-containing cells. A discrepancy can be seen at the terminal stage of tumor growth between the
number of cells showing intracytoplasmic IgG and cells possessing sur-
face-associated IgG. More work on B-cell maturation and differentiation as well as IgG synthesis and secretion needs to be done. In this
last phase, the tumor-bearing hamster resembles a thymectomized animal
in which the capacity to produce IgG_2-class antibodies is not lost.
It is known that the level of IgG_2 is normal, or nearly so, in thymectomized hamsters (11-14). The abrupt disappearance of T-lymphoid cells
is difficult to interpret, but may be related to involution of the
thymus. We have no explanation for the invasion of the spleen and

thymus by a population of immature lymphoblasts with intracytoplasmic IgG, which in the case of $ZDCl_{25}$ tumors are synthesizing antibodies. Possibly the tumor cells secrete factors not yet identified that favor thymic involution and lymphoblastic proliferation.

REFERENCES

1. Eddy, B.E. et al. J Natl Cancer Inst 20 (1958) 777.
2. Stocker, M.; McPherson, I. Virology 14 (1961) 359.
3. McPherson, I.; Stoker, M. Virology 16 (1962) 147.
4. Sachs, I. et al. Virology 17 (1962) 491.
5. Loisillier, F. et al. Br J Exp Pathol 58 (1977) 533.
6. de Vaux St. Cyr, C. et al. Ann Microbiol (Inst Pasteur) 128B (1977) 385.
7. Zuinghedau, J. et al. Bull Cancer (Paris) 66 (1979) 383.
8. Sainte-Marie, G. J Histochem Cytochem 10 (1962) 250.
9. Laurell, C.B. Anal Biochem 15 (1966) 45.
10. Zuinghedau, J. et al. Br J Cancer 39 (1979) 594.
11. Arnason, B.G. et al. J Immunol 93 (1964) 915.
12. Fayey, J.L. et al. J Natl Cancer Inst 35 (1965) 663.
13. Humphrey, J.H. et al. Immunology 7 (1964) 419.
14. Tyan, M.L.; Herzenberg, L.A. J Immunol 101 (1968) 446.

C-TYPE PARTICLES IN THYMIC DEVELOPMENT: A CORRELATION WITH THYMIC FUNCTION

Pamela L. Witte, J. Wayne Streilein, and W. A. Shannon, Jr.

Department of Cell Biology, University of Texas Health
Science Center at Dallas, Dallas, TX 75235
and Veterans Administration Hospital, Dallas, TX 75216

INTRODUCTION

Endogenous C-type retroviruses are expressed morphologically and antigenically in embryos of many mammalian species (1,2). Viral DNA is inserted into the host genome and thus can be vertically transmitted from parent to offspring. In addition, the expression of these viruses is highly regulated by host genes (1). In both inbred and feral mice, C-type particles are seen consistently in developing lymphoid organs during fetal life, but disappear prior to birth (3,4). It has been reported (5) that in fetal murine thymus, C-type particles are first seen budding from reticular epithelial cells and later from thymocytes. Consequently, it has been suggested that the expression of these particles may play a role in the differentiation of normal T lymphocytes.

Certain features of differentiation and function of the thymus-dependent immune system in Syrian hamsters are unusual when compared with those of other rodents:

1. Autoradiography shows that few lymphocytes migrate from thymus to spleen in the first three weeks after birth (6).
2. Thymectomy as late as four weeks after birth can still produce a wasting syndrome (7).
3. No definitive evidence is available for existence of suppressor and killer T-cell populations.
4. High susceptibility to carcinogenic agents and oncogenic viruses in hamsters may reflect a deficiency in T cell-mediated immune surveillance (8).

If C-type particles are important in thymic ontogeny, the Syrian hamster could be an interesting model to examine the possible relationship. Results of previous studies of C-type particle expression in fetal hamsters have been contradictory. Some researchers (9) found no evidence of viral expression in pooled fetal organs from 8 or 9 and 14 or 15 day hamster fetuses. Others, however, using a radioimmunoassay for viral p30 antigen, found positive expression in spleen and liver of late gestation hamster fetuses (10).

We have examined thymic development and C-type particle expression by light and electron microscopy, using LSH hamsters and C57BL/6 mice. The results indicate that virus expression in murine thymus coincides with a time of increased proliferation of thymocytes and rapid morphologic development into cortical and medullary compartments. No comparable phenomenon is found in fetal or neonatal hamster thymus, and the development of cortex and medulla in the hamster is delayed compared to murine thymic development.

MATERIALS AND METHODS

Female LSH hamsters and C57BL/6 mice from our colony were mated with syngeneic males. Evidence of sperm in a vaginal smear or a vaginal plug counted as day 0 of gestational term. Embryos and neonates were selected at various times after conception: from fetal day 13 through the day of birth for mouse embryos and from fetal day 10 through seven days after birth for hamster embryos.

Thymic lobes were dissected out, minced, if larger than 0.5 mm, and fixed in 4% glutaraldehyde in Millonig's phosphate buffer (0.12M) overnight. The lobes were washed in phosphate buffer, postfixed in 1% osmium tetroxide, and dehydrated in graded alcohols before embedding in epon. One- or two-micron survey sections were stained with toluidine blue and studied by light microscopy. For electron microscopy, 50- to 70-mm thin sections were made approximately midway through each lobe in random areas. When a cortex and medulla were visible, thin sections were made of both areas. Sections were mounted on 300-mesh copper grids, stained with uranyl acetate and lead citrate, and observed in a Philips 301 electron microscope.

Expression of C-type particles was determined by electron microscopy. Sections were mounted on 300-mesh copper grids; 75 to 100 grid squares were examined for each developmental day. Thymic lobes from three to five animals were examined for each time sampled.

RESULTS AND DISCUSSION

Morphological events during thymic development can be grouped into phases through which both hamster and mouse embryonic thymuses

Table 1. Characteristics of Morphological Events in Thymus Development

Event	Characteristics
1. Formation of the thymic anlage	Pharyngeal epithelium outpockets and migrates posteriorly ad medially forming the thymic rudiment.
2. Invasion of the anlage by lympho-blasts	The rudiment is infiltrated by large lymphoblasts that, by light microscopy, are not easily distinguished from the numerous reticular epithelial cells. Reticular epithelial cells are light staining, have numerous cytoplasmic inclusions, and large euchromatic nuclei with centrally located nucleoli. Lymphoblasts are large cells with dense cytoplasm containing many mitochondria, developed Golgi, some RER, and irregularly shaped nuclei.
3. Differentiation into mature lymphocytes and reticular epithelial cells	Reticular epithelial cells, with dendritic processes, form a stroma that surrounds large rounded thymocytes. Large lymphocytes can be distinguished from lymphoblasts by their round, somewhat condensed nuclei and decreased content of cytoplasmic organelles.
4. Differentiation of cortex and medulla	Small lymphocytes appear primarily in the cortex. The cortex now also contains numerous lymphocytes of various sizes and few elongate reticular cells stretched between thymocytes. The differentiating medulla, on the other hand, contains few lymphocytes at this stage but is composed primarily of large reticular epithelial cells.
5. Adult morphology	The cortex is characterized by its great density of small lymphocytes, numerous mitotic figures, and few reticular epithelial cells. The medulla, while containing many reticular epithelial cells, also has thymocytes of various sizes. A fully differentiated cortico-medullary junction has formed.

progress.   Characteristics of these events are outlined in Table 1.
As shown in Fig. 1, chronological development of the thymus proceeds
at a comparable rate in mice and hamsters until the organ is infiltrated with lymphocytes and the reticular epithelial cells have gained
a mature, dendritic appearance.   The fetal mouse thymus then rapidly
differentiates (within three days) into the two compartments, cortex
and medulla; the hamster thymus reaches this highly differentiated
state more slowly, within six days.   At birth, the mouse thymus has
reached an adult morphology, nine days after the appearance of the
thymic anlage.   The hamster thymus does not reach an adult-like morphology until one week after birth, fourteen days after the thymic
anlage forms.   Thus, hamster and mouse thymuses undergo differentiation events comparable by morphologic criteria; the mouse thymus, however, attains a mature morphology in less time, by several days, than

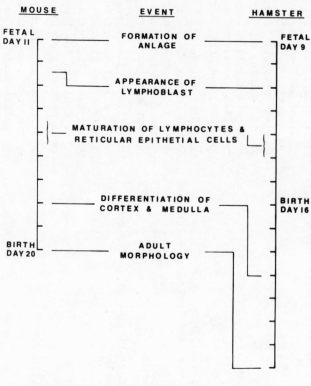

COMPARISON OF MORPHOLOGICAL EVENTS
IN THYMUS DEVELOPMENT

Fig. 1:   Chronological development of murine and hamster thymus.

the hamster thymus. This developmental lag in the hamster appears between the time the embryonic thymus becomes recognized as lymphoid
and the time a cortex and medulla differentiate (Fig. 1).

Proliferation rates may correlate with chronological differentiation events. Apparent frequency of observed mitotic figures among

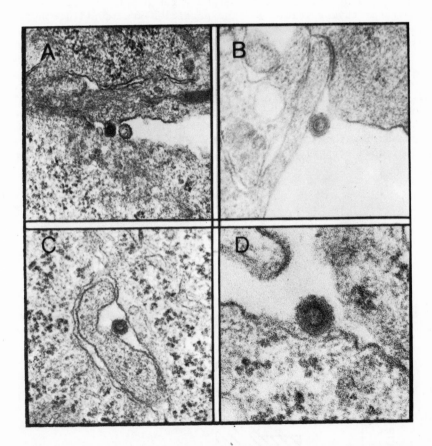

Fig. 2: C-type virus particles in fetal murine thymic tissue. C-
type particles can be identified by EM as enveloped with
dense central cores. The particles are characteristically
100 nm in diameter. C-type particles can be seen extra-
cellularly or budding from mouse fetal thymic cells.
A. Budding virus particle. Magnification x33,000.
B. Budding virus particle. Magnification x44,000.
C. Extracellular virus particle. Magnification x44,000.
D. Extracellular virus particle. Magnification x100,000.
(Reduced 14% for reproduction.)

lymphocytes indicates that the proliferative rate within the mouse thymus peaks and is maintained at 15 to 16 days of fetal life, but intense proliferation within the hamster thymus is delayed until three to five days after birth. Intense proliferation of murine thymocytes, therefore, begins a few days before a cortico-medullary demarcation appears, whereas intense proliferation is not seen in hamster thymus until cortex and medulla form.

As reported by others (3,4), C-type virus particles are expressed in murine fetal thymus (Fig. 2). The particles are identified by electron microscopy as 100-nm, dense-core enveloped virions. If the expression of C-type virus particles in murine thymus is followed through gestation, they are first seen on day 13, then the number of particles peaks around fetal day 15, and the particles gradually disappear before birth (Fig. 3). The appearance and quantitative expression of C-type particles in fetal C57BL/6 thymus correspond temporally to an increase in lymphocyte proliferation and subsequent compartmentalization of the mouse thymus, from fetal days 15 to 18. In contrast, at no time during thymic development in LSH hamsters are C-type particles expressed morphologically within reticular epithelial cells or

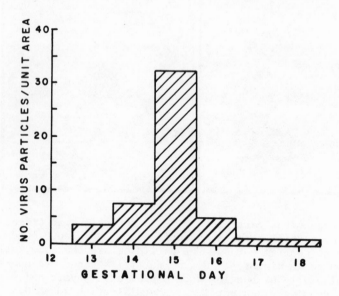

Fig. 3:   Quantitation of C-type particles during murine thymic development. Number of C-type virus particles for 10 grid squares (0.1 mm^2) is reported for each gestational day.

thymocytes, and peak proliferation of hamster thymocytes appears to be delayed until three to five days after birth when the cortex and medulla are formed.

In summary, our results indicate that:

1. Maturation of hamster and mouse thymuses occurs at a comparable rate in early stages.
2. Fetal mouse thymus rapidly attains an adult morphology, while hamster thymus matures at a slower pace.
3. Rapid development of murine thymus appears shortly after peak expression of C-type virus particles and intense cellular proliferation.
4. No similar phenomenon appears in developing hamster thymus.

We suggest the possibility that delayed thymic maturation in the hamster is related to the failure of C-type particle expression, which implies that mice may use these viral sequences, inserted in their genome, as physiologic differentiation signals. The increased proliferation around days 15 to 16 in fetal murine thymus may begin with a mitogenic stimulus present at that time; this signal may be delayed or absent in hamster thymus. It has been suggested (11) that murine C-type retroviruses provide mitogenic signals to murine thymocytes, and in this way, may induce T-cell lymphomas in adult mice. More recent work (12) shows that thymoma-specific monoclonal antibodies can block binding of virus in vitro and cause an inhibition of cell growth. Some of the inhibiting monoclonal antibodies bind specifically to the Thy-1 molecule. Thy-1 appears in high density on immature thymocytes and is less dense on mature thymocytes and peripheral T cells. Thy-1 also appears during murine fetal life at a time that coincides with virus expression (13,14). The possibility exists that binding of the Thy-1 surface molecules by C-type virus acts as a mitogenic signal; the subsequent increased proliferation of thymocytes may speed differentiation in fetal murine thymus as a normal developmental event. This expression of C-type particles in adult thymus, however, may lead to morbidity.

As several papers in this symposium have reported, the hamster has been successfully employed for the study of numerous disease models involving immunity, oncogenesis and infectious agents. Failure to reject virus-transformed tumor cells, enhanced susceptibility to carcinogenic agents, and ease of infection with bacterial, parasitic and virus agents, all characterize the Syrian hamster, and may reflect aberrations in T lymphocyte-mediated immune surveillance. Our studies demonstrate that by morphological criteria, the tempo of development of the hamster thymus is slow, and maturation of this organ is delayed in comparison to the mouse. The delay corresponds with an apparent lack of expression of histologically identifiable C-type particles during thymic development, suggesting that endogenous viruses do not express themselves (by non-serologic criteria) in this species.

Whether aberrations in thymic maturation and C-type particle expression are interrelated or important in the putative defect of the hamster thymus immune system is not known. It is not unreasonable to suggest, however, that delayed and perhaps incomplete thymic development may relate to the very T-cell deficiencies that have made the hamster the animal model of choice in the studies reported in this symposium.

ACKNOWLEDGMENTS

Supported by N.I.H. grant 5 RO1 RR01133-02.

REFERENCES

1.   Aaronson, S.A.; Stephenson, J.R. Biochim Biophys Acta 458 (1976) 323.
2.   Huebner, R.J. et al. Proc Natl Acad Sci USA 67 (1970) 366.
3.   Mandel, T. Z Zellforsch 106 (1970) 498.
4.   Vernon, M.L. et al. J Natl Cancer Inst 51 (1973) 1171.
5.   Koppenheffer, T.L. et al. Am J Anat 153 (1978) 165.
6.   Linna, T.J. Blood 31 (1968) 727.
7.   Adner, M.M. et al. Blood 25 (1965) 511.
8.   Berman, L.D.; Black, P.H. Prog Exp Tumor Res 16 (1972) 497.
9.   Freeman, A.E. et al. J Natl Cancer Inst 52 (1974) 1469.
10. Charman, H.P. et al. J Virol 14 (1974) 910.
11. McGrath, M.S.; Weissman, I.L. Cell 17 (1979) 65.
12. McGrath, M.S. et al. Nature 285 (1980) 259.
13. Jenkinson, E.J. et al. Nature 284 (1980) 177.
14. Owen, J.J.T. et al. In: Developmental Immunobiology, ed. Solomon and Horton. Elsevier/North Holland Biomedical Press (1977) 131.

SUMMATION

J. Wayne Streilein

Department of Cell Biology
University of Texas Health Science Center at Dallas
Dallas, TX   75235

In the grand schema of biomedical research, any species that is used as a laboratory animal will be judged ultimately on its ability to shed light on human disease: causes, pathogenesis, and therapy. Since its introduction into research more than 50 years ago, the Syrian hamster has been utilized in numerous model systems. The thesis of this symposium, as well as that of its predecessor three years ago has been that hamsters can be profitably employed to investigate infectious and oncologic diseases with immunologic overtones. At this symposium, several important, and quite unique, experimental systems have been described in the Syrian hamster, model systems that represent reasonably faithful replicas of human disease counterparts. Most turn on the extraordinary susceptibility of adult hamsters to infections with agents that are taxonomically identified with other species. For example, Dr. Niklaus Weiss has described in remarkable detail the infectious disease in hamsters caused by Dipetalonema viteae, a filarial parasite that causes a disorder that resembles the human disease, filariasis. A meticulous survey of the effect of this parasite on hamster immune responses, especially responses directed specifically at antigens expressed on the parasite, has been achieved. Infections of hamsters with bacterial agents also has been amply described with both Mycoplasma pneumoniae and Treponema pallidum. In fact, respiratory infections in hamsters with Mycoplasma pneumoniae and the human influenza virus are remarkably similar to the human diseases caused by these agents. Once again, the hamster proves to be uniquely susceptible to infection with these agents, which allows for an experimental analysis of the role of the immune system and other defense mechanisms in the pathogenesis and resolution of these diseases.

Hamsters have also been shown to respond to infection with measles virus by developing a central nervous system disorder resem-

463

bling subacute sclerosing panencephalitis. What is intriguing is the observation by Johnson and his colleagues that among the viral-dependent proteins that attend measles infections, an alteration in the M protein occurs simultaneously with the appearance of a host immune response. This event also coincides with the time of onset of chronic infection of central nervous system cells with the viral agent. Several laboratories have turned to the Syrian hamster in order to study unconventional virus agents, scrapie being the most common. The rapidity with which the scrapie agent is able to cause clinical signs of infection in hamsters, and the multiplicity of infectious units that can be harvested from infected hamster nervous tissue, undoubtedly will hasten the description, identification and, hopefully, isolation of the causative agent; the single most important discovery that is needed in the field of unconventional viral agents is identification of the organism.

Finally, exposing the respiratory tract of hamsters to carcinogens such as benzopyrene induces respiratory cancers that are quite similar to those found in man. Thus unique models described in this symposium with Syrian hamsters involve parasites, bacteria, viruses, and oncogenic agents.

Exploitable Features of the Syrian Hamster

In the presentations in this symposium, several features of hamsters were described that account, in part, for the expanding usefulness of this species to the biomedical research community. The most dramatic is the extraordinary capacity of hamsters to sustain the replication of the scrapie agent. While the pathophysiologic basis of this capacity of hamsters remains essentially unexplored, the animals ultimately will prove useful not only for the rapid production of the scrapie agent but also for an experimental dissection of the cause of their peculiar susceptibility.

Several investigators attested to the extremely "clean" nature of the hamster lung and pulmonary tract. In comparison with other laboratory rodents, where respiratory infections with a variety of agents are endemic in domestic colonies, virtually no chronic, endogenous pulmonary disease exists among laboratory hamsters. This undoubtedly accounts, at least in part, for the successful exploitation of hamsters in the study of Mycoplasma pneumoniae and influenza A virus infection. The "clean" character of hamster lungs permits the use of this tissue for the study of inflammation-inducing agents which, when studied in other laboratory rodents, usually result in a pneumonitic process that obscures the agent's primary pharmacologic action.

Hamster cell lines transformed with SV40 in vitro are able to establish tumors regularly in hamsters, even in adult hamsters. This is almost unprecedented among laboratory animals. This unique capacity

of hamsters to accept in vitro transformed cells has allowed Lewis and
Cook to begin to make significant inroads into our understanding of
the SV40 transformational event and its relationship to the expression
of cell-surface molecules.

The concentration of mast cells in the thoracic and peritoneal
cavities of hamsters is considerably greater than in mice and rats.
As Sullivan and his colleagues have shown, this enrichment of mast
cells will allow for an accelerated description of the IgE antibody
system in the hamster and will offer a readily available source of
large numbers of mast cells for immunopharmacologic studies. Therefore,
four classes of immunoglobulins have now been described in the Syrian
hamster--IgM, IgG, IgA, and now IgE, leaving only the hamster IgD-equivalent molecule to be defined. In that regard, a likely candidate for
this important Ig class has been suggested by studies on cell-surface
immunoglobulins.

Numerous isogenic lines of Syrian hamsters are available commercially. The increasing use of different inbred lines in experimental
models has allowed the description and analysis of host responses to
infectious and oncogenic agents in this species to reach a new level
of sophistication.

Newly Described Immune Capabilities in the Hamster

Several significant new discoveries of hamster immune capabilities were reported at this symposium.

1. Hm-1, the hamster major histocompatibility complex (MHC) equivalent, has now been defined on the basis of serologic, immunochemical,
and lymphocyte-activating criteria. The Hm-1 locus (loci) has at least
six independent alleles, two of which are serologically active. Hamster homologues of murine and human class I and class II MHC cell-
surface determinants have now been described.
2. Strong circumstantial evidence for the presence of hamster IgE
was found through the study of hamster mast cells. Now four isotypes
of immunoglobulin have been identified: IgM, IgG, IgA and IgE.
3. Functional evidence for the presence of all components of the
classical complement system have been identified in serum from normal
hamsters.
4. Alpha-2 macroglobulin isolated from hamster serum has been shown
to have a potential place in regulation of immune responses, either
through its native role as a protease inhibitor, or when complexed
with protease.
5. Contact hypersensitivity in hamsters was reported to be mediated
by T cells representing the hamster homologues of murine Lyl^+23^- cells.
6. Functional subsets of alveolar macrophages have been identified
and methods for their induction described.

7. The so-called female protein, a sex-related serum protein, has tentatively been identified as the hamster homologue of C-reactive protein.

Unusual Features of Hamster Immune Capabilities

As the functional, cellular, and molecular descriptions of the hamster immune system improve, a number of specific aberrations appear to have been identified.

1. Hm-1, the hamster major histocompatibility complex, displays a significant number of allelic forms, most of which are serologically silent. In addition, despite the availability of at least six Hm-1 allodisparate strains, no evidence exists for polymorphism at a putative hamster class I locus (analogous to murine H-2 K/D or human HLA-A,B,C).

2. At least two inbred strains of hamsters, PD4 and CB, appear to be deficient in the sixth component of complement (undetectable levels); these two strains also have reduced serum levels of C4 and C2, the evidence suggesting that this situation results from increased serum concentrations of inhibitors of these complement components.

3. Maturation of the hamster thymus during ontogeny is considerably delayed compared to mice and rats, the adult histologic state not being identifiable until approximately 7 to 10 days after birth. Unlike those in mice, ultrastructurally identifiable C-type viral particles never are seen in thymic epithelium or lymphocytes throughout the course of hamster fetal and postnatal development.

4. In an SV40 tumor system and in response to intratracheal infection with parainfluenza virus, circumstantial evidence was produced to suggest that suppressor and cytotoxic T cells can be generated in hamsters. In systems designed to optimize the finding of functional T lymphocytes that are cytotoxic and that suppress, however, no such lymphocyte subpopulations were defined. Resolution of these conflicting results are important to our understanding of hamster immunobiology.

Effector Systems in Hamster Immune Responses

Numerous laboratories have now reported that under most experimental situations in which immune cytotoxic effector cells are produced, the responsible cells are natural killers (NK) or the reactivity is mediated by antibody-dependent mechanisms. NK cells appear to dominate hamster responses to tumors, and to many virus infected tissues. Nonetheless, Henderson and colleagues reported at this symposium strong circumstantial evidence for the presence in hamsters of cytotoxic T cells induced by parainfluenza infection. Whether it is possible for hamsters to generate cytotoxic T cells in response to antigenic challenge is an important matter to resolve. Unequivocal

demonstration of cytotoxic T cells in hamsters, however, will not
eclipse the natural proclivity of this species to use alternative
cytotoxic mechanisms such as NK and antibody-dependent cell-mediated
cytotoxicity in response to many noxious and antigenic agents.

Requisites for Further Development of Hamsters as Models of Infectious and Oncologic Diseases

Although a good deal has been learned about the hamster immune
response and much has been done to relate the specifics of hamster immune responses to the susceptibility of this species to many infectious and oncogenic agents, much still remains unknown. By far the
most pressing need would appear to be development of highly selective
and specific reagents capable of identifying the cell-surface markers
of T- and B-lymphocyte subsets, macrophage populations, NK cells, etc.
Functional studies are too imprecise to provide unequivocal answers
concerning participation of individual types of lymphoreticular cells
in hamster immune reactions. In addition, readily available and dis-
criminant reagents able to recognize heavy chains of the various hamster immunoglobulin isotypes and subisotypes are essential. Reagents
need to be developed that distinguish hamster light chains of immunoglobulin and to identify other serum proteins relevant to immune reactivities.

As expressions of how important the development of these reagents
is, two examples will be cited. Several laboratories have now developed antisera that are reputed to be able to identify hamster T cells.
The discrepancies in results from laboratories using these reagents
suggest that: 1. the Thy-1 molecular homologue in hamsters must be
unusually distributed among lymphoid cells; or 2. there is another
species of cell-surface molecules on T cells, unrelated to murine
Thy-1, that contaminates anti-T cell reagents and gives conflicting
and confusing answers. In the second example, the availability of
cross-reacting heterologous anti-immunoglobulin antisera and isotype-
specific hamster antisera has not allowed an accurate description to
this date of the IgD-equivalent molecule on hamster B lymphocytes, or
in hamster serum.

The other development crucially important to continuing work with
hamsters is the introduction into laboratory strains of more samples
of hamster genes from the wild. Partially inbred lines that are being
developed at the University of Texas Health Science Center at Dallas
are proceeding toward a coefficient of inbreeding that will allow
their dissemination to other laboratories in the near future. It seems
clear that some (although surely not all) of the unusual characteristics of the laboratory hamster can be ascribed to the extremely restricted gene pool from which all domesticated hamsters appear to be
derived. Finally, there is a commercial impediment to the development
of hamsters as models in experimental biology. Only a very few commer-

cial vendors are willing to maintain the inbred lines that are of crucial importance to contemporary research, and even they do not maintain breeding stocks and production lines of sufficient magnitude to
meet the rapidly increasing demands of the scientific community. This
matter needs to be addressed individually and collectively, at the
earliest possible moment, by the community of investigators working
with hamsters.

A new legitimacy is descending upon the Syrian hamster as a model
system for numerous investigations, especially the relationship between unusual aspects of hamster immune responses and the extraordinary susceptibility of the hamster to a variety of infectious and oncogenic agents. The goal of this symposium has been admirably realized
and the significant advances in our knowledge represent good omens for
the future.

ADCC, Antibody Dependent Cell-
    Mediated Cytotoxicity,
    146
Adenovirus, 177, 417, 436
Adherent lymphoid cells, 158,
    331, 360
Adoptive Transfer Of
  tumor immunity, peritoneal
    exudate cells, 167
  tumor immunity, spleen cells,
    167
  tumor immunity, thymocytes,
    167
  Contact hypersensitivity, 48
Aggregation, Scrapie-induced, 385
Alloantisera, 26, 75
Alpha globulins, 111
Alpha 2-Macroglobulin, 111
  isolation of, 113
  antibody to, 112, 114
  regulation of lymphocyte
    activation, 111
  and protease complexes, 115
Alveolar macrophages, 205
Antibody responses to
  Pichinde virus, 332
  Vesicular Stomatitis virus,
    345
  tumors, 445
  alpha-2 macroglobulin, 112,
    114
Antigen stimulation of lympho-
    cytes, 7, 10
  modulation by proteases, 13
  modulation by ions, 16
  modulation by protease
    inhibitors, 13

Anti hamster immunoglobulin
    sera, 54, 445
Anti hamster T lymphocyte
    sera, 48, 124, 144, 445

BCG, Bacillus Calmette-Gurein,
    179, 206
Behavioral changes in Scrapie,
    376
B lympyocytes, 8, 23, 49, 62, 69,
    87, 111, 417, 450
  and Treponema infection 295,
    296
B cell lymphoma, 69, 143
Bioassay, for Scrapie, 359
Bone marrow cells, 7, 74
Bone marrow reconstitution, 124

Carageenan, 156
CB hamster strain, 23, 46, 103,
    124, 145, 179, 218, 342,
    442
  tumors of, 124
Cell fusion, Scrapie agent, 369
Cell surface immunoglobulin, 87
Cell mediated immunity, 43, 59,
    123, 135, 153, 165, 215,
    291, 327, 433, 445
Cell surface alloantigens, 71
Cheek pouch, 45
Chemotactic responses, polymor-
    phonuclear leukocytes,
    225
Chemotactic factors and lung
    injury, 225
[51]Chromium release assay, 136,
    216

Class I MHC products, 23, 71, 144
Class II MHC products, 23, 73
Clinical symptoms in Scrapie, 388
Complement, 103
  levels of, 103
  components, 103, 222
  deficiency of, 103
  synthesis of, 228
  isolation of, 222
Concanavalin A, 8, 123, 438
Contact hypersensitivity, 43, 59
  regulation of, 43, 59
  T lymphocytes in, 48
  antibody in, 54
  adoptive transfer of, 52
  immunopotentiation of, 61
  T suppressor cells in, 62
  flare reaction in, 63
  induction of, 46
Cortisone, 419
Cricetulus, 95, 96
  migratorius, 96
  griseus, 96
  cricetus, 96
C-type particles, 455
Cytotoxicity, 215
Cytotoxic effector cells, 123
Cytotoxic T cells, 123, 145, 153, 216
Cyclophosphamide, 60, 156, 419

DFW hamster strain, 26
Dextran sulfate, 9
Defective interfering viral
    particles, 341, 347, 353
DNP-BSA, 13
Deficiency of complement, 103
Dipetalonema viteae
  infection in hamsters, 253
  life cycle in hamsters, 254
  immune respones to, 256
  cellular immune reponse to, 257
  humoral immune response to, 256
  model for human disease, 253
  and immune competence, 258

ELISA (enzyme-linked immuno-
    absorbent assay)
  in Scrapie, 405
Encephalopathies
  spongiform, 385
Electron microscopy, of thymus, 455, 460
Estrone, 428

Female protein in contact hyper-
    sensitivity, 63
Female mortality in Herpes
    Simplex Virus infection, 311
Fibrosarcoma, 417, 445
(5) Five hydroxytryptophan in
    Scrapie, 375
Flare reaction in contact hyper-
    sensitivity, 63
f-Met-Leu-Phe, chemotactic re-
    sponses, 222
Foot pad swelling assay
  Pichinde virus infection, 332
  Herpes Simplex virus infec-
    tion, 332

Genetic control
  of foot pad swelling to virus
    infection, 332
  limitation of virus replica-
    tion, 327
Genetic resistance
  to Pichinde virus infection, 327
  to Vesicular Stomatitis virus, 339
  to bone marrow transplantation, 155
Gonadectomy, 417
GVHR, Graft-versus-host reactions, 25
  graft-versus-host disease, 43

Hamster strains
  CB, 23, 44, 103, 124, 143, 177, 215, 340, 435
  DFW, 24
  inbred lines, 23
  LHC, 24, 60, 103, 192

LSH, 23, 44, 136, 154, 166, 177, 192, 291, 327, 340, 435, 456

LVG, random bred, 60, 103, 136, 154, 215, 234, 327

MHA, 8, 23, 34, 44, 72, 103, 111, 124, 136, 143, 192, 215, 327, 340

MIT, 24, 75, 143, 340

PD4, 23, 60, 103

SYR, 24

TX, 24, 143

UT1, 24, 136, 340

UT2, 24, 340

UT, undefined, 143

ZDC$_{125}$, 445

ZO, 24

Haplotypes, MHC, 23, 44

Herpes Simplex virus, 135, 311
  immunosuppression in, 311
  clinical signs, 313
  histopathology, 315
  placental infection, 315
  fetal mortality and, 322

Hilar lymph nodes, immune response in, 192

Histopathology in
  Herpes Simplex virus infection, 315
  Vesicular Stomatitis virus infection, 340
  SV40 tumor growth, 434

Histamine
  release of, 33

HLA, 71

Hm-1, 23, 44

Ileal hyperplasia, 267
  causative organism, 275
  serodiagnostic test, 279
  clinical signs, 267
  epizootiology, 268
  pathology, 271
  control of disease, 280

Immune response to
  allografts, 23, 43
  chemical contactants, 44, 60
  Dipetalonemia vitae, 253
  Mycoplasma pneumonia, 233, 241

Treponema pallidum, 291

tumors, 43, 123, 135, 153, 165, 177, 210, 417, 434, 445

unconventional virus agents, 359, 401

viruses, 43, 135, 143, 192, 303, 311, 327, 339, 353

Immune surveillance, 461

Immunocrossreactivity, 95

Immunofluorescence
  Herpes Simplex virus, 312
  lymphoid tissue, 446
  tumor tissue, 446

Immunoglobulins, hamster
  IgM, 87, 95
  IgG1, 87, 95, 446
  IgG2, 95, 446
  IgA, 87, 95
  IgE, 34, 87
  IgD, 87

Immunosuppression, 418
  in virus infection, 311, 332
  with cyclophosphamide, 61, 311

Immunopotentiation
  of contact hypersensitivity, 61

Immunoprecipitation, 35, 69

Inbred hamster strains, 103

Incubation period of Scrapie, 359, 385

Induction of contact hypersensitivity, 44, 59

Infectious centers, virus infections, 327

Inflammatory response in Scrapie, 401

Influenza virus, 192, 215

Interferon, 340, 353

Intratracheal inoculation
  of antigen, 192

Ions, lymphocyte activation, 7

Jerne plaque assay, 193

KLH, Keyhole limpet hemocyanin, 11

Langerhans cells of epidermis, 45

Lethal virus infection, 327, 339,
      353
   Pichinde virus, 327
   vesicular stomatitis virus, 339
LiCl, modulation of lymphocyte
      stimulation, 71
LHC hamsters, 68, 103, 192, 387
Listeria monocytogenes, 206
LPS, lipopolysaccharide, 7, 111,
      206
LSH hamsters, 23, 44, 136, 154,
      177, 192, 291, 327, 340,
      435, 456
Lung inflammation, 221
Lung lavage, 206, 216
LVG hamsters (see random bred),
      61, 339
Lymphocytes, 7, 89, 123, 136
   see B cells
   lymph node cells, 7, 89
   peripheral blood cells, 123,
      136
   see splenocytes
   see T cells
   see thymocytes
Lymphocyte derived chemotactic
      factor (LDCF), 206
Lymphocyte proliferation, 7, 11,
      123, 194, 436, 459

M protein, measles virus, 307
Macrophages, 124, 165, 177, 205,
      359
   activated, 177, 359
   alveolar, 205
   migration inhibition, 124
   tumor cell killing, 177
Mast cells, 33
Measles virus, M protein, 307
Membrane IgD, 87
Membrane IgM, 87
Mesocricetus brandti, 95
Mesocricetus newtoni, 95
MHA, hamster, 23, 34, 44, 69,
      103, 124, 136, 143, 192,
      215, 327, 340
MHC, major histocompatibility
      complex, 23, 44, 69,
      143, 339

   tissue distribution of de-
      terminatants, 71
MIT, hamsters, 24, 75, 143
Mitogen stimulation, 7
   modulation by ions, 7
   modulation by LiCl, 7
MLR, mixed lymphocyte reaction,
      23
Mucosal hyperplasia, intestinal,
      267
Mycobacterium bovis, 205
Mycoplasma pneumoniae, 233, 241
   avriulent strains, 234
   disease, 233
   hamster tracheal rings, 242
   HA+ and HA⁻ in vivo, 242
   HA⁻ mutants and virulence, 242
   hemadsorption mutants, 242
   humoral immune response to, 235
   immunopathology, 236
   pathology, 236
   protective immunity to, 236
   two-dimensional gel analysis,
      242
   vaccinogens, 233, 241

NK cells and newborn hamsters,
      169
NK cell characteristics, compari-
      son with murine NK, 153
NK cells, natural killer cells,
      135, 148, 153, 162, 328
Non adherent lymphoid cells, 359
Nylon wool fractionation of
      lymphoid cells, 216

Oncogenesis, 153, 417, 434
Ovalbumin, 11

Parainfluenza type 3 virus infec-
      tion, 215
Peripheral blood lymphocytes, 126,
      136, 436
Peritoneal exudate cells (PEC),
      126, 166, 360, 436
   adoptive transfer of tumor
      immunity, 165

Peritumoral response, 447
PD4, hamster strain, 23, 68, 103
Persistent virus infection, 303,
    354, 359, 365, 375
PHA, phytohemagglutinin, 7, 123
Pichinde virus, 327
Placenta, virus infection of,
    311
Pneumocytes
  complement synthesis by, 224
  culture of, 223
Pokeweed mitogen, 125
Polymorphism
  of complement components, 103
  of female protein, 95
  of MHC, 23, 69, 143
PPD, purified protein derivative
    of tubercle bacillus, 206
Prostaglandins, 33
Proteases, 7
Protease inhibitors, 7, 111
Protection, against VSV infec-
    tion, 339
Proteolytic lability of IgM and
    IgD, 87

Quipazine maleate, in Scrapie,
    376

Radioiodination of cells, 34, 69,
    88
Random bred hamsters, 154, 215,
    234
Regulation of contact hypersen-
    sitivity, 44
Resistance to tumor development,
    153, 434
Reticular epithelial cells of
    thymus, 455
Retroviruses, 457
Reversed anaphylaxis, 37
Role of cell surface Ig in immune
    responsiveness, 87
Route of infection
  Pichinde, 327
  VSV, 339

Scrapie, 359, 365, 375, 385, 401
  aggration induced by, 385
  behaviorial changes, 375
  bioassay for, 359, 385
  clinical symptoms, 385
  inactivation, 365
  incubation period, 359, 385
  inflammatory response in, 401
  immunoreactivity in, 401
  serotonin levels in the brain,
      375
  spongiform pathology, 365
  quipazine maleate in, 376
Sendai virus, 218
Serosal cells, peritoneal, 35
Serotonin, in brain with Scrapie,
    376
Sheep erythrocytes, 7, 192
Skin graft rejection, 23
Silica, 159
Simian virus 40 (SV40), 177, 417,
    434, 445
  SV40 adenovirus 7 hybrid virus,
      136
Spleen, 8
  cells, 165, 434, 123
  cells, adoptive transfer of
      tumor immunity, 165
  virus infection of, 329
Splenectomy, 196
SRS-A, slow reactive substance of
    anaphylaxis, 33
Subacute sclerosing panencephalitis
    (SSPE), 303
  defective measles virus, 303
  hamster pathology, 305
  human pathology, 303
  and immune responses, 306
Susceptibility to
  Pichinde virus, 327
Suppression
  of immune response, 44
  of NK activity, 161
Suppressor T cells, 123
SYR, hamster strain, 24

T-antigen, 436
T-cells, 28, 43, 59, 123, 143,
    165, 215, 291, 417, 438,
    445, 455
  and Treponema infection, 291
  proliferation, 111, 194
  subsets of, 44, 123
Testosterone, 418
Thy 1 antigen, 461
Thymectomy, 124, 144, 418,
    436, 456
Thymic maturation, 43, 455
  C-type particles in, 455
  corticomedullary demarcation,
    459
Thymocytes, 167, 455
  adoptive transfer of tumor
    immunity with, 167
Thymus, 7, 455
Thymus dependent immune re-
    sponses, 123, 435, 455
Tissue distribution of MHC de-
    terminants, 69
TNP-Brucella abortus, 8
Transformation
Treponema pallidum, 291
  strain Bosnia A, 292
  and intradermal infection,
    292
  T-lymphocytes and resistance
    to, 296
  B-lymphocytes and resistance
    to, 296
  resistance to infection, 291
  protection with cell transfer,
    291
Toxoplasma gondii, 179
Tumor cells, killing, 124, 206

Tumor immunity, 165
Tumor specific transplantation
    antigens(TSTA), 123,
    165, 418, 446

UT1 hamster strain, 24, 136, 340
UT2 hamster strain, 24, 340
UT, undefined hamster strain,
    24, 143
Ultraviolet light irradiation,
    47
Vaccinia virus infection, 138,
    143, 153
  and cell-mediated cytotoxicity,
    143
Vertical transmission, virus,
    311, 455
Viral interference, 339, 353
Virus infection, 135, 215, 327,
    339, 353
  Herpes simplex, 135, 311, 327
  Influenza virus, 192
  Measles virus, 303
  of placenta, 311
  of spleen, 329
  Parainfluenza-3, 215
  Pichinde virus, 327
  Scrapie agent, 359, 365, 375,
    385, 401
  Vaccinia virus, 143, 359

YAC-1 tumor cell line, 153

ZDC$_{125}$, hamster strain, 445
Zinc, Zn^{+2}, 7
Zymosan, 206